Register Now f____ ____ss to You____

SPRINGER PUBLISHING COMPANY
CONNECT™

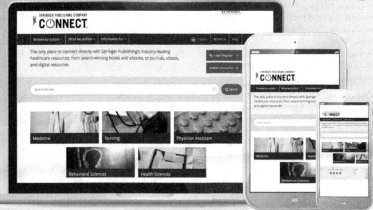

Digital Access to **PODCASTS** Included!

Your print purchase of *Physical Activity and Public Health Practice,* **includes online access to the contents of your book**—increasing accessibility, portability, and searchability!

Access today at:

http://connect.springerpub.com/content/book/978-0-8261-3459-2
**or scan the QR code at the right with your smartphone
and enter the access code below.**

J4H4EUH4

*Scan here for
quick access.*

SPRINGER PUBLISHING COMPANY
View all our products at springerpub.com

Daniel B. Bornstein, PhD, is an associate professor in the Department of Health and Human Performance at The Citadel, the Military College of South Carolina, in Charleston, South Carolina. Dr. Bornstein has held national leadership positions in the physical activity and public health field, including project coordinator for the U.S. National Physical Activity Plan from 2009 to 2014, and chair of the American Public Health Association's (APHA) Physical Activity Section from 2015 to 2016. Dr. Bornstein serves on several national committees including the U.S. Department of Health and Human Services' Committee on Physical Activity Communications, the American Heart Association's Expert Advisory Group on Physical Education and Physical Activity Policy in Schools, and the National Physical Activity Plan's Communications Committee. Locally, Dr. Bornstein is a member of the City of Charleston's Mayor's Health and Wellness Committee, and he is chair of The Citadel's Fitness Pillar. Dr. Bornstein has 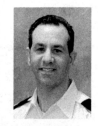 published extensively in the areas of physical activity monitoring, physical activity coalitions, physical activity communication and messaging, and physical activity as it relates to military readiness and national security. Dr. Bornstein's research has been featured in hundreds of national and international media outlets, including *USA Today, Newsweek, Stars and Stripes*, and *National Public Radio*. Dr. Bornstein's research has also been the focus of federal congressional briefings and senior military briefings. Prior to his academic career, Dr. Bornstein owned and operated fitness companies in the southwestern region of the United States. Dr. Bornstein received his BS in psychology from Hobart College in Geneva, New York, and his doctoral degree in Exercise Science from the University of South Carolina in Columbia, South Carolina.

Amy A. Eyler, PhD, CHES, is an associate professor in the graduate program of public health in the Brown School at Washington University in St. Louis. She currently chairs the public health sector standing committee of the U.S. National Physical Activity Plan. She was the past chair of the physical activity section of the American Public Health Association (APHA), a member of the American College of Sports Medicine (ACSM), and is a Certified Health Education Specialist. For over a decade, she served as principal investigator for the Physical Activity Policy Research Network (PAPRN), a national network of researchers to study the influence of policy on population physical activity. Dr. Eyler also served as senior associate editor for the *Journal of Physical Activity and Health*. She remains actively involved in physical activity promotion at the local and national level. Locally, she serves on the university's wellness steering committee and volunteers with several community organizations such as *TrailNet* and *Girls on* 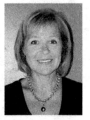 *the Run*. She has an extensive publication record, including the 2016 book titled *Prevention, Policy, and Public Health*, and was an author on the Institute of Medicine report *Educating the Student Body*. She also contributed to the 2017 U.S. National Physical Activity Plan Walking and Walkability Report Card. Dr. Eyler's main research interests are health promotion through community policy and environmental interventions, with a focus on physical activity and obesity prevention. She has a master's degree in Physical Education and Adult Fitness from Ohio University and a doctorate in Public Health from Oregon State University.

Jay E. Maddock, PhD, FAAHB, is a dean and professor at the Department of Environmental and Occupational Health, School of Public Health at Texas A&M University. Dr. Maddock assumed the leadership of the School of Public Health in 2015. He also serves as the Senior Academic Advisor for the President George H. W. Bush China–U.S. Relations Foundation and is on the Board of Directors for the Texas Health Institute and the Well-Connected Communities Initiative. Dean Maddock previously served as the director and chair of the University of Hawaii Public Health Program and was named the Bank of Hawaii Community Leader of the Year in addition to receiving the Award of Excellence from 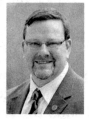 the American Public Health Association (APHA), Council on Affiliates. He has chaired the Hawaii state board of health and served as President of the American Academy of Health Behavior and Honorary Secretary of the Asia-Pacific Academic Consortium for Public Health. His research has been featured in several national media outlets including *The Today Show, Eating Well, Prevention*, and *Good Housekeeping*, and he has authored over 100 scientific articles, which have been cited over 4,000 times. He is internationally recognized for his research in social ecological approaches to increasing physical activity and has given invited lectures in numerous countries including Australia, South Korea, Japan, China, Taiwan, Indonesia, El Salvador, Austria, and Brazil, and has held honorary professorships at two universities in China. He has served as principal investigator on over $18 million in extramural funding. Dean Maddock received his undergraduate degree in Psychology and Sociology, magna cum laude, from Syracuse University and his master's and doctoral degrees in Experimental Psychology from the University of Rhode Island.

Justin B. Moore, PhD, MS, FACSM, is an associate professor in the Departments of Family and Community Medicine, Epidemiology and Prevention, and Implementation Science at the Wake Forest School of Medicine in Winston-Salem, North Carolina. Dr. Moore also serves as the director of the Implementation Science Affinity Group within the Wake Forest Clinical and Translational Science Institute. He has served as the chair of the editorial board of the *American Journal of Public Health* and is the associate editor of the *Journal of Public Health Management and Practice*. Dr. Moore is also an active member of the American College of Sports Medicine (ACSM) and the American Public Health Association (APHA). He was named 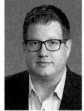 a fellow in the ACSM in 2010 and was a founding member of the Physical Activity Section of the APHA. He served as the chair of the Physical Activity Section and later as the section's representative on the APHA Governing Council. He conducts community-engaged research focused on the dissemination and implementation of evidence-based strategies for the promotion of healthy behaviors. He also conducts epidemiological research examining the determinants of health behaviors and related comorbidities in youth and adults. In addition to his leadership at the national, state, and local levels, he has published more than 120 peer-reviewed articles and has received funding as principal investigator for his research from the National Institutes of Health, the U.S. Centers for Disease Control and Prevention, the Robert Wood Johnson Foundation, and the de Beaumont Foundation, among others. Dr. Moore is a graduate of Texas A&M University—Corpus Christi (BS), the University of Mississippi (MS), and the University of Texas at Austin (PhD). He also holds a certificate of competencies in Epidemiology from the University of Michigan School of Public Health.

PHYSICAL ACTIVITY AND PUBLIC HEALTH PRACTICE

Editors

Daniel B. Bornstein, PhD

Amy A. Eyler, PhD, CHES

Jay E. Maddock, PhD, FAAHB

Justin B. Moore, PhD, MS, FACSM

SPRINGER PUBLISHING COMPANY

Springer Publishing Company, LLC
11 West 42nd Street
New York, NY 10036
www.springerpub.com

Acquisitions Editor: David D'Addona
Compositor: diacriTech, Chennai

ISBN: 978-0-8261-3458-5
ebook ISBN: 978-0-8261-3459-2
DOI: 10/1891/9780826134592

Instructor's Materials: Qualified instructors may request supplements by emailing textbook@springerpub.com:
Instructor's Manual: 978-0-8261-3506-3
Instructor's Test Bank: 978-0-8261-3507-0
Instructor's PowerPoints: 978-0-8261-3508-7

19 20 21 22 23 / 5 4 3 2 1

Library of Congress Cataloging-in-Publication Data
Names: Bornstein, Daniel Benjamin, editor.
Title: Physical activity and public health practice / [edited by] Daniel B. Bornstein, PhD, Associate Professor, Department of Health and Human Performance, The Citadel, The Military College of SouthCarolina, Charleston, South Carolina, Amy A. Eyler, PhD, CHES, Associate Professor, Brown School, Prevention Research Center, Washington University in St. Louis, St. Louis, Missouri, Jay E. Maddock, PhD, FAAHB, Dean and Professor, Department of Environmental and Occupational Health, School of Public Health, Texas A&M University, College Station, Texas, Justin B. Moore, PhD, MS, FACSM, Associate Professor, Department of Family and Community Medicine, Wake Forest School of Medicine, Winston-Salem, North Carolina.
Description:Danvers, MA : Springer Publishing Company, LLC, [2019] | Includes bibliographical references and index.
Identifiers: LCCN 2018048563 | ISBN 9780826134585
Subjects: LCSH: Exercise—Physiological aspects. | Public health.
Classification: LCC RA781 .P496 2019 | DDC 613.7/1–dc23 LC record available at https://lccn.loc.gov/2018048563

Daniel B. Bornstein ORCID: https://orcid.org/0000-0001-9948-1876
Amy A. Eyler ORCID: https://orcid.org/0000-0001-8417-1656
Jay E. Maddock ORCID: https://orcid.org/0000-0002-1119-0300
Justin B. Moore ORCID: https://orcid.org/0000-0003-4059-0538

Printed in the United States of America.

We would like to dedicate this book to those who work tirelessly to promote physical activity through policy, practice, and research. We thank you for the work you do to increase physical activity and improve public health.

CONTENTS

PHYSICAL ACTIVITY AND PUBLIC HEALTH PRACTICE PODCASTS

The Editors of *Physical Activity and Public Health Practice* have recorded 10 podcasts featuring interviews with local and national public health experts. Featuring discussions of real-world physical activity programs with insider perspectives on lessons learned and obstacles that affect an interventions' effectiveness, each podcast provides an auditory lens to the challenges and promises of physical activity research and practice. It is our hope that they are not only used as a basis for classroom discussions, but they also inspire public health initiatives and greater physical activity in communities across the country and globe. We have numbered the podcasts to align with topics featured in associated chapter numbers and hope you enjoy listening. You can access the podcasts by scanning the QR code or following this link to Springer Connect™:   http://connect.springerpub.com/content/book/978-0-8261-3459-2/front -matter/fmatter9.

Podcast 4.1 Physical Activity Messaging and Framing
Dan Bornstein with *Michelle Segar*

Podcast 6.1 Coalitions
Jay Maddock with *Bev Brody*

Podcast 7.1 Developing Physical Activity Plans
Jay Maddock with *Heid Hansen Smith*

Podcast 8.1 Physical Activity Policy
Dan Bornstein with *Laurie Whitsel* and *Amy Eyler*

Podcast 12.1 Physical Activity in Schools
Justin Moore with *Dave Gardner*

Podcast 13.1 Physical Activity in Out-of-School Time Settings
Justin Moore with *Michael Beets*

Podcast 18.1 Walkable Communities
Jay Maddock with *Mark Fenton*

Podcast 18.2 Physical Activity Equity and Advocacy
Amy Eyler with *Grace Kyung*

Podcast 19.1 Physical Activity in Rural Communities
Jay Maddock with *M. Renée Umstattd Meyer*

Podcast 22.1 Evidence-based Physical Activity Interventions
Amy Eyler with *Ross Brownson*

CONTRIBUTORS

Melissa Bopp, PhD
Associate Professor
Department of Kinesiology
The Pennsylvania State University
University Park, Pennsylvania

Daniel B. Bornstein, PhD
Associate Professor
Department of Health and Human Performance
The Citadel, the Military College of South Carolina
Charleston, South Carolina

Danielle R. Brittain, MPH, PhD
Associate Professor and Chair
Community Health Program, Colorado School of Public Health
University of Northern Colorado
Greeley, Colorado

Russell L. Carson, PhD
Professor
School of Sport and Exercise Science, Colorado School of Public Health
Founding Director, Active Schools Institute
Research and Health & Wellness Advisor, PlayCore
University of Northern Colorado
Greeley, Colorado

Morgan N. Clennin, PhD, MPH
Postdoctoral Research Fellow
Partners in Evaluation & Research Center
Institute for Health Research
Kaiser Permanente of Colorado
Aurora, Colorado

Angie L. Cradock, ScD, MPE
Senior Research Scientist
Department of Social and Behavioral Sciences
Harvard T.H. Chan School of Public Health
Boston, Massachusetts

Alicia A. Dahl, PhD, MS
Assistant Professor
Department of Public Health Sciences
University of South Carolina at Charlotte
Charlotte, South Carolina

Brian D. Dauenhauer, PhD
Associate Professor
School of Sport and Exercise Science
Director, Active Schools Institute
University of Northern Colorado
Greeley, Colorado

William J. Davis, PhD, PE
D. Graham Copeland Professor of Civil Engineering
Civil and Environmental Engineering, Construction Engineering
The Citadel, the Military College of South Carolina
Charleston, South Carolina

Michael B. Edwards, PhD
Associate Professor
Department of Parks, Recreation and Tourism Management
College of Natural Resources
North Carolina State University
Raleigh, North Carolina

Laura A. Esparza, MS, MCHES, PAPHS
Assistant Director
Latino Research Initiative
The University of Texas at Austin
Austin, Texas

Amy A. Eyler, PhD, CHES
Associate Professor
Brown School, Prevention Research Center
Washington University in St. Louis
St. Louis, Missouri

Casey Foster, MS, ACSM-CPT
Exercise and Activity Specialist
Brenner Children's Hospital
Wake Forest Baptist Medical Center
Winston-Salem, North Carolina

George L. Grieve, PhD
Assistant Professor
College of Nursing and Health Sciences
Valdosta State University
Valdosta, Georgia

Brook E. Harmon, PhD, RD
Assistant Professor
Division of Social and Behavioral Sciences
University of Memphis School of Public Health
Memphis, Tennessee

Morgan Hughey, PhD, MPH
Assistant Professor
Department of Health and Human Performance
College of Charleston
Charleston, South Carolina

Danielle E. Jake-Schoffman, PhD
Assistant Professor
Department of Health Education and Behavior
University of Florida
Gainesville, Florida

Lindsay Elliott Jorgenson, MSW, MPH
Community Food Systems Agent
Johnson County K-State Research and Extension
Kansas State University
Olathe, Kansas

Andrew T. Kaczynski, PhD
Associate Professor
Department of Health Promotion, Education, and Behavior
Arnold School of Public Health
University of South Carolina
Columbia, South Carolina

Jay E. Maddock, PhD, FAAHB
Dean and Professor
Department of Environmental and Occupational Health
School of Public Health
Texas A&M University
College Station, Texas

Jaimie McMullen, PhD
Associate Professor
School of Sport and Exercise Science
University of Northern Colorado
Greeley, Colorado

Justin B. Moore, PhD, MS, FACSM
Associate Professor
Department of Family and Community Medicine
Department of Epidemiology and Prevention
Department of Implementation Science
Wake Forest School of Medicine
Winston-Salem, North Carolina

Andrew Mowen, PhD
Professor
Department of Recreation, Park, and Tourism Management
The Pennsylvania State University
University Park, Pennsylvania

Theresa M. Oniffrey, MPH, EMT-P
Senior Associate
Cerus Consulting, LLC
Winston-Salem, North Carolina

Marcia G. Ory, PhD, MPH, FAAHB, FGSA
Regents Distinguished Professor
Center for Population Health and Aging
Department of Environmental and Occupational Health
School of Public Health, Texas A&M University
College Station, Texas

Greg J. Petrucci Jr.
Graduate Research and Teaching Assistant
University of Massachusetts Amherst
Amherst, Massachusetts

Nicolaas P. Pronk, PhD, MA, FACSM, FAWHP
President, HealthPartners Institute
Chief Science Officer, HealthPartners
Adjunct Professor, Harvard T.H. Chan School of Public Health
Boston, Massachusetts

Barbara Resnick, PhD, CPRN, FAAN, FAANP
Professor
Department of Organizational Systems and Adult Health
School of Nursing, University of Maryland
Baltimore, Maryland

Elizabeth A. Richards, PhD, MSN, RN, CHES
Assistant Professor
School of Nursing
Purdue University
West Lafayette, Indiana

Jonathan J. Ruiz-Ramie, MS
Doctoral Student
Department of Exercise Science
Arnold School of Public Health
University of South Carolina
Columbia, South Carolina

Mark A. Sarzynski, PhD, FAHA, FACSM
Assistant Professor
Department of Exercise Science
Arnold School of Public Health, University of South Carolina
Columbia, South Carolina

Michelle M. Segar, PhD, MPH
Director, Sport, Health, and Activity Research and Policy Center
Researcher, Institute for Research on Women and Gender
University of Michigan
Ann Arbor, Michigan

Bianca Shulaker
Senior Federal Grants Program Manager
Trust for Public Land
Washington, DC

Camelia R. Singletary, MPH
Project Manager
Department of Family and Community Medicine
Wake Forest School of Medicine
Winston-Salem, North Carolina

John R. Sirard, PhD
Assistant Professor
Department of Kinesiology and Commonwealth Honors College
University of Massachusetts Amherst
Amherst, Massachusetts

Joseph A. Skelton, MD, MS
Associate Professor
Department of Pediatrics
Department of Epidemiology and Prevention
Wake Forest School of Medicine
Winston-Salem, North Carolina

Matthew Lee Smith, PhD, MPH, CHES, FAAHB, FGSA
Associate Professor and Co-Director
Center for Population Health and Aging
Department of Environmental and Occupational Health
School of Public Health, Texas A&M University
College Station, Texas

Mark Stoutenberg, PhD, MSPH
Associate Professor and MPH Program Director
Department of Health and Human Performance
University of Tennessee at Chattanooga
Chattanooga, Tennessee

Kiley J. Tyler, PhD
Assistant Professor of Exercise Science
Loyola University Chicago
Marcella Niehoff School of Nursing
Chicago, Illinois

M. Renée Umstattd Meyer, PhD, MCHES
Associate Professor
Department of Public Health
Baylor University
Waco, Texas

Benjamin L. Webb, PhD
Assistant Professor
Department of Applied Health
Southern Illinois University Edwardsville
Edwardsville, Illinois

Laurie Whitsel, PhD
Director of Policy Research
American Heart Association
Washington, DC

Kaela Yates, MD
Resident
Department of Pediatrics
Wake Forest School of Medicine
Winston-Salem, North Carolina

Aya Yoshikawa, PhD
Postdoctoral Fellow
Center for Population Health and Aging
Texas A&M University
College Station, Texas

FOREWORD

Over the past half century, the scientific foundation for addressing physical activity (PA) in public health settings has advanced exponentially. Early epidemiological studies of the health benefits of PA led to more recent research on interventions. To describe the evolution of the science underpinning PA promotion, our team (led by Andrea Ramirez Varela) recently mapped the history of research on PA and public health (1). *Etiologic research* on health outcomes began in the 1950s, most notably with Morris's landmark study of coronary heart disease and PA among transport workers in London (2). From 1953 to 2015, there were nearly 70,000 studies of PA and health outcomes.

Four more recent types of research form the basis for promotion of PA in public health settings. *Measurement research* allows us to track levels of PA, providing the framework for large-scale surveillance systems. Studies of *determinants and correlates* (often with cross-sectional designs) build knowledge of the reasons for activity or sedentariness in various population subgroups. As a key focus for this text, studies of *interventions* (including *policy change*) provide an array of effective approaches for increasing population-level rates of PA. Compared with other types of research, the body of literature on PA interventions remains the smallest (approximately 7,200 studies from 1996 to 2015) (1). The number of intervention studies is likely to be quite small if limited to rigorous investigations (i.e., those with a strong design and strong execution).

Intervention research in the 1990s focused largely on individual-level approaches (e.g., the effects of health provider counseling on PA). It was increasingly recognized that in order to be effective, interventions need to span levels of the ecological framework (i.e., individual, social, organizational, environmental, and policy). This multilevel approach is particularly important given that our modern world provides very few opportunities to be active in daily life, which in turn has contributed to epidemic rates of obesity and related chronic diseases. Changing the environment and related policies begins to address health equity and may also provide necessary conditions for implementation of related interventions (e.g., a social support intervention for walking will be ineffective if there are no safe places to walk). This critical focus on comprehensive, multilevel intervention, with particular attention to policy and the built environment, is well-covered in this book.

Knowing which PA interventions work (*the what*, as outlined in the *Community Guide*) (3) is only the beginning. There has been sparse attention to understanding the contextual conditions within which interventions are implemented and how they are adapted and evaluated, thus informing *the how* of PA promotion. Studies to date have tended to overemphasize internal validity (e.g., well-controlled trials) while giving sparse attention to external validity (e.g., the translation of intervention science to the various circumstances of practice). Much of this contextual evidence is described in Part III in this volume, highlighting intervention challenges and opportunities in multiple settings (e.g., schools, worksites) and among populations at particular risk experiencing inequalities (e.g., persons with disabilities, rural residents).

Our ability to successfully deploy and evaluate PA interventions is enhanced by transdisciplinary, team science (4, 5). In nearly all cases, planning, implementing, and evaluating interventions require a wide range of skills and ability to build nontraditional partnerships with people and organizations not working directly in public health. For example, to address the barriers to PA in cities, urban planners, transportation experts, and persons working in parks and recreation are essential in developing environments and policies to make communities friendly toward PA. Transdisciplinary practice and research can benefit the cooperating partners in multiple ways. A key element, as noted in Chapter 4, is finding common ground and mutual benefits. For example, public health officials pursue comprehensive, school-based physical education to benefit the health of youth. Yet school officials may be motivated more by improving academic achievement, which shows a direct relationship with PA.

As the tactics in this book are applied, they will contribute to our understanding of practice-based evidence—the process of deriving or determining the effectiveness and implementation of evidence-based interventions from evaluation in real-world practice (6). This practice-oriented focus requires more consistent evaluation of natural experiments (e.g., a new PA policy), additional "real-world" research that responds better to practitioners' needs, and reliance on so-called "tacit knowledge" or "colloquial evidence" (pragmatic information based on direct, practice-based experience).

Given that practitioners are the end users for this book, its many lessons and strategies provide a springboard for workforce development. We know that many public health practitioners lack formal training in one or more core public health disciplines (e.g., epidemiology, health education). Therefore, without a stronger commitment to hands-on, workforce training and leadership development, it is unlikely that aspirations to translate research to PA practice can be attained. A model program to build the workforce is the *Physical Activity and Public Health Course for Practitioners*, which has shown positive benefits in building capacity to design, implement, and evaluate interventions (7).

This timely and exciting new how-to guide for PA practitioners is long overdue. If every practitioner and applied researcher studies and applies the lessons in this book, our goal of higher rates of PA and health equity will be realized more quickly.

Ross C. Brownson, PhD
Washington University School of Medicine in St. Louis
St. Louis, Missouri

■ References

1. Varela AR, Pratt M, Harris J, et al. Mapping the historical development of physical activity and health research: a structured literature review and citation network analysis. *Prev Med.* 2018;111:466–472. doi:10.1016/j.ypmed.2017.10.020
2. Morris JN, Heady JA, Raffle PA, et al. Coronary heart-disease and physical activity of work. *Lancet.* 1953;265(6796):1111–1120. doi:10.1016/S0140-6736(53)91495-0
3. Task Force on Community Preventive Services. Guide to community preventive services. https://www.thecommunityguide.org Accessed July 1, 2018
4. Hall KL, Vogel AL, Stipelman B, et al. A four-phase model of transdisciplinary team-based research: goals, team processes, and strategies. *Transl Behav Med.* 2013;2(4):415–430. doi:10.1007/s13142-012-0167-y

5. Vogel AL, Stipelman BA, Hall KL, et al. Pioneering the transdisciplinary team science approach: lessons learned from National Cancer Institute grantees. *J Transl Med Epidemiol.* 2014;2(2):1027.

6. Brownson RC, Fielding JE, Green LW. Building capacity for evidence-based public health: reconciling the pulls of practice and the push of research. *Annu Rev Public Health.* 2018;39:27–53. doi:10.1146/annurev-publhealth-040617-014746

7. Evenson KR, Brown DR, Pearce E, . Evaluation of the physical activity and public health course for practitioners. *Res Q Exerc Sport.* 2016;87(2):207–213.

PREFACE

The overall goal of this book is to provide you, the reader, with the practical guidance required to design, deliver, and evaluate physical activity (PA) interventions across a range of settings and populations. Research in PA and public health is rather new. The field gained a lot of momentum in the 1980s and 1990s when the link between daily movement and health outcomes was solidified and codified in the 1995 PA recommendations put forth by the American College of Sports Medicine. Since then, the recommendations for adult PA have remained fairly consistent at 30 minutes of moderate-intensity PA most days of the week. Even though the recommendations are established, there is still a lot of knowledge to be discovered to quantify the impact on health and to determine the best ways to get people to be physically active throughout their life. For example, discoveries continue to be published of the effects of PA on dementia, diabetes, cancer, mental health, and heart disease. Two things in our field are clear: (a) PA has a strong positive effect on health and well-being and (b) population levels of PA remain perilously low.

While the first generation of PA researchers effectively demonstrated the link between PA and health, the second generation of researchers has expanded this work to focus on the importance of policies, practices, and environments in changing individual-level PA behavior. Despite widespread knowledge about the importance of PA, fewer than a quarter of U.S. adults meet PA guidelines. However, when communities and organizations plan, implement, and evaluate comprehensive interventions to increase PA, they often get positive results. It is for this reason that we have dedicated our careers to developing effective strategies for promoting PA and training leaders for the future. In this capacity, all four of us have served as chair of the Physical Activity Section of the American Public Health Association. Through our collective experiences, we have found a lack of comprehensive knowledge about what it takes to get communities and organizations set up to support active lifestyles for the individuals living, working, playing, learning, praying, or commuting in those communities and organizations. As we looked for resources to recommend to public health educators and professionals interested in improving population PA, we realized that we would have to recommend dozens of readings from different sources. Therefore, the impetus for this book was the need for a single, comprehensive, practical, and evidence-based guide for current and future public health professionals that will enable them to take the field of PA and public health to the next level.

We believe that this book, written by the leading experts from different subdisciplines of PA and public health, provides a highly practical guide to creating and maintaining communities and organizations that support active living. We hope that it will be an invaluable tool in increasing PA and improving the health of the population.

Before we describe our approach to the scope, we would like to acknowledge Elena Vidrascu for her role in assisting us during the development of this book, including its distinguishing features and accompanying instructional materials.

Scope—The book is divided into four parts: An Introduction to the Science of Physical Activity and Public Health, Planning Your Physical Activity Intervention, Implementing Physical Activity Interventions in Specific Communities and Settings, and Evaluating Your Intervention and Disseminating the Results. The first part is written for individuals who have had limited exposure to the field of PA and health prior to reading this book. In the first chapter, the state of the evidence around PA and chronic disease is reviewed. In the second chapter, the different methods for measuring PA along with their strengths and weaknesses are explored. In the third chapter, important milestones in the field are explored, including the evolution of PA guidelines, which are reviewed and explained. The final chapter in the first part looks at how to increase the value of PA for different stakeholders. Developing a strong value proposition is important since many in the public health field look solely at health outcomes, not realizing that nonhealth-related outcomes related to PA are often what motivate others to act.

In Part II, we examine what needs to happen before you launch an intervention. Implementing a program without sufficient planning is one of the biggest reasons that programs fail. In Chapter 5, the steps taken to develop policy and environmental interventions are explored. These are powerful tools since changes in policy and environments can change behavior without people even thinking about it. In Chapter 6, we examine how to build and maintain a coalition. No one is the expert in everything. Coalitions support the bringing together of people with similar goals but different jobs and expertise to create a comprehensive campaign. In Chapter 7, we detail the process of developing a PA plan. Plans are essential for keeping on track and maximizing resources and efficiency. A well-developed plan can be the difference between success and failure. In the final chapter of this part, we examine how policies actually move into action. Once a policy is adopted, how it is implemented and enforced can change greatly. In this chapter, we explore factors that can help ensure effective implementation of policies.

Part III examines implementing interventions in specific communities and populations. There are important considerations in developing interventions across diverse areas and varied populations. Settings explored in this part include worksites, faith-based organizations, healthcare, schools, out-of-school areas, and parks and recreation. Populations examined include families, older adults, individuals with disabilities, and urban and rural populations.

The final part (IV) is devoted to evaluating interventions. Evaluation is essential to assessing the effectiveness of your intervention and Disseminating the Results. The first chapter explores implementation monitoring. This involves how the program was implemented, with whom it was implemented, and any unanticipated changes along the way. The second chapter describes outcome and impact evaluation as well as cost-effectiveness. This chapter helps to answer questions such as: Did your intervention work? Did it actually change health? How much did it cost relative to how effective it was? In the final chapter, dissemination is explored. Here, you will be given tools on how to share the news of what worked and what did not, and how to encourage and ensure adoption in other settings and communities.

Distinguishing Features/Learning Tools—This book is written as a "how to" guide for planning, implementing, and evaluating interventions. It includes hands-on activities and exercises to encourage applying the content knowledge and informing group work. Essential information is highlighted in every chapter to reinforce the main points.

Instructor's Resources—We have designed resources to facilitate teaching and to encourage active learning in class. We have provided a set of PowerPoint slides for each of the chapters to make lecturing easier. A series of resources is provided at the end of each chapter to encourage further research of and guidance for the topic. Discussion questions at the end of each chapter can be used in small group settings or for homework exercises. Ancillary materials include in-class group projects, discussion questions, and a test bank of multiple-choice questions to provide easy exam creation **(to access these ancillary materials, qualified instructors should email *textbook@springerpub.com*)**.

This book is an ideal textbook for advanced undergraduate classes or first year master's degree classes in public health, kinesiology, or nutrition, with a focus on PA where students are preparing for careers in health and wellness. It is also intended for anyone working to make their communities or organizations more active. This includes practitioners in state and local health departments; voluntary organizations like the American Heart Association, American Cancer Society, and The Y; local governments; those working in corporate wellness; and anyone else concerned about health.

For those working to improve population health through PA, consider this book your guide. Enjoy the exploration!

Daniel B. Bornstein
Amy A. Eyler
Jay E. Maddock
Justin B. Moore

I

AN INTRODUCTION TO THE SCIENCE OF PHYSICAL ACTIVITY AND PUBLIC HEALTH

PHYSICAL ACTIVITY AND CHRONIC DISEASE

JONATHAN J. RUIZ-RAMIE | MARK A. SARZYNSKI | GEORGE L. GRIEVE

LEARNING OBJECTIVES

By the end of this chapter, the student should be able to

1. Define what chronic disease is and then use prevalence data to discuss the public health burden associated with the different chronic diseases discussed.

2. Support the argument that physical activity (PA) is an effective form of prevention and/or treatment for different types of cardiovascular disease based on evidence from different types of scientific studies.

3. Construct a figure that demonstrates the dose–response relationship between PA and chronic disease.

4. Argue for why a doctor should prescribe PA over medication as an effective form of type 2 diabetes prevention based upon evidence from experimental studies among individuals with impaired glucose tolerance.

5. Design an intervention for a workplace aimed at reducing sedentary time, based on emerging evidence on the relationship between chronic diseases and being sedentary.

◼ Introduction

Chronic diseases of long duration (i.e., 3 months or more) generally progress slowly. About half of U.S. adults had one or more chronic diseases as of 2012, with the prevalence increasing to 86% in adults 65 years or older (1). Furthermore, both in the United States and in developed countries worldwide, seven of the top 10 causes of death are chronic diseases. Heart disease and cancer have been the top two causes of death in the United States for the past 40 years, accounting for over 45% of all deaths in 2015 (2). Stroke (5.2%

© Springer Publishing Company DOI: 10.1891/9780826134592.0001

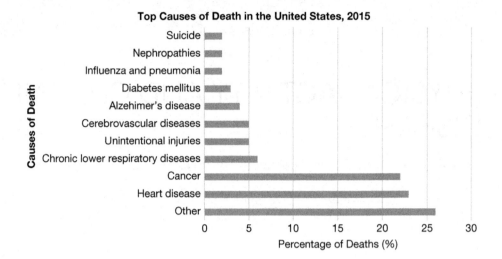

FIGURE 1.1 Top causes of death in the United States in the year 2015.

SOURCE: Adapted from Centers for Disease Control and Prevention. Leading causes of death in 1975 and 2015: United States, 1975–2015 (Figure 8). Health, United States, 2016. https://www.cdc.gov/nchs/data/hus/hus16.pdf#019.

of deaths) and diabetes (2.9%) were the fifth and seventh leading causes of death in the United States (Figure 1.1). It is estimated that 86% of the nation's $2.7 trillion annual healthcare expenditures are for people with chronic and mental health conditions (3). It is well known that modifiable health risk behaviors, particularly **physical inactivity**, poor nutrition, and tobacco use, are major contributors to these leading chronic diseases. Thus, modifying these behaviors is critical for both the prevention and management of chronic diseases.

Physical activity (PA) is defined by the Centers for Disease Control and Prevention (CDC) as "[a]ny bodily movement produced by the contraction of skeletal muscle that increases energy expenditure above a basal level" (4). For the purposes of this chapter, PA generally refers to the subset of PA that enhances health. PA includes occupational, leisure-time, household, and transportation activities, as well as planned exercise and sports. Physical inactivity may be defined as PA levels insufficient to meet present recommendations or PA levels less than those required for optimal health and prevention of premature death. The current global and U.S. PA guidelines both recommend that adults perform at least 150 minutes per week of moderate-intensity PA, or at least 75 minutes per week of vigorous PA, or an equivalent combination of moderate and vigorous PA. Furthermore, muscle-strengthening activities should be done involving major muscle groups on two or more days a week (5, 6). The World Health Organization (WHO) estimates that one in four adults is not active enough (7). In 2015, 50% of U.S. adults aged 18 years or older did not meet recommendations for aerobic PA and 79% did not meet recommendations for both aerobic and muscle-strengthening physical PA (8).

According to WHO, physical inactivity is the fourth leading risk factor for global mortality and has been associated with 35 diseases/conditions (9). Lee et al. (10) estimated that physical inactivity caused 9% of premature mortality that occurred worldwide in 2008, as well as 6% of the disease burden of coronary heart disease (CHD), 7% of type 2 diabetes, and 10% each of breast and colon cancer. The authors estimated that elimination of physical inactivity would increase the life expectancy of the world's population by 0.68 years. These worldwide estimates are very similar to those for the United States, with studies finding physical inactivity being responsible for 10% to 11% of all deaths (10, 11). The costs related to physical inactivity are also enormous, with conservative estimates showing physical inactivity costing healthcare systems $53.8 billion worldwide in 2013, and an additional $13.7 billion due to productivity losses (12).

It is evident that increasing PA levels worldwide would have a major global economic and public health impact. Therefore, the remaining sections of this chapter will provide more detailed information on the association between PA and specific chronic diseases, namely cardiovascular disease (CVD), hypertension, diabetes, and cancer. We have chosen to focus on these four diseases based on their public health burden, as well as the quality and quantity of evidence of their association with PA.

▮ Physical Activity and Cardiovascular Disease

The WHO defines CVD as the group of disorders of heart and blood vessels, which includes hypertension, CHD, cerebrovascular disease (stroke), peripheral vascular disease, heart failure, rheumatic heart disease, congenital heart disease, and cardiomyopathies. Risk factors that promote the development of CVD include behavioral, metabolic, socioeconomic, age, psychological, and genetic influences, among others. Though some risk factors are nonmodifiable (e.g., age and genetics), metabolic risk factors (e.g., hypertension, diabetes, high cholesterol, and overweight and obesity) are largely modifiable through behavioral changes (e.g., tobacco use, physical inactivity, unhealthy diet, and excessive alcohol use) (13).

CVD is the leading cause of death among American adults, responsible for one in every seven deaths. Approximately 92.1 million American adults are living with CVD or the results of stroke, and by 2030, CVD prevalence is projected to be 40.5%. Additionally, CVD is responsible for 17% of national health expenses, totaling more than $316 billion in direct and indirect costs (14, 15). Therefore, effective treatment and prevention of CVD is a national public health priority.

Observational Studies

PA can aid in the control of metabolic risk factors, such as hypertension, diabetes, high cholesterol, and overweight and obesity (6, 16, 17). There is an inverse association between PA and CVD and it was first discovered in the early 20th century through **observational studies**. In the late-1940s, Morris et al. observed that among transport workers in London, the mortality rate of the double decker bus drivers was higher than that of the conductors (18). After examining autopsies of the drivers and observing behavioral patterns, Morris et al. showed that the drivers had a much higher prevalence of CHD than the conductors, which was likely due to the conductors performing greater amounts of PA during their shifts (18).

In the early 1950s in the United States, Paffenbarger (19) initiated the California Longshoreman Study, a longitudinal cohort study from 1951 to 1961 that examined the occupational PA levels of over 6,000 oceanside dockworkers in California. It was shown that among the longshoremen, those that performed light and moderate work had 1.8 and 1.7 times increased risk of CHD, respectively, compared to the reference group that performed strenuous work (19). Thus, the California Longshoreman Study was one of the first studies to show an inverse dose–response relationship between occupational PA levels and the risk of CHD.

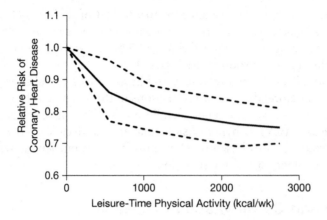

FIGURE 1.2   Dose–response association between LTPA and incident CHD. CHD, coronary heart disease; LTPA, leisure-time physical activity.

SOURCE: Adapted from Sattelmair J, Pertman J, Ding EL, et al. Dose response between physical activity and risk of coronary heart disease: a meta-analysis. *Circulation.* 2011;124:789-795. doi:10.1161/circulationaha.110.010710.

Subsequent population-based cohort studies found similar associations between PA and CVD (20–24). In a meta-analysis of 21 prospective cohort studies ($n > 650,000$) examining the association between PA and CVD, Li and Siegrist (22) showed a 24% and 27% reduction in the risk of developing CVD in men and women, respectively, who performed a high level of **leisure-time physical activity (LTPA)** compared to the reference group who performed a low level of LTPA. In addition to the protective effect of LTPA on CVD, the meta-analysis also found a similar protective effect of occupational PA on CVD, though not as strong as that of LTPA. Additionally, in a meta-analysis of 32 **randomized controlled trials (RCTs)** examining the effect of walking on CVD risk factors in sedentary individuals, Murtagh et al. (17) showed significant reductions in systolic blood pressure (SBP) and diastolic blood pressure (DBP), weight and body fat, and significant increases in aerobic fitness.

The 2010 WHO Global Recommendations on PA for Health state that risk for CVD decreases by approximately 30% with the accumulation of 150 minutes per week of moderate PA (13). In a meta-analysis of nine epidemiological PA studies from 1995 to 2009, Sattelmair et al. (24) demonstrated a protective dose–response between LTPA and CHD. They found that individuals who performed 150 and 300 minutes per week of moderate-intensity LTPA had a 14% and 20% lower risk of CHD, respectively, than individuals who performed no LTPA (Figure 1.2). Furthermore, the meta-analysis showed that individuals with LTPA levels of half the recommended 150 minutes per week of moderate-intensity PA also had a 14% lower risk of CHD compared to those who performed no LTPA (24). These results support the 2008 National PA Guidelines statements of "some PA is better than none" and "additional benefits occur with more PA" (5).

Summary of PA and CVD

CVD is a highly prevalent and growing problem among American adults that carries a large economic burden. There is a strong body of evidence that PA is an effective tool for the management and prevention of CVD, ranging from large-scale observational studies to numerous RCTs. The 2008 PA Guidelines and 2010 WHO Global Recommendations on PA for health both provide PA recommendations for the management and prevention of CVD.

▣ PA and Hypertension

A subcategory of CVD, hypertension affects an estimated 33.5% of American adults 20 years of age or older, and 15.9% of those with hypertension are unaware of their condition (14). Hypertension is associated with an increased risk for all-cause and CVD mortality (25). When considering all subcategories of CVD, which include hypertension, CHD, heart failure, and stroke, hypertension is the most prevalent and is subsequently responsible for the greatest healthcare costs. By 2030, hypertension prevalence is projected to increase to 37.3% with a projected total of $200.3 billion in healthcare costs (14). Therefore, effective treatment and prevention of hypertension is a national public health priority.

Hypertension is defined as a SBP $\geq$140 mmHg or a DBP $\geq$90 mmHg, self-reported antihypertensive medicine use, or having been told previously, at least twice, by a physician or other health professional that one has high blood pressure (BP) (26). Risk factors for hypertension are similar to those for CVD and include age, race, genetic factors, socioeconomic status, overweight/obesity, physical inactivity, tobacco use, psychosocial stressors, sleep apnea, and dietary factors. Furthermore, hypertension is itself an independent risk factor for CVD (13). Although some of the risk factors for hypertension are nonmodifiable, modifiable risk factors include weight, PA levels, tobacco use, and diet. PA is an effective nonpharmacologic treatment for hypertension and can aid in weight control as well (6).

Observational Studies

Early epidemiological studies provided evidence for the inverse relationship between PA and hypertension. In the Harvard Alumni Health Study, which followed male alumni (n = 14,998) from Harvard University after graduation, Paffenbarger et al. observed the relationship between PA levels and the incidence of hypertension. Males in the study who did not regularly perform vigorous sports following graduation had a 35% greater risk of hypertension than those that did, independent of sports participation in college (27). In a meta-analysis examining lean and obese participants across 68 epidemiological studies and RCTs (n = 2,674) that examined PA as a treatment for hypertension, Fagard (28) showed an inverse relationship between PA and hypertension, independent of weight loss. The meta-analysis showed that PA was responsible for a slight lowering of BP in normotensive individuals, but a more pronounced lowering of BP in hypertensive individuals (28). Additionally, in a meta-analysis of 13 prospective cohort studies (n = 136,846), Huai et al. (29) showed an inverse dose–response relationship between PA levels and risk of hypertension. The meta-analysis showed that those that performed high and moderate levels of PA had a 19% and 11% reduced risk of developing hypertension, respectively, compared to those that performed low levels of PA (29). Moreover, in a meta-analysis of 29 cohort studies (n = 330,222), Liu et al. (30) examined the association between LTPA and hypertension in 24 studies and showed an inverse dose–response association between LTPA and hypertension. They found that individuals who met the recommended 150 minutes per week of PA (10 MET-hours per week) had a 6% lower risk of developing hypertension than individuals who did not meet the PA recommendations. Furthermore, those that performed two- and six-times the recommendations had a 12% and 33% lower risk of developing hypertension, respectively (Figure 1.3) (30).

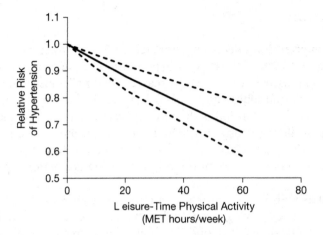

FIGURE 1.3 Dose–response association between LTPA and incident hypertension.
LTPA, leisure-time physical activity; MET, metabolic equivalent.

SOURCE: Adapted from Liu X, Zhang D, Liu Y, et al. Dose–response association between physical activity and incident hypertension: a systematic review and meta-analysis of cohort studies. *Hypertension*. 2017;69:813-820. doi:10.1161/hypertensionaha.116.08994.

BOX 1.1

What is a MET?

A MET is an absolute measure of energy expenditure during PA. For example, sitting is equivalent to one MET and brisk walking is equivalent to approximately three METs. An entire compendium of MET values for many types of PA is available as a resource.

SOURCE: Ainsworth BE, Haskell WL, Herrmann SD, et al. Compendium of physical activities: a second update of codes and MET values. *Med Sci Sports Exerc*. 2011;43(8):1575–1581. doi: 10.1249/MSS.0b013e31821ece12.

   MET, metabolic equivalent; PA, physical activity.

Experimental Studies on Hypertension and PA

Numerous nonrandomized trials and RCTs have demonstrated a strong association between increased PA levels and reduced hypertension risk (31–35). A meta-analysis examining 24 RCTs (*n* = 1,128) from 1971 to 2004 showed that previously sedentary individuals who began regular PA in the form of walking experienced a significant decrease in DBP of -1.54 mmHg (34). Furthermore, a meta-analysis examining 16 RCTs and nonrandomized trials (*n* = 650) from 1966 to 1998 showed significant decreases of 2% in both SBP (-3 mmHg) and DBP (-2 mmHg) (35). Additionally, a meta-analysis examining 27 RCTs (*n* = 1,480) from 1980 to 2014 with moderate- to vigorous-intensity physical activity (MVPA) as the treatment showed an average decrease of 11 mmHg of SBP and 5 mmHg of DBP among individuals with hypertension (31). These meta-analyses of RCTs further strengthen the clinical evidence of inverse associations between PA and hypertension that have been shown in numerous observational studies (27, 36).

Summary of PA and Hypertension

Hypertension is a highly prevalent and growing problem among American adults that carries a large and growing economic burden. There is a strong body of evidence that PA is an effective tool for the management and prevention of hypertension, ranging from large-scale observational studies to numerous RCTs. The CDC and American College of Sports Medicine (ACSM) state that just moderate amounts of PA can effectively treat hypertension (37). As such, the 2008 National PA Guidelines and 2010 WHO Global Recommendations on PA for Health both provide PA recommendations for the management and prevention of hypertension.

■ PA and Diabetes

Recently ranked as the seventh leading cause of death in the United States, diabetes mellitus is a major public health concern (2). Type 2 diabetes mellitus (hereafter referred to as diabetes), a chronic condition in which the body ineffectively uses insulin, results in increased blood glucose levels, and represents the majority of diabetes cases around the world (38). A strong independent risk factor for mortality, diabetes additionally serves as a leading cause of blindness (due to diabetic retinopathy) and kidney disease (nephropathy) in the United States. Increased risk of CVD and nerve damage (neuropathy), primarily of the lower leg and foot, are also associated complications from diabetes. The prevalence of diabetes continues to increase, with it being estimated that over 10% of the global population will have diabetes by 2040 (39). This increased global diabetes prevalence is associated with the global prevalence of physical inactivity (40). Thus, while more expensive medical therapies such as oral medications and insulin injections may be used to control or prevent diabetes, PA represents a low-cost approach that may aid in diabetes management and prevention.

Observational Studies on PA and Diabetes

Multiple prospective cohort studies have investigated the association between PA and diabetes. Smith et al. (41) recently published a meta-analysis of 28 prospective cohort studies dating from 1991 to 2015. Pooled analysis revealed a risk reduction for diabetes of 13% per 10 MET-hours per week increment of PA (41). For the same PA increment, LTPA resulted in a larger risk reduction (17%) than total PA (5%) (41). Risk reduction for vigorous PA accumulation was much larger (56%) per 10 MET-hours per week. Achieving the recommended 150 minutes per week of MVPA (11.25 MET-hours per week) was associated with a 26% reduced risk of developing diabetes relative to completely inactive individuals. Doubling this activity level to 22.5 MET-hours per week resulted in a 10% greater reduction in risk. Interestingly, no plateau effect of obtained benefit was found, with up to a 53% risk reduction at a PA dosage of 60 MET-hours per week (41).

Experimental Studies on PA and Diabetes

While observational cohort studies have been able to provide associations between PA and diabetes, RCTs have tested these associations to further tease out causal inferences. A landmark intervention study on the role of lifestyle in diabetes prevention, the Diabetes Prevention Program (DPP), compared metformin, a popular antihyperglycemic medication, to a lifestyle modification program in subjects with impaired glucose tol-

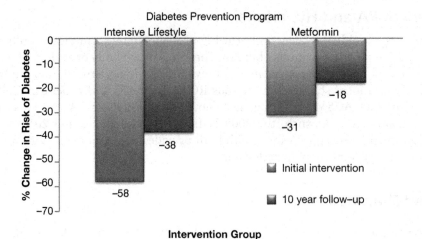

FIGURE 1.4   Reduction in risk of type 2 diabetes in the DPP. DPP, Diabetes Prevention Program.

SOURCE: Adapted from Knowler WC, Barrett-Connor E, Fowler SE, et al. Reduction in the incidence of type 2 diabetes with lifestyle intervention or metformin. *N Engl J Med.* 2002;346:393-403. doi:10.1056/NEJMoa012512; Diabetes Prevention Program Research Group; Knowler WC, Fowler SE, et al. 10-year follow-up of diabetes incidence and weight loss in the Diabetes Prevention Program Outcomes Study. *Lancet.* 2009;374:1677-1686. doi:10.1016/s0140-6736(09)61457-4.

erance (42). Prior interventions had already exposed the benefits of diet, exercise, and their interaction in reducing the incidence of diabetes (43, 44). However, the DPP was one of the first to examine the potential benefit of medications in diabetes prevention, as well as comparing these effects to that of an intensive lifestyle modification within the same study. Participants were randomized to three different groups: placebo (control), metformin, or lifestyle intervention, which included diet and exercise. The lifestyle intervention consisted of the goal of at least 7% weight loss, as well as a minimum of 150 minutes per week of PA, in line with current national recommendations. After an average follow-up of 2.8 years (range, 1.8–4.6), the metformin group reduced the incidence of diabetes by 31%, whereas the lifestyle modification group reduced diabetes incidence by 58% (Figure 1.4) (42). While both intervention groups significantly reduced diabetes incidence, lifestyle modification was significantly more effective than metformin in diabetes incidence reduction.

Results from the 10-year follow-up of the DPP study show that both the metformin and lifestyle intervention group maintained a level of reduced risk of diabetes. While the initial weight loss of the lifestyle group was not maintained over the course of follow-up, these participants still showed a reduction in risk for diabetes of 38% as compared to an 18% reduction in the metformin group (Figure 1.4) (45). These outcomes are supported by follow-up data from the Finnish Diabetes Prevention Study, showing that participants randomized to a similar lifestyle intervention maintained an improved level of glucose tolerance, as well as a reduced incidence of diabetes over a follow-up of 7 years (46).

Just as PA can be beneficial in the prevention of diabetes, it can also be used as a therapy for persons with diabetes. PA has been shown to improve glucose tolerance and increase insulin sensitivity in individuals with diabetes (47). Along with its benefits on glucose metabolism, PA has been associated with increased cardiorespiratory fitness (48), lower BP (49), improved blood lipid profiles (50), weight loss (51), and increased overall quality of life for individuals with diabetes (52). Consequently, these benefits are also associated with reduced risk of comorbidities such as retinopathy, nephropathy, neuropathy, and CVD, as well as reduced risk for all-cause mortality (53). A joint position stand by the American Diabetes Association and ACSM recommends that individuals with diabetes engage in a minimum of 150 minutes per week of MVPA most days of the week and maintain these PA levels over many years to maintain risk reduction and prevent complications and/or comorbidities (54).

Summary of PA and Diabetes

There is a strong body of literature, both epidemiological and interventional, supporting the benefits of regular PA in preventing or delaying the onset of diabetes. Similarly, PA has also been shown to be beneficial for individuals with diabetes. The major benefits of PA are thought to be attributable to improved glucose metabolism, which therefore decreases the deleterious effects of high plasma glucose.

PA and Cancer

Cancer, a condition of uncontrolled growth of abnormal cells, is a global concern and the second leading cause of death in the United States, trailing only deaths from heart disease (55). In 2014, 23% of the 2.6 million overall deaths in the United States were attributable to cancer (55). The three most common fatal cancers in 2014 for U.S. men were estimated (in order of frequency) to be cancers of the lung, prostate, and colorectal. For women, the most fatal cancers were lung, breast, and colorectal (55). Given the public health burden of cancer, much attention has been given to identifying possible cures and preventive measures. PA has recently emerged as a modifiable risk factor for cancer incidence and mortality. Overall, PA confers a 7% reduction in risk of cancer when comparing high (90th percentile) to low (10th percentile) levels of PA (56). This risk reduction can vary substantially when analyzing individual types of cancer. For this reason, we will focus on the association between PA and the four leading causes of cancer mortality in the United States: lung, prostate, breast, and colorectal (55).

Lung Cancer

Lung cancer is the leading cause of cancer mortality in the United States for both males and females, accounting for over 26% of cancer deaths in 2014 (55). Multiple studies have documented the associations between PA and lung cancer, with consistent positive results. The meta-analysis by Moore et al. (56) found that high levels (90th percentile) of LTPA were associated with a 27% decreased risk of lung cancer when compared to low levels (10th percentile) of LTPA. In terms of mortality, results from the NIH-AARP Diet and Health Study (n = 293,511; 42% female) reported a 15% decreased risk of lung cancer death in persons who achieved greater than 1 hour of MVPA a week, with minimal increased benefit at higher activity levels (57).

Prostate Cancer

The reported associations between PA and risk of prostate cancer have been largely inconsistent. While individual studies may indicate a benefit of PA, meta-analysis suggests a slight, if not insignificant, benefit. Moore et al. meta-analysis data suggest no benefit of LTPA on prostate cancer risk (56). An earlier report of 19 cohort and 24 case control

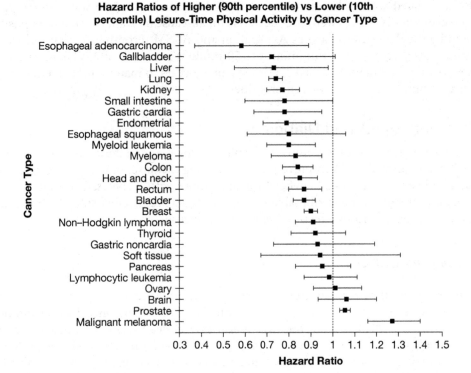

FIGURE 1.5 Hazard ratios for 26 types of cancer. Ratios compared 90th (high) with 10th (low) percentile of leisure-time physical activity.

SOURCE: Adapted from Moore SC, Lee IM, Weiderpass E, et al. Association of leisure-time physical activity with risk of 26 types of cancer in 1.44 million adults. *JAMA Intern Med.* 2016;176:816-825. doi:10.1001/jamainternmed.2016.1548.

studies suggests a modest 10% risk reduction when comparing the most active to least active individuals (58). In terms of mortality, men with prostate cancer in the Health Professionals Follow-Up Study ($n = 2,705$) who achieved ≥ 3 hours per week of vigorous activity had a 61% lower risk of prostate-cancer-specific mortality when compared with men that achieved less than 1 hour per week (59). Another study of 4,623 Swedish men diagnosed with prostate cancer reported a 39% reduced risk of prostate-cancer-specific mortality in men who walked/biked ≥ 20 minutes per day as compared to those achieving less than 20 minutes per day (60).

Breast Cancer

Breast cancer is the second leading cause of all cancer deaths in U.S. women (55). PA has been shown to be beneficial for both breast cancer morbidity and mortality. The meta-analysis by Moore et al. (56) found that high levels (90th percentile) of LTPA were associated with a 10% decreased risk for breast cancer (relative to low levels; 10th percentile) while another dose–response meta-analysis of 31 prospective cohort analyses estimated a 5% risk reduction for every 2 hours per week increment in moderate plus vigorous PA (61). Based on this dose–response analysis, a woman achieving the recommended 150 minutes of MVPA would have a 6.25% reduced risk for breast cancer compared to a sedentary woman. Schmid and Leitzmann (62) performed a meta-analysis of 16 studies on breast cancer survivors. The analyses showed a 23% and 28% reduction in risk of breast cancer mortality associated with the highest versus the lowest pre- and postdiagnosis PA levels, respectively (62).

Colorectal Cancer

Colorectal cancer is the third leading cause of cancer deaths in the United States among both men and women (55). The associated benefits of PA with colorectal cancer include both lowered risk of development and colorectal-cancer-specific mortality. In their meta-analysis, Moore et al. (56) found that high levels of LTPA (90th percentile) were associated with risk reductions of 16% and 13% for colon and rectal cancers, respectively, when compared to low LTPA (10th percentile). In another meta-analysis of seven studies of colorectal cancer survivors, the highest prediagnosis levels of PA were associated with a 25% reduced risk of colorectal cancer mortality when compared to the lowest PA levels (8). In the same meta-analysis, postdiagnosis recreational PA was associated with a 39% reduced risk for colorectal cancer mortality when comparing subjects with the highest PA levels to those with the lowest PA (62).

Summary of PA and Cancer

Multiple studies have examined the association of PA in cancer prevention and management. Recent studies suggest that increased levels of PA are associated with reduced risk of developing lung, breast, and colorectal cancers, with prostate cancers showing inconsistent results. PA has also been associated with decreased risk of cancer-specific mortality for lung, prostate, breast, and colorectal cancers. The ACSM recognizes exercise as generally safe for cancer survivors and stands by the U.S. Department of Health and Human Services' general recommendation of 150 minutes of MVPA, or 75 minutes of vigorous PA per week, for cancer survivors and the general population alike (63). It is recognized that these recommendations may need to be adapted to individual survivors, their health status, treatments received, and anticipated disease trajectory (63). Aside from prevention and treatment of cancer, PA is associated with benefits such as improvements in quality of life, fatigue, and depression (64).

Current Issues in PA and Chronic Disease Research: Sedentary Behavior

Emerging epidemiological evidence strongly suggests that sedentary behavior is associated with increased cardiovascular morbidity and mortality (65). The word *sedentary* is defined as "characterized by or requiring a sitting posture." Operationally, sedentary behavior is defined as waking activities performed while sitting or reclining that require energy expenditure less than 1.5 metabolic equivalents (METs), while physical inactivity is defined as insufficient amounts of MVPA (i.e., not meeting current PA guidelines) (66). One MET is defined as the energy expended while sitting at rest (equivalent to 3.5 mL of oxygen per kilogram of body weight per minute), while MVPA is defined as activities that expend at least 3.0 METs (67). Thus, sedentary behavior is distinct from both lack of MVPA and physical inactivity. As such, each behavior is thought to have its own determinants and health consequences (65).

According to objectively measured sedentary time in the National Health and Nutrition Examination Survey (NHANES) 2005 to 2006, U.S. adults spend an average of almost

8 hours per day sitting (68), with this number increasing in older adults (69, 70). Overall, NHANES data show that two thirds of an average day is spent sleeping or sitting, with another 7.8 hours in light activity (68, 71). In terms of occupational energy expenditure, data from the U.S. Bureau of Labor Statistics show a steep decline in occupation-related PA energy expenditure across the past several decades, as almost half the jobs in the early 1960s required at least moderate-intensity PA, while less than 20% of jobs required this level of energy expenditure in 2008 (72).

There is accumulating evidence from prospective cohort studies that sedentary behavior is positively associated with risk of CVD, type 2 diabetes, and all-cause CVD mortality (65). For example, objective data from over 1,900 NHANES (2003–2004) participants aged 50 and older followed over an average of 2.8 years showed that participants in the third (8.7–10.1 hours women, 9.2–10.8 hours men) and fourth quartile (>10.1 hours women, >10.8 hours men) of daily sedentary time had four and six times increased risk of death, respectively, compared to those in the lowest quartile, independent of MVPA levels and other confounding factors (73). Systematic reviews and meta-analyses show mostly consistent findings for the association of sedentary behavior and all-cause and CVD mortality, whereas the findings for cancer mortality are less consistent (65).

There is accumulating evidence from prospective cohort studies that sedentary behavior is positively associated with risk of CVD, type 2 diabetes, and all-cause and CVD mortality (65). For example, objective data from over 1,900 NHANES (2003–2004) participants aged 50 and older followed an average of 2.8 years showed that participants in the third (8.7–10.1 hours women, 9.2–10.8 hours men) and fourth quartile (>10.1 hours women, >10.8 hours men) of daily sedentary time had four and six times increased risk of death, respectively, compared to those in the lowest quartile. A systematic review and meta-analysis of studies through August 2014 found that greater sedentary time was positively associated with an increased risk for all-cause mortality, CVD mortality, cancer mortality, CVD incidence, cancer incidence, and type 2 diabetes incidence, independent of PA levels (74). Additionally, the effects of sedentary time on all-cause mortality appeared to be 30% lower among individuals with high levels of PA compared to those with low levels of PA. Although increased levels of PA and MVPA appear to attenuate the detrimental effects of sedentary behavior on mortality and CVD outcomes, sedentary behavior appears to be an independent risk factor.

In 2012, Katzmarzyk and Lee estimated that U.S. population life expectancy would be 2 years higher if adults reduced their usual sitting to less than 3 hours per day, and 1.38 years higher if they reduced their television-watching behaviors to less than 2 hours per day (75). Additionally, recent analyses have attempted to estimate the benefits of replacing sedentary behaviors with other PA behaviors. A study of over 150,000 older adults in one study found that replacing 1 hour per day of sitting with an equal amount of exercise or nonexercise activities (e.g., household chores, walking) was associated with 42% and 30% lower all-cause mortality, respectively (76). Similarly, estimates from NHANES 2005 to 2006 data showed that replacing 30 minutes per day of sedentary time with equal time of sleep, light-intensity PA, or MVPA were associated with improved CVD risk factor levels (e.g., insulin, triglycerides, high-density lipoprotein cholesterol, waist circumference) (77). Although several studies have performed interventions designed to reduce sedentary behaviors, further RCTs are needed to examine the effects of reduced sedentary time on health outcomes.

Overall, the preponderance of evidence suggests greater sedentary behavior is an independent risk factor for CVD morbidity and mortality and all-cause mortality.

Current PA guidelines do not include recommendations for sedentary behavior, although sedentary behavior guidelines have been developed in several countries. However, existing sedentary guidelines are vague and nonquantitative (65). For example, Australia and the United Kingdom have public health guidelines stating that adults should minimize the amount of time spent being sedentary (sitting) for extended periods (78, 79). A recent position statement from the American Diabetes Association recommended that all adults, particularly those with diabetes, should reduce the amount of time spent in daily sedentary behavior and that prolonged sitting should be interrupted with bouts of light activity every 30 minutes for blood glucose benefits (80).

Further evidence is needed to identify the amount of sedentary behavior required to maximize health outcomes. As such, the recent American Heart Association Science Advisory concluded that "Given the current state of the science on sedentary behavior and in the absence of sufficient data to recommend quantitative guidelines, it is appropriate to promote the advisory, 'Sit less, move more.'"(65)

▧ Summary

The beneficial effects of habitual PA on chronic disease prevention and control are well-known and have been demonstrated in epidemiological studies for over 60 years. The extensive evidence for the inverse dose–response association between volume of PA and all-cause mortality is strong, with a curvilinear dose–response curve where a larger decrease in risk is observed at the lower end of the PA spectrum compared to the higher end; hence the expression "some PA is better than none, more is better." There is also a clear, strong evidence base from prospective cohort studies and case–control studies showing an inverse dose–response association between PA volume and CVD. Similarly, extensive evidence from RCTs or meta-analyses shows a clear inverse relationship between PA and both hypertension and diabetes. Lastly, pooled analyses of large prospective cohort studies found that high levels of PA were associated with lower risk of 13 different cancers, including lung, colorectal, and breast. Importantly, all of the aforementioned associations exist for both men and women and individuals of all ages. There is no evidence for sex-specific, age-specific, or race/ethnic-specific effects when volume is the exposure rather than relative intensity. Furthermore, the inverse association of PA and all-cause mortality and several of these traits are independent of body mass index (BMI). Taken together, the current evidence highlights the importance of performing regular PA across the life span for its beneficial effects on numerous health outcomes.

▧ Things to Consider

- PA reduces risk of many of the chronic diseases including CVD, hypertension, diabetes, and cancer.
- There are many types of studies (e.g., observational, RCT) that demonstrate the reduction in chronic disease risk with PA.
- Since sedentary behavior is a risk factor for many chronic diseases, it needs to be addressed in interventions in addition to promoting PA.

■ References

1. Ward BW, Schiller JS, Goodman RA. Multiple chronic conditions among US adults: a 2012 update. *Prev Chronic Dis.* 2014;11:E62. doi:10.5888/pcd11.130389
2. Centers for Disease Control and Prevention. Leading Causes of Death in 1975 and 2015: United States, 1975–2015 (Figure 8). Health, United States. 2016. Available at: https://www.cdc.gov/nchs/data/hus/hus16.pdf{#}019
3. Gerteis J, Izrael D, Deitz D, et al. *Multiple Chronic Conditions Chartbook.* AHRQ Publications No. Q14–0038. Rockville, MD: Agency for Healthcare Research and Quality; 2014.
4. Centers for Disease Control and Prevention. Physical Activity for Everyone. 2011. Available at: http://www.cdc.gov/physicalactivity/everyone/glossary/indexhtml
5. Physical Activity Guidelines Advisory Committee. *Physical Activity Guidelines Advisory Committee Report.* Washington, DC: Department of Health and Human Services; 2008.
6. World Health Organization. *Global Recommendations on Physical Activity for Health.* Geneva, Switzerland: World Health Organization; 2010.
7. World Health Organization. *Physical Activity Fact Sheet.* 2017.
8. U.S. Department of Health and Human Services. Healthy People 2020: Physical Activity. Available at: https://www.healthypeople.gov/2020/topics-objectives/topic/physical-activity/objectives
9. Booth FW, Roberts CK, Laye MJ. Lack of exercise is a major cause of chronic diseases. *Compr Physiol.* 2012;2:1143–1211. doi:10.1002/cphy.c110025
10. Lee IM, Shiroma EJ, Lobelo F, et al. Effect of physical inactivity on major non-communicable diseases worldwide: an analysis of burden of disease and life expectancy. *Lancet.* 2012;380:219–229. doi:10.1016/S0140-6736(12)61031-9
11. Danaei G, Ding EL, Mozaffarian D, et al. The preventable causes of death in the United States: comparative risk assessment of dietary, lifestyle, and metabolic risk factors. *PLOS Med.* 2009;6:e1000058. doi:10.1371/journal.pmed.1000058
12. Ding D, Lawson KD, Kolbe-Alexander TL, et al. The economic burden of physical inactivity: a global analysis of major non-communicable diseases. *Lancet.* 2016;388:1311–1324. doi:10.1016/S0140-6736(16)30383-X
13. World Health Organization. *Global Atlas on Cardiovascular Disease Prevention and Control;* 2011.
14. Benjamin EJ, Blaha MJ, Chiuve SE, et al. Heart disease and stroke statistics—2017 update: a report from the American Heart Association. *Circulation.* 2017;135:e146–e603.
15. Heidenreich PA, Trogdon JG, Khavjou OA, et al. Forecasting the future of cardiovascular disease in the United States. *Circulation.* 2011;123:933–944. doi:10.1161/CIR.0b013e31820a55f5
16. Grundy SM, Pasternak R, Greenland P, et al. Assessment of cardiovascular risk by use of multiple-risk-factor assessment equations. *Circulation.* 1999;100:1481. doi:10.1161/01.cir.100.13.1481
17. Murtagh EM, Nichols L, Mohammed MA, et al. The effect of walking on risk factors for cardiovascular disease: an updated systematic review and meta-analysis of randomised control trials. *Prev Med.* 2015;72:34–43. doi:10.1016/j.ypmed.2014.12.041
18. Morris JN, Heady J, Raffle P, et al. Coronary heart-disease and physical activity of work. *The Lancet.* 1953;262:1111–1120. doi:10.1016/s0140-6736(53)91495-0
19. Paffenbarger RSJ, Hale WE. Work activity and coronary heart mortality. *N Engl J Med.* 1975;292:545–550. doi:10.1056/nejm197503132921101
20. Kannel WB, Sorlie P. Some health benefits of physical activity: the Framingham study. *Arch Intern Med.* 1979;139:857–861. doi:10.1001/archinte.139.8.857
21. Sesso HD, Paffenbarger RS, Lee IM. Physical activity and coronary heart disease in men. *Circulation.* 2000;102:975. doi:10.1161/01.cir.102.9.975
22. Li J, Siegrist J. Physical activity and risk of cardiovascular disease—a meta-analysis of prospective cohort studies. *Int J Environ Res Public Health.* 2012;9:391–407. doi:10.3390/ijerph9020391

23. Oguma Y, Shinoda-Tagawa T. Physical activity decreases cardiovascular disease risk in women: review and meta-analysis. *Am J Prev Med.* 2004;26:407–418. doi:10.1016/j.amepre.2004.02.007

24. Sattelmair J, Pertman J, Ding EL, et al. Dose response between physical activity and risk of coronary heart disease: a meta-analysis. *Circulation.* 2011;124:789–795. doi:10.1161/circulationaha.110.010710

25. Pescatello LS, Franklin BA, Fagard R, et al. American College of Sports Medicine position stand. Exercise and hypertension. *Med Sci Sports Exerc.* 2004;36:533–553.

26. Crim MT, Yoon SS, Ortiz E, et al. National surveillance definitions for hypertension prevalence and control among adults. *Circ Cardiovasc Qual Outcomes.* 2012;5:343–351.

27. Paffenbarger RS Jr, Wing AL Jr, Hyde RT Jr, et al. Physical activity and incidence of hypertension in college alumni. *Am J Epidemiol.* 1983;117:245–257. doi:10.1093/oxfordjournals.aje.a113537

28. Fagard R. Physical activity in the prevention and treatment of hypertension in the obese. *Med Sci Sports Exerc.* 1999;31:S624–S630. doi:10.1097/00005768-199911001-00022

29. Huai P, Xun H, Reilly KH, et al. Physical activity and risk of hypertension. *Hypertension.* 2013;62:1021–1026.

30. Liu X, Zhang D, Liu Y, et al. Dose-response association between physical activity and incident hypertension: a systematic review and meta-analysis of cohort studies. *Hypertension.* 2017;69:813–820. doi:10.1161/hypertensionaha.116.08994

31. Börjesson M, Onerup A, Lundqvist S, et al. Physical activity and exercise lower blood pressure in individuals with hypertension: narrative review of 27 RCTs. *Br J Sports Med.* 2016;50:356–361. doi:10.1136/bjsports-2015-095786

32. Whelton SP, Chin A, Xin X, et al. Effect of aerobic exercise on blood pressure: a meta-analysis of randomized, controlled trials. *Ann Intern Med.* 2002;136:493–503. doi:10.7326/0003-4819-136-7-200204020-00006

33. Wen H, Wang L. Reducing effect of aerobic exercise on blood pressure of essential hypertensive patients: a meta-analysis. *Medicine.* 2017;96:e6150. doi:10.1097/md.0000000000006150

34. Murphy MH, Nevill AM, Murtagh EM, et al. The effect of walking on fitness, fatness and resting blood pressure: a meta-analysis of randomised, controlled trials. *Prev Med.* 2007;44:377–385. doi:10.1016/j.ypmed.2006.12.008

35. Kelley GA, Kelley KS, Tran ZV. Walking and resting blood pressure in adults: a meta-analysis. *Prev Med.* 2001;33:120–127. doi:10.1006/pmed.2001.0860

36. Paffenbarger RS, Jung DL, Leung RW, et al. Physical activity and hypertension: an epidemiological view. *Ann Med.* 1991;23:319–327. doi:10.3109/07853899109148067

37. Pate RR, Pratt M, Blair SN, et al. Physical activity and public health: a recommendation from the Centers for Disease Control and Prevention and the American College of Sports Medicine. *JAMA.* 1995;273:402–407. doi:10.1001/jama.1995.03520290054029

38. Alberti KG, Zimmet PZ. Definition, diagnosis and classification of diabetes mellitus and its complications. Part 1: diagnosis and classification of diabetes mellitus provisional report of a WHO consultation. *Diabet Med.* 1998;15:539–553. doi:10.1002/(sici)1096-9136(199807)15:7<539:: aid-dia668>3.0.co;2-s

39. International Diabetes Federation. *IDF Diabetes Atlas.* 7th ed. International Diabetes Federation; 2015.

40. Oggioni C, Lara J, Wells JC, et al. Shifts in population dietary patterns and physical inactivity as determinants of global trends in the prevalence of diabetes: an ecological analysis. *Nutr Metab Cardiovasc Dis.* 2014;24:1105–1111. doi:10.1016/j.numecd.2014.05.005

41. Smith AD, Crippa A, Woodcock J, et al. Physical activity and incident type 2 diabetes mellitus: a systematic review and dose-response meta-analysis of prospective cohort studies. *Diabetologia.* 2016;59:2527–2545. doi:10.1007/s00125-016-4079-0

42. Knowler WC, Barrett-Connor E, Fowler SE, et al. Reduction in the incidence of type 2 diabetes with lifestyle intervention or metformin. *N Engl J Med.* 2002;346:393–403. doi:10.1056/NEJMoa012512

43. Pan XR, Li GW, Hu YH, et al. Effects of diet and exercise in preventing NIDDM in people with impaired glucose tolerance. The Da Qing IGT and Diabetes Study. *Diabetes Care.* 1997;20:537–544. doi:10.2337/diacare.20.4.537

44. Tuomilehto J, Lindstrom J, Eriksson JG, et al. Prevention of type 2 diabetes mellitus by changes in lifestyle among subjects with impaired glucose tolerance. *N Engl J Med.* 2001;344:1343–1350. doi:10.1056/nejm200105033441801

45. Diabetes Prevention Program Research Group, Knowler WC, Fowler SE, et al. 10-year follow-up of diabetes incidence and weight loss in the Diabetes Prevention Program Outcomes Study. *Lancet.* 2009;374:1677–1686. doi:10.1016/s0140-6736(09)61457-4

46. Lindstrom J, Ilanne-Parikka P, Peltonen M, et al. Sustained reduction in the incidence of type 2 diabetes by lifestyle intervention: follow-up of the Finnish Diabetes Prevention Study. *Lancet.* 2006;368:1673–1679. doi:10.1016/s0140-6736(06)69701-8

47. Winnick JJ, Sherman WM, Habash DL, et al. Short-term aerobic exercise training in obese humans with type 2 diabetes mellitus improves whole-body insulin sensitivity through gains in peripheral, not hepatic insulin sensitivity. *J Clin Endocrinol Metab.* 2008;93:771–778. doi:10.1210/jc.2007-1524

48. Boule NG, Kenny GP, Haddad E, et al. Meta-analysis of the effect of structured exercise training on cardiorespiratory fitness in type 2 diabetes mellitus. *Diabetologia.* 2003;46:1071–1081. doi:10.1007/s00125-003-1160-2

49. Schneider SH, Khachadurian AK, Amorosa LF, et al. Ten-year experience with an exercise-based outpatient life-style modification program in the treatment of diabetes mellitus. *Diabetes Care.* 1992;15:1800–1810. doi:10.2337/diacare.15.11.1800

50. Verity LS, Ismail AH. Effects of exercise on cardiovascular disease risk in women with NIDDM. *Diabetes Res Clin Pract.* 1989;6:27–35. doi:10.1016/0168-8227(89)90054-5

51. Look Ahead Reseach Group. Eight-year weight losses with an intensive lifestyle intervention: the look AHEAD study. *Obesity (Silver Spring).* 2014;22:5–13. doi:10.1002/oby.20662

52. Thiel DM, Sayah FA, Vallance J, et al. Physical activity and health-related quality of life in adults with type 2 diabetes: results from a prospective cohort study. *J Phys Act Health.* 2017;14:368–374. doi:10.1123/jpah.2016-0271

53. Blomster JI, Chow CK, Zoungas S, et al. The influence of physical activity on vascular complications and mortality in patients with type 2 diabetes mellitus. *Diabetes Obes Metab.* 2013;15:1008–1012. doi:10.1111/dom.12122

54. Colberg SR, Sigal RJ, Fernhall B, et al. Exercise and type 2 diabetes: the American College of Sports Medicine and the American Diabetes Association: joint position statement. *Diabetes Care.* 2010;33:e147–e167. doi:10.2337/dc10-9990

55. Siegel RL, Miller KD, Jemal A. Cancer statistics, 2017. *CA Cancer J Clin.* 2017;67:7–30. doi:10.3322/caac.21387

56. Moore SC, Lee IM, Weiderpass E, et al. Association of leisure-time physical activity with risk of 26 types of cancer in 1.44 million adults. *JAMA Intern Med.* 2016;176:816–825. doi:10.1001/jamainternmed.2016.1548

57. Arem H, Moore SC, Park Y, et al. Physical activity and cancer-specific mortality in the NIH-AARP Diet and Health Study cohort. *Int J Cancer.* 2014;135:423–431. doi:10.1002/ijc.28659

58. Liu Y, Hu F, Li D, et al. Does physical activity reduce the risk of prostate cancer? A systematic review and meta-analysis. *Eur Urol.* 2011;60:1029–1044. doi:10.1016/j.eururo.2011.07.007

59. Kenfield SA, Stampfer MJ, Giovannucci E, et al. Physical activity and survival after prostate cancer diagnosis in the health professionals follow-up study. *J Clin Oncol.* 2011;29:726–732. doi:10.1200/jco.2010.31.5226

60. Bonn SE, Sjolander A, Lagerros YT, et al. Physical activity and survival among men diagnosed with prostate cancer. *Cancer Epidemiol Biomarkers Prev.* 2015;24:57–64. doi:10.1158/1055-9965.epi-14-0707

61. Wu Y, Zhang D, Kang S. Physical activity and risk of breast cancer: a meta-analysis of prospective studies. *Breast Cancer Res Treat.* 2013;137:869–882. doi:10.1007/s10549-012-2396-7

62. Schmid D, Leitzmann MF. Association between physical activity and mortality among breast cancer and colorectal cancer survivors: a systematic review and meta-analysis. *Ann Oncol.* 2014;25:1293–1311. doi:10.1093/annonc/mdu012

63. Schmitz KH, Courneya KS, Matthews C, et al. American College of Sports Medicine roundtable on exercise guidelines for cancer survivors. *Med Sci Sports Exerc.* 2010;42:1409–1426. doi:10.1249/mss.0b013e3181e0c112

64. Desnoyers A, Riesco E, Fulop T, et al. Physical activity and cancer: update and literature review. *Rev Med Interne.* 2016;37:399–405. doi:10.1016/j.revmed.2015.12.021

65. Young DR, Hivert MF, Alhassan S, et al. Sedentary behavior and cardiovascular morbidity and mortality: a science advisory from the American Heart Association. *Circulation.* 2016;134:e262–e279. doi:10.1161/cir.0000000000000440

66. Sedentary Behaviour Research Network. Letter to the editor: standardized use of the terms "sedentary" and "sedentary behaviours". *Appl Physiol Nutr Metab.* 2012;37:540–542. doi:10.1139/h2012-024

67. Strath SJ, Kaminsky LA, Ainsworth BE, et al. Guide to the assessment of physical activity: clinical and research applications: a scientific statement from the American Heart Association. *Circulation.* 2013;128:2259–2279. doi:10.1161/01.cir.0000435708.67487.da

68. Schuna JM Jr, Johnson WD Jr, Tudor-Locke C. Adult self-reported and objectively monitored physical activity and sedentary behavior: NHANES 2005–2006. *Int J Behav Nutr Phys Act.* 2013;10:126. doi:10.1186/1479-5868-10-126

69. Harvey JA, Chastin SF, Skelton DA. Prevalence of sedentary behavior in older adults: a systematic review. *Int J Environ Res Public Health.* 2013;10:6645–6661. doi:10.3390/ijerph10126645

70. Gorman E, Hanson HM, Yang PH, et al. Accelerometry analysis of physical activity and sedentary behavior in older adults: a systematic review and data analysis. *Eur Rev Aging Phys Act.* 2014;11:35–49. doi:10.1007/s11556-013-0132-x

71. Matthews CE, Chen KY, Freedson PS, et al. Amount of time spent in sedentary behaviors in the United States, 2003–2004. *Am J Epidemiol.* 2008;167:875–881. doi:10.1093/aje/kwm390

72. Church TS, Thomas DM, Tudor-Locke C, et al. Trends over 5 decades in U.S. occupation-related physical activity and their associations with obesity. *PLOS ONE.* 2011;6:e19657. doi:10.1371/journal.pone.0019657

73. Koster A, Caserotti P, Patel KV, et al. Association of sedentary time with mortality independent of moderate to vigorous physical activity. *PLOS ONE.* 2012;7:e37696. doi:10.1371/journal.pone.0037696

74. Biswas A, Oh PI, Faulkner GE, et al. Sedentary time and its association with risk for disease incidence, mortality, and hospitalization in adults: a systematic review and meta-analysis. *Ann Intern Med.* 2015;162:123–132. doi:10.7326/m14-1651

75. Katzmarzyk PT, Lee IM. Sedentary behaviour and life expectancy in the USA: a cause-deleted life table analysis. *BMJ Open.* 2012;2:e000828. doi:10.1136/bmjopen-2012-000828

76. Matthews CE, Moore SC, Sampson J, et al. Mortality benefits for replacing sitting time with different physical activities. *Med Sci Sports Exerc.* 2015;47:1833–1840. doi:10.1249/mss.0000000000000621

77. Buman MP, Winkler EA, Kurka JM, et al. Reallocating time to sleep, sedentary behaviors, or active behaviors: associations with cardiovascular disease risk biomarkers, NHANES 2005-2006. *Am J Epidemiol.* 2014;179:323–334. doi:10.1093/aje/kwt292

78. Australian Government Department of Health. *Australia's Physical Activity and Sedentary Behaviour Guidelines for Adults (18–64 years).* Canberra, Australia: Australian Government Department of Health; 2014.

79. UK Department of Health. *Start Active, Stay Active: A Report on Physical Activity for Health From the Four Home Countries' Chief Medical Officers.* London, England: Crown Copyright; 2011.

80. Colberg SR, Sigal RJ, Yardley JE, et al. Physical activity/exercise and diabetes: a position statement of the American Diabetes Association. *Diabetes Care.* 2016;39:2065–2079. doi:10.2337/dc16-1728

81. Ainsworth BE, Haskell WL, Herrmann SD, et al. Compendium of physical activities: a second update of codes and MET values. *Med Sci Sports Exerc.* 2011;43(8):1575–1581. doi:10.1249/MSS.0b013e31821ece12

MEASUREMENT OF PHYSICAL ACTIVITY AND SEDENTARY BEHAVIORS

JOHN R. SIRARD | GREG J. PETRUCCI JR.

LEARNING OBJECTIVES

By the end of this chapter, students should be able to

1. Define validity and reliability as they relate to different instruments for measuring physical activity (PA).

2. Compare the validity and reliability of objective instruments versus subjective instruments based on the context in which PA is being measured.

3. Critique the pros and cons of research-grade accelerometers versus commercial-grade activity trackers for measuring PA.

4. Compare the utility of a step counter versus a self-report instrument for measuring population levels of PA across the country.

5. Select a highly appropriate instrument for measuring PA based on: the population being measured, the setting and context in which PA is occurring, and the goals of the intervention.

■ Introduction

Physical activity (PA) and sedentary behavior (SB) are distinct and complex behaviors. They are distinct because individuals can perform regular vigorous exercise but also spend the rest of their free time and the bulk of their workday being sedentary. Just because a person is meeting or exceeding PA recommendations, we cannot assume the person is accumulating only small amounts of sedentary time.

If we consider PA to be any movement produced by skeletal muscle that results in energy expenditure (1), then a purely mechanical analysis of the frequency, intensity, and duration of those movements would be sufficient. Indeed, this type of assessment is

© Springer Publishing Company DOI: 10.1891/9780826134592.0002

what motion sensors, like pedometers and accelerometers, excel at providing. However, PA and SB are complex behaviors and there are many ways to be active and many ways to be sedentary. PA could include walking or bicycling to work, playing tag, or structured exercise routines like jogging or resistance training, just to name a few. SBs can include, but are not limited to, a wide variety of screen-time behaviors (computer use, TV viewing, smartphone, or tablet). For many interventions, being able to discern the specific type of PA or SB is critical to the intervention process and outcomes.

For many interventions, the context in which PA and SB are happening may also be important, which means attempting to understand these behaviors beyond just identifying frequency, intensity, and duration of movements. People do not live and make decisions about their behavior in a vacuum. Therefore, our PA and SB interventions also need to consider the multilevel influences on each of these behaviors. Researchers will typically adopt an ecological perspective and consider individual, social, cultural, physical, environmental, and policy issues that directly or indirectly steer people toward one behavior versus another. Although these contextual factors are not the focus of this chapter, there may be situations, when obtaining data about the "with whom" and "where" of PA and SB, that would be important to help understand these behaviors and to help explain intervention success or failure. A number of self-report tools directly ask about activity type. Only recently have researchers started to explore the use of ecological momentary assessment (EMA) to simultaneously collect PA and SB, along with important contextual information.

Because PA and SB are so complex, a number of assessment tools are already available and more are always being developed, each with its own strengths and weaknesses. Therefore, the goals for this chapter are for the reader to identify the important factors to consider when deciding on which PA and/or SB assessment tool to use, the strengths and weaknesses of these tools, understanding the difference between an assessment tool and an intervention tool, and lastly, providing the reader with online and print resources to find existing PA and SB assessment tools and the supporting research.

■ Finding the Right Tool for the Job

Unfortunately, there is no best tool that fits all situations and needs for measuring PA and SB. For this chapter, we use the terms "tool" and "instrument" synonymously to refer to all methods of PA and SB assessment, whether a paper-and-pencil survey or a sophisticated research-grade accelerometer. Each tool comes with its own strengths and limitations that need to be weighed against the needs of the research or intervention program that is being conducted. For example, using a self-report instrument to assess the change in time spent standing and walking in older adults with dementia (or other cognitive limitation) may not yield reliable or valid estimates, due to challenges with memory. Therefore, an objective motion sensor that is sensitive to changes in posture and stepping would be a better choice for this specific application.

This chapter will identify a number of objective and self-report instruments that are currently available and have acceptable reliability and validity. However, this is not an exhaustive list and there are new surveys and devices being developed and tested all of the time. Therefore, this section provides a very brief overview of the concepts and considerations that will empower the reader to work through these issues and use a data-driven approach to identify the best tool to assess PA and SB for an intervention project.

Reliability

For this discussion, reliability has to do with the tool's ability to produce the same output, given that the person is doing the same behaviors or the device is moving in the same way; how reproducible is the output from the questionnaire or device from one time to the next?

The reliability of self-report instruments is most often assessed with test–retest reliability. Researchers will have participants complete the same questionnaire within a relatively short time span. The goal is to have the participant recall the same time period at each administration. For example, an approach may be to have participants complete the same 7-day PA recall twice, with several hours or 1 day between administrations. The output from the repeated assessments should not be significantly different from one another and they should be highly correlated.

For motion sensors, the reader should look for a device's intra- and interinstrument reliability. Intrainstrument (within device) reliability will typically be tested by having the device mechanically shaken or moved in a controlled way on two or more separate trials. The values produced by the device should be very similar across trials. From an applied perspective, if a person walks a 3-mile loop every morning, the device should record very similar output for that walk each morning. Interinstrument (between devices) reliability is typically assessed by having two (or more) of the same device (i.e., at least two identical accelerometer devices) put through the same movements. For example, if two identical accelerometers are put on the same part of a person's body (e.g., hip), they should produce very similar estimates of the person's movement. Making sure that each device produces the same output, given a certain movement, allows researchers and interventionists some assurance that each participant's movements will be appropriately recorded and someone's device is not significantly over- or underestimating movement. Low reliability, whether for a self-report or device, will lead to potentially misleading interpretations of an intervention's effectiveness.

For reliability, comparisons of means should indicate that there is no statistically significant difference between the repeated measures (*t*-test or ANOVA [analysis of variance] *p* value $>.05$), and correlation coefficients (Pearson, Spearman, or Intraclass) should be $r \geq 0.80$, which is a common threshold for acceptable reliability.

Validity

In general, validity has to do with the tool measuring what it is supposed to measure. In our context, validity can be considered the degree to which your PA and SB measurement tool actually measures what it is supposed to. While a given tool may be reliable, it may not be valid. That is, the tool may give you consistently incorrect (over- or underestimated) levels of PA and SB. To be truly validated, a given tool must demonstrate both acceptable reliability *and* validity. Usually, a new tool is compared to an existing tool (concurrent validity) and/or a criterion measure of PA (criterion validity). Sometimes, researchers will demonstrate that the outcomes from the PA or SB measurement tool are related to variables that should, theoretically, be associated with PA or SB (construct validity). For example, aerobic fitness or weight status should be associated with PA and/or SB to some extent. Therefore, if the measurement tool can demonstrate a significant association in the hypothesized direction, the tool would have acceptable construct validity. Criterion validity provides the greatest support for a given measurement tool, construct validity the weakest.

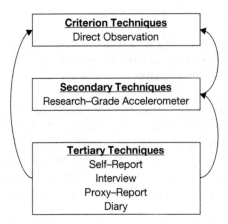

FIGURE 2.1 Validation scheme for PA and sedentary assessment tools. PA, physical activity.

Source: Adapted from Sirard JR, Pate RR. Physical activity assessment in children and adolescents. *Sports Med.* 2001;31(6):439-454. (2)

A frequently cited validation scheme is presented in Figure 2.1, with direct observation (DO) as the primary criterion measure of PA and SB. However, DO is very labor intensive and only feasible for several hours at a time. Therefore, it has been used rarely as a criterion measure. Often, researchers will use a measure of energy expenditure (oxygen consumption) as a criterion technique during short duration laboratory-based protocols when validating new devices. Using DO to validate a 3- or 7-day recall instrument would not be feasible since the researcher would need to follow the participant nearly constantly during that time period. One of the key elements of Figure 2.1 is that a survey tool should not be used as the criterion measure when evaluating a new accelerometer device. This paradigm has been generally accepted in the research community since all of the tertiary techniques rely on a participant to recall or record behavior, while secondary techniques avoid this aspect of human error.

Researchers will often assess an instrument's validity using correlation coefficients. The standard for demonstrating validity depends on the tool being validated and what the tool is being compared to. For example, it is common to find correlation coefficients of $r = 0.30$ to 0.40 when comparing estimates from a PA self-report questionnaire, compared with a research-grade accelerometer. This level of validity is often considered acceptable since the instruments are typically assessing slightly different constructs and the self-report relies on often faulty recall. However, such measures of association do not tell the full story. One must look beyond these tests of association and include other evaluations of the tool's ability to assess PA and SB (e.g., t-test, or equivalence testing). A t-test or other direct comparison of means should also be considered. Figure 2.2 shows a high level of association between minutes of moderate-to-vigorous PA (MVPA) measured by a self-report survey and research accelerometer ($r = 0.95$). Despite a strong correlation coefficient, the paired t-test for the difference in means shows that measures from the two methods are significantly different. In addition to the very important concepts of reliability and validity, interventionists also need to consider a number of other considerations to choose the right PA and/or SB assessment tool for each project.

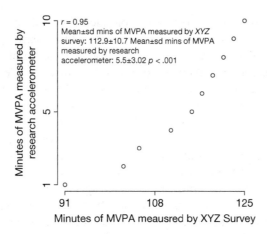

FIGURE 2.2 High association but low comparison of means (survey tool consistently underestimates compared to criterion measure). MVPA, moderate-to-vigorous physical activity.

▉ Other Considerations

This section introduces a number of factors to consider when deciding on which PA or SB measure to use. A more detailed description of these issues can be found elsewhere (3). Careful consideration of these issues up front can prevent costly or irreversible missteps.

Goals

What is the goal of the intervention? Increasing steps per day in order to achieve 10,000 steps per day? Increasing minutes of MVPA per day? Increasing the proportion of people meeting the MVPA recommendation? Increasing use of a pedestrian/cyclist trail? Or, is the intervention goal to decrease sedentary or sitting time? Many community-based PA intervention programs focus on the promotion of walking, since this is the most common form of PA for adults, and walking is usually the easiest PA for sedentary people to adopt. However, other interventions may encourage the adoption of any type of activity (e.g., gardening) or structured exercise (e.g., bicycling, resistance training). Therefore, it is essential that the PA and SB tool be able to capture the movements and behaviors you are trying to improve.

Clearly defined goals and specified PA and SB outcome variables will help narrow the choices for measurement tools. For example, the amount of time spent sitting each day can be hard for people to recall on a self-report instrument. However, the ActivPal accelerometer, worn on the thigh, is able to distinguish lying and sitting from standing and stepping. Such a device allows for the quantification of total sitting time, breaks from sitting, and daily patterns. However, compared to a self-report, using a research-based accelerometer will be more expensive and does introduce additional participant and investigator burden.

A research-grade accelerometer, like the ActivPal mentioned earlier, provides a rich source of data. But, how much detail is needed to demonstrate intervention success? In the earlier example, a self-report tool may be able to categorize individuals into high, moderate, or low amounts of time spent sitting, based on general work duties or work classifications (4). If the goal, however, is to reduce prolonged bouts of sitting by incorporating short activity breaks throughout the workday, an objective measurement tool (accelerometer) would be better able to capture the number and duration of those breaks—details that might be difficult for participants to remember. In fact, research-grade accelerometers are able to collect and store movement data up to 100 times per second for up to 2 weeks. This amount of detailed data may be overwhelming for some intervention efforts. Collecting research-grade accelerometer data can be fairly straightforward. Knowing what to do with all of that data once it is collected is an important consideration that should be thoroughly explored before using any research-grade accelerometer. Self-reports (surveys, logs/diaries) can also provide very rich data in other ways; they provide detailed contextual information (e.g., specific activities performed, where, with whom) but will not have the time granularity of the accelerometer for quantifying frequency, intensity, and duration of movement. Again, the choice of measurement tool depends heavily on the goals of the study. Additional considerations related to the participants, setting, and other contextual factors are presented in the text that follows.

Participants

Who are the individuals that will make up your intervention group? Children, adolescents, adults, or older adults? Families? Clinical populations? Self-report questionnaires are not recommended for children under 9 or 10 years old (5) due to cognitive limitations, especially due to recall and when trying to report the duration of events. Therefore, research-grade accelerometers have become the standard measurement tool for studies involving younger children (6, 7). Current research is even exploring the use of accelerometers in infants and toddlers (8). The widest array of measurement tools exists for adolescents and the general adult population, with many options for questionnaires and several research-grade accelerometers. The subsequent section lists a number of these assessment tools (see Measurement Techniques section).

Measuring PA and SB in older adults presents several of the same challenges faced by those working with young children, such as faulty memory. Unfortunately, using accelerometers in this population can be problematic due to the wide variability in how older adults move. Some 85-year-old adults move much like someone 20 to 30 years younger, while others are very functionally limited and have altered gait patterns, making the use of hip-worn accelerometers more problematic. As an active area of research, there are no definite solutions to these issues. One option for older clinical populations, who may have functional limitations, is to have the participants wear a research-grade accelerometer during a baseline functional walking test, like the 6-minute walk test. Using the accelerometer output during this test would allow one to identify a threshold (i.e., cut point) to discriminate walking activity from less intense movement. These participant-specific cut points are one option that requires additional research to support their use in older adults and various clinical populations.

Setting

Closely related to "participants," the settings (or communities) in which interventions are conducted represent the structure of how individuals are grouped together. These settings are very diverse and would include organizations such as preschools, schools, and work sites; geographically defined neighborhoods or towns/cities; and communities based around similar physical needs (e.g., assisted living facilities) or similar belief structures (e.g., churches/faith-based groups). On a larger scale, these settings may represent different geographical areas within a country (e.g., Northeast vs. Southwest United States) or different countries. In our increasingly electronically connected world, settings would also include online groups or communities.

When participants are physically close to each other (e.g., schools or worksites), questionnaires can be administered or accelerometers distributed to a group of participants, allowing for relatively efficient data collection. When participants are more geographically disbursed, other methods need to be considered. Obviously, a paper-and-pencil questionnaire can be mailed anywhere, and several research groups have successfully implemented this approach when collecting accelerometer data. That is, participants are mailed the device along with instructions and a self-addressed stamped (padded) envelope for its return once the data collection period is over (6).

Online survey tools are increasingly common, although not all electronic versions of surveys have been tested for reliability and validity. An assumption can be made that if the wording of the online version stays the same as the paper-and-pencil version, the output should be very similar. However, assumptions can be dangerous, and this issue has been tested with only several instruments (9). The use of an online versus a paper-and-pencil questionnaire is also related to the participants. Older adults, who may be less familiar with online technology, may be more comfortable with a paper-and-pencil method, whereas younger groups may prefer the online version since so much of their time is now spent on screen-based technology.

Context

Measuring the contextual factors related to PA and SB as part of an intervention is slightly outside the scope of this chapter. However, context can be critically important for PA and SB interventions that are conducted outside of a lab or clinic setting. Some assessment tools or combination of tools may be able to capture contextual elements, which could help explain the success or failure of the intervention. Are there contextual factors that could help explain the variability in success of the intervention? For your intervention, is it important to know when people are performing their prescribed activity? Do you need to know who they are with or where they are when they are active and/or sedentary? Is it important to know their emotional state or mood before, during, or after an activity session? Research-grade accelerometers will not be able to provide much of this contextual information while a self-report instrument may include many of these elements. One self-report example is EMA administered via text messaging or smartphone app, to periodically assess a participant's PA and/or SB along with contextual information (10, 11).

Practical Considerations

There are strengths and weaknesses with each measurement tool. Ideally, you will be able to use the tool that best allows you to assess whether or not the goal of the intervention was achieved. In reality, resources are often limited so one needs to weigh the benefits of the assessment tool versus its cost, including money for things (e.g., devices and related software, paper and copying fees, postage for mailings), money for people (e.g., data collection staff, interviewers), and time to get all of the data collected. Expenses like postage may seem nominal, but it can add up if there are hundreds of participants in the intervention. Research-grade accelerometers are a more expensive initial investment but can be used repeatedly for the same study, as long as the research design allows for successive waves at each data collection time point, or if there is a rolling recruitment into the intervention. In this type of data collection plan, accelerometers can be used in relatively large intervention studies. And they can be used for future studies as well. One caveat is that not all of the accelerometers distributed will "survive." Some will get lost and never returned, they may get damaged and need repair, or they may be broken beyond repair. It would be wise to factor in the replacement of devices into a budget, if possible.

■ Specific PA and SB Measurement Techniques

Now that you are familiar with some of the primary constructs and considerations related to PA and SB measurement, this section introduces some commonly used tools to assess PA and SB. This section is designed to give a brief overview of the three major PA assessment techniques used in intervention research: DO, secondary measurement techniques, and subjective measurement techniques. Tables 2.2 through 2.4 work to show the capabilities of *some* specific secondary and subjective measurement tools. The definitions in Table 2.1 are provided to clarify the headings used in the other tables. These tables are not meant to be a comprehensive list of all available measurement tools. Rather, readers are encouraged to use this list and the related resources as a starting point for independent research to identify the most appropriate PA and SB assessment tool for your needs.

Direct Observation

First, and most powerful for assessing participant behavior, is DO. DO is powerful because it provides a method for researchers to evaluate many of the distinct and complex features of PA and SB. However, this powerful assessment technique comes with several drawbacks. DO is very labor intensive, requiring researchers to observe (in real time) and code activities (either in real time or retrospectively using video playback). This process can be very time-consuming, especially if using a comprehensive DO system that assesses the main behaviors but also contextual information. In addition to time spent observing and coding, researchers using DO should be aware of the amount of time required to train observers. To obtain accurate and reliable estimates of behavior, observers/coders must be trained to use the DO system. To assess validity and reliably, most DO systems calculate intercoder reliability (e.g., percent agreement) compared with a "master-coder," in addition to comparisons among several other coders. Intracoder reliability can be calculated if participants are videotaped and a coder watches the same video twice. In all, training to achieve passing scores (inter- and intracoder reliability of ≥ 0.80) can take many hours.

In addition to properly training coders, it is important to select a DO system that is appropriate for your study population. A variety of DO systems have been developed/validated for both pediatric and adult populations. Most systems require researchers to observe a participant during a specific time period (defined amount of time, in a particular setting). Depending on the system, activities are coded for their intensity, duration, and type (e.g., vigorous, 10 minutes, basketball). The comprehensiveness of DO systems is variable. Some systems code only the highest intensity activity over a 15-second interval, while others that use video recordings may note each activity that lasts longer than 1 second. For most DO systems, the

TABLE 2.1. Definitions

LABEL	DEFINITION
Primary pop	The primary population that the PA assessment tool is used with (youth, adults, older adults)
Time frame	The time of activity the tool assesses, such as: usual, past 24 hours, past week, past 3 months, past year, historical
Domain	The domain(s) activity was performed in, such as: household, occupation, transportation, or leisure time
Intensity	Absolute or relative intensity per session or activity
Duration	Minutes or hours spent in activity intensity or time spent per PA bout
Frequency	Number of sessions or bouts per unit time (day/week/month/year)
Volume	Frequency x intensity x duration expressed at MET-minutes or other metric
EE	TEE or PAEE in kcals
Strength	Resistance exercise, weight training
Flex	Activities that target flexibility or balance
Type	The type of activity performed (specific sports, activity or exercise classes, activities of daily living)
Location	Where the PA was performed
Timing	Specific time of day when the activity was performed (e.g., morning, during school, evening)
Walk	Assessment of walking
SB	Assessment of SB (including, but not limited to, sitting and screen time)
Sit	Assessment of time spent sitting

NOTE: EE, energy expenditure; MET, metabolic equivalent; PA, physical activity; PAEE, physical activity energy expenditure; SB, sedentary behavior; TEE, total energy expenditure.

main outcome is the intensity category of the activity (i.e., sedentary, light, moderate, vigorous). Additional variables could include the specific activity types, an estimate of energy expenditure, and contextual information like who the participant was with and where he or she was. Readers interested in learning more about DO should find the primary references that accompany Table 2.2.

Research-Grade Accelerometers

In many situations, assessing participant behavior with DO is not feasible. In those situations, secondary measurement techniques are next best (26). Secondary measurement techniques are made up of motion sensors that use different mechanical and analytical approaches to measure movement. For this chapter, we include all research-grade accelerometers in this category. This does not include pedometers or the increasingly

TABLE 2.2. DO and secondary PA measurement tools

TOOL	PRIMARY POP	TIME FRAME	DOMAIN	INTENSITY	DURATION	FREQUENCY	VOLUME	EE	STRENGTH	FLEX	TYPE	LOCATION	TIMING	WALK	SB	SIT
DO (12–15)	All ages	1–2 hr	+	+	+	+	+	−	+	+	+	+	+	+	+	+
Accelerometer—hip worn (7,16–18)	3+ y	1–2 wk	−	+	+	+	+	+	−	−	−	−	+	+	+	−
Accelerometer—thigh worn (19–22)	5+ y	1–2 wk	−	+	+	+	+	+	−	−	−	−	+	+	+	+
Combo—Accelerometer + GPS (23–25)	10+ y	Days to weeks	+	+	+	+	+	+	−	−	−	+	+	+	+	+

NOTE: D0, direct observation; EE, energy expenditure; GPS, global positioning system; PA, physical activity.

popular activity trackers, which are discussed in a separate section. The most widely embraced secondary measurement tool is the ActiGraph accelerometer (ActiGraph, LLC, Pensacola, FL) (27). The ActiGraph, traditionally worn on an elastic band at the hip, captures acceleration of whole-body human movements, which interventionists can use to quantity the frequency, intensity, and duration of a participant's PA, or lack thereof.

Due to the technology and data processing involved, we recommend that if you have the resources to use a research-grade accelerometer, consult an expert in PA and SB assessment to determine the best way to process and interpret the data. You should consult this expert before you collect your data, as he/she may have valuable advice for data collection, not just data processing. In addition to requiring some experience and knowledge of data processing methods, accelerometers are relatively more expensive than most subjective techniques. The cost of the units may vary up to several hundred dollars and there is usually a cost for the software needed to initialize, download, and process the data.

BOX 2.1

Technically Speaking

Each brand of research-grade accelerometer will collect data slightly differently, and there are a wide variety of methods to process accelerometer data into more meaningful variables (i.e., translating raw acceleration values from the device into minutes spent in activity intensity categories). In-depth information about specific data processing methods for accelerometers is outside the scope of this chapter; however, you should be aware that different data processing methods exist and they can significantly affect the output.

In Figure 2.3, intensity category cut points are presented for several ActiGraph data processing algorithms from the literature. One can see that movement that registers as 750 counts/minute from the ActiGraph (red line) may be considered sedentary, light, moderate, or vigorous intensity, depending on which method is used to process the data.

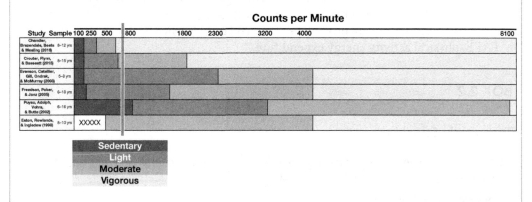

FIGURE 2.3 Different ActiGraph cut points for school-aged children.

In addition, different protocols exist for discriminating times when the device was not worn versus times when the device was worn but the participant was just very sedentary. Once nonwear time is removed from the accelerometer data, one must decide on how many hours of wear time per day are required to represent a usual or valid day of data. There are currently no standard guidelines for processing accelerometer data that are accepted across all studies.

Subjective Techniques

Subjective measurement techniques offer a lower cost alternative for assessing PA and SB in interventions. Self-report surveys and interviewer-administered surveys are both considered subjective measurement techniques because they rely on responses from the participant. Apart from the cost of paper and pencils (and paying staff for interviewer-administered surveys), self-report surveys are relatively inexpensive. Surveys are useful because they can provide some information that secondary measures cannot. For example, motion sensors cannot specifically detect strength training or flexibility/balance activities, and most devices need to be removed during swimming. However, many surveys can capture these specific activities (28–31). Also, most surveys ask questions about activity in certain domains (e.g., occupational, leisure time, household, and active transportation). This information might be particularly useful for informing process evaluations of your intervention. Table 2.3 lists the attributes for several commonly used tools for adult populations; Table 2.4 contains tools for children and adolescents. The citations in parentheses will take the reader to reliability and validation studies while the links will take the reader to the actual survey tool.

Despite the benefits, surveys are subject to different types of error. One type of error is called *social desirability bias*, which occurs when the participants; responses are influenced by what the participants think the researchers want them to report. For example, if the interviewer praises the health benefits of PA before the interview, participants will likely respond by overestimating their activity level. This type of bias can also occur if a self-report survey has a heading on it for "The Physical Activity and Health Lab" (or something similar), which may cue participants to respond favorably to questions about participating in PA. Another type of error is called *recall bias*, which relates to the differences in accuracy and completeness in recalling events from the past. Participants who have developed type 2 diabetes may search their memory more thoroughly, compared with a healthy person, when trying to recall exposure to factors they know are related to the etiology of their condition, such as low levels of PA.

Data processing is an additional consideration for using subjective measurement techniques. Although not as complex as data processing for accelerometers, most self-report surveys require some basic calculations to compute outcome variables. Scoring protocols for each survey are provided in the primary reference for the survey.

PAEE, physical activity energy expenditure

BOX 2.2

Technically Speaking

An example of survey data processing using the Paffenbarger alumni study questionnaire to calculate an estimate of total **PAEE** per week.
  Participants report:
  20 flights of stairs/d; 10 blocks walked/d; 2 days of basketball for 60 min/d.
  Calculations:
  20 flights/d × 4 kcal/flight = 80 kcals/d × 7 d/wk = 560 kcal/wk for stairs
  10 blocks/d × 8 kcal/block = 80 kcal/d × 7 days/wk = 560 kcal/wk for walking
  60 min/d basketball × 2 d/wk × 10 kcals/min = 1,200 kcal/wk for basketball
  PAEE = 560 + 560 + 1,200 kcals = 2,320 kcals/wk

TABLE 2.3. Subjective techniques for adult populations

TOOL	PRIMARY POP	TIME FRAME	DOMAIN	INTENSITY	DURATION	FREQUENCY	VOLUME	EE	STRENGTH	FLEX	TYPE	LOCATION	TIMING	WALK	SB
Paffenbarger Alumni Study Questionnaire (29, 32)	Adult, 18+ y	Past week or year	Leisure	+	+	+	+	+	–	–	–	–	–	+	+
Modifiable Activity Questionnaire (33, 34)	Age 10+ y	Past year	Leisure, occupational	+	+	+	+	+	–	–	–	–	–	+	+
Baecke Physical Activity Survey (29, 35)	Adult, 20+ y	Past week or year	Occupational	+	–	+	–	–	–	–	–	–	–	+	+
			Sport	+	+	+	+	–	–	–	–	–	–	–	–
			Nonsport leisure	+	+	+	+	–	–	–	–	–	–	+	+
7-d PAR (28, 29)	Age 11+ y	Past week	All	+	+	+	+	+	+	+	–	–	–	–	–
IPAQ (short form) (36)	Age 15–69 y	Past week	All	+	+	+	+	+	–	–	–	–	–	+	–
Vital Signs Survey (37)	Adult, 18+ y	Past week	All	+	+	+	+	–	–	–	–	–	–	–	–
NHANES	Age 2+ y	Historical (typical week)	Leisure, occupational, active transit	+	+	+	+	–	–	–	–	–	–	+	+
BRFSS	Adult, 18+ y	Past month	Leisure	–	+	+	+	–	+	–	+	–	–	–	–
CHAMPS (30)	Age 65–90 y	Past week	Leisure, occupational, household	+	+	+	+	+	+	+	+	–	–	+	–
Godin-Shephard (38)	5th grade +	Past week	Leisure	+	–	+	–	–	–	–	–	–	–	–	–

References/Links to find the full survey:
Paffenbarger Alumni Study Questionnaire: (39)
Modifiable Activity Questionnaire: (33)
Baecke Physical Activity Survey: (4) **7-d PAR:** (40)
IPAQ: Retrieved from: https://sites.google.com/site/theipaq/home **Vital signs survey:** (41)
CHAMPS: (42) **Godin-Shephard:** (43)
NHANES: Retrieved from: https://wwwn.cdc.gov/nchs/nhanes/continuousnhanes/questionnaires.aspx?BeginYear=2017.
BRFSS: Retrieved from: https://www.cdc.gov/brfss/questionnaires/pdf-ques/2017_BRFSS_Pub_Ques_508_tagged.pdf

NOTE: BRFSS, Behavior Risk Factor Surveillance System; EE, energy expenditure; IPAQ, International Physical Activity Questionnaire; NHANES, National Health and Nutrition Examination Survey

TABLE 2.4. Subjective techniques for children and adolescents

TOOL	PRIMARY POP	TIME FRAME	DOMAIN	INTENSITY	DURATION	FREQUENCY	VOLUME	EE	STRENGTH	FLEX	TYPE	LOCATION	TIMING	WALK	SB
PAQC (44, 45)	8–14 y	Previous week	Leisure, school, evening, weekend	–	–	+	–	–	–	–	–	–	–	–	+
PAQ-A (46)	14–19 y	Previous week	Leisure, school, evening, weekend	–	–	–	–	–	–	–	–	–	–	–	+
Modifiable Activity Questionnaire for Adolescents (31)	15–18 y	Previous 2 weeks, previous year	Leisure, PE, sports	+	+	+	+	+	+	–	–	–	–	–	–
Youth Activity Profile (9)	4th–12th grade	Previous week	School, home	+	–	+	–	–	–	–	–	–	+	–	+
3DPAR	8th and 9th grade females	Previous 3 d	All	+	+	+	+	+	–	–	+	–	+	+	+
YRBSS (47)	Middle and high school students	Previous week, previous year	Leisure, school, home	–	+	+	+	–	–	–	–	–	–	–	–

References/Links to find the full survey:
PAQ-C and PAQ-A:
The Physical Activity Questionnaire for Older Children (PAQ-C) and Adolescents (PAQ-A) Manual. https://www.researchgate.net/profile/Peter_Crocker/publication/228441462_The_Physical_Activity_Questionnaire_for_Older_Children_PAQ-C_and_Adolescents_PAQ-A_Manual/links/00b7d51a37fe869464000000.pdf.
Modifiable Activity Questionnaire From Adolescents: (48)
3DPAR: Retrieved from: http://www.asph.sc.edu/USC_CPARG/pdf/tool_3daypar.pdf
YRBSS: Retrieved from: https://www.cdc.gov/healthyyouth/data/yrbs/questionnaires.htm
+, the tool assesses the given construct
–, the tool does not assess this construct

NOTE: PAQ-A, physical activity questionnaire for adolescents; PAQ-C, physical activity questionnaire for older children; YRBSS, Youth Risk Behavior Surveillance System

Pedometers and Activity Trackers

Activity trackers (e.g., Fitbit, Misfit, VivoFit, Apple Watch) and many pedometers are direct to consumer devices. All of these devices have a display or are linked to a smartphone app or online website that provides the user with immediate or on-demand feedback. Research-grade accelerometers lack such displays or feedback mechanisms. This behavioral feedback mechanism is an important distinction and is the reason why these devices are presented separately and not with the rest of the assessment tools. We consider activity tracker devices to be potentially powerful *intervention tools*, used to guide and support behavior change *during* the intervention, *not* to be used as assessment tools (e.g., for baseline, midpoint, and postintervention time points) to determine intervention effectiveness.

Because pedometers and consumer activity trackers all have a behavioral feedback function, the behavior of the participants can be altered simply by wearing the device. If the goal is to get a true sense of what participants are actually doing for PA and SB, providing the participants with feedback on those behaviors could lead to an increase in PA and decrease in SB, just from wearing the device (49). For example, if the goal of an intervention is to increase the number of steps per day and participants are given an activity tracker that provides this information directly, the baseline value for steps per day may be greater than what it would normally be without such feedback. In essence, the intervention has already started during those first days of data collection, due to the behavioral feedback from the device. Without a true baseline from which to start, the effect of the intervention is unclear and could lead to the intervention actually improving behavior but not being able to detect that change when the data is analyzed.

Pedometers have been used as intervention tools and, as mentioned earlier, can induce additional steps just from wearing the device. Others have also used pedometers as assessment tools by physically preventing the participant from opening the device using tape or stickers (50, 51), and a healthy dose of trust. Traditional pedometers are devices that count steps using a mechanical lever to accumulate the number of times the lever moves. Newer, more sophisticated models are based on accelerometer technology (the same technology used in research-grade accelerometers). Still, the main function of pedometers is to count steps, although they may provide additional outputs like cadence and time spent being active (52).

Interestingly, the accelerometer technology in newer pedometers is the same technology found in today's consumer activity trackers that have gained such wide popularity over the past few years. A growing number of research studies are being conducted to validate these activity trackers (53–57), the Fitbit devices being the ones studied most (58–62). Interestingly, the one output that all of these activity trackers provide, and the variable that has the strongest validation support, is step counts (63). Comparison of step counts from several types of activity trackers ranged from -753 to -757, compared to a criterion measure of videotaped DO of adults in free-living settings (64). Validation of other variables produced by activity trackers indicates greater variability in the validation estimates. For example, estimates of energy expenditure (i.e., calories burned) from activity trackers are underestimated anywhere from about -100 to -900 kcals per day. The questionable validity for these other output metrics from activity trackers makes it impossible to say that one device provides highly accurate and precise estimates for all of its output. So, if the one metric we can consider to be valid from most activity trackers is steps, are today's activity trackers really just pedometers with more sophisticated feedback mechanisms and a great deal of slick marketing and packaging? In addition, device manufacturers update models and can change device firmware without notifying users, which may include changes in the algorithms used to create their output. Having such an update occur in the middle of an intervention could affect the output and make the interpretation of the results very unclear. Therefore, these activity tracker devices are attractive as intervention tools, but the current state of the science does not support their use as outcome assessment tools.

■ Summary

The complexity of PA and SB has resulted in a proliferation of assessment tools, with no clear all around "winner" since each tool comes with strengths and weaknesses. Reliability and validity should be of paramount concern when choosing an assessment tool, while also weighing the additional factors presented here. Interventionists should pay careful attention in this selection process, especially regarding whether or not the outcome variables produced by the tool will directly relate to the goals of the intervention. Along with the tables and resource links, the reader should be able to explore these, and other assessment tools, and feel confident in selecting the best assessment tool for any planned intervention.

■ Things to Consider

- PA and SB are complex behaviors, so the tools to measure these behaviors will, ideally, capture that complexity.
- There is no "one size fits all" option for measuring PA and SB. The tool you use will depend on many factors, including the goals of the program and the population of interest.
- Reliability and validity are distinct concepts; measurement tools should have acceptable reliability and validity.
- Research-grade accelerometers are powerful measurement tools but critical decisions in data collection and data processing should be carefully considered before the project begins.
- Based on the specifics of your project, a subjective measure of PA or SB may be most appropriate, especially if a major concern is the social and physical context of these behaviors.

■ References

1. Caspersen CJ, Powell KE, Christenson GM. Physical activity, exercise, and physical fitness: definitions and distinctions for health-related research. *Public Health Rep.* 1985;100:126–131.
2. Sirard JR, Pate RR. Physical activity assessment in children and adolescents. *Sports Med.* 2001;31(6):439–454. doi:10.2165/00007256-200131060-00004
3. Sternfeld B, Goldman-Rosas L. A systematic approach to selecting an appropriate measure of self-reported physical activity or sedentary behavior. *J Phys Act Health.* 2012;9(suppl 1):S19–S28. doi:10.1123/jpah.9.s1.s19
4. Baecke JA, Burema J, Frijters JE. A short questionnaire for the measurement of habitual physical activity in epidemiological studies. *Am J Clin Nutr.* 1982;36(5):936–942. doi:10.1093/ajcn/36.5.936
5. Sallis JF. Self-report measures of children's physical activity. *J Sch Health.* 1991;61(5):215–219. doi:10.1111/j.1746-1561.1991.tb06017.x

6. Trost SG, McIver KL, Pate RR. Conducting accelerometer-based activity assessments in field-based research. *Med Sci Sports Exerc.* 2005;37(suppl 11):S531–S543. doi:10.1249/01.mss.0000185657.86065.98

7. Freedson P, Pober D, Janz KF. Calibration of accelerometer output for children. *Med Sci Sports Exerc.* 2005;37(suppl 11):S523–S530. doi:10.1249/01.mss.0000185658.28284.ba

8. Johansson E, Ekelund U, Nero H, et al. Calibration and cross-validation of a wrist-worn Actigraph in young preschoolers. *Pediatr Obes.* 2015;10(1):1–6. doi:10.1111/j.2047-6310.2013.00213.x

9. Saint-Maurice PF, Welk GJ. Web-based assessments of physical activity in youth: considerations for design and scale calibration. *J Med Internet Res.* 2014;16(12):e269. doi:10.2196/jmir.3626

10. Liao Y, Skelton K, Dunton G, et al. A systematic review of methods and procedures used in ecological momentary assessments of diet and physical activity research in youth: an adapted STROBE checklist for reporting EMA studies (CREMAS). *J Med Internet Res.* 2016;18(6):e151. doi:10.2196/jmir.4954

11. Dunton GF, Liao Y, Intille SS, et al. Investigating children's physical activity and sedentary behavior using ecological momentary assessment with mobile phones. *Obesity (Silver Spring).* 2011;19(6):1205–1212. doi:10.1038/oby.2010.302

12. Brown WH, Pfeiffer KA, McLver KL, et al. Assessing preschool children's physical activity: the observational system for recording physical activity in children-preschool version. *Res Q Exerc Sport.* 2006;77(2):167–176. doi:10.1080/02701367.2006.10599351

13. Lyden K, Swibas T, Catenacci V, et al. Estimating energy expenditure using heat flux measured at a single body site. *Med Sci Sports Exerc.* 2014;46(11):2159–2167. doi:10.1249/MSS.0000000000000346

14. McKenzie TL. The use of direct observation to assess physical activity. In: Welk G, ed. *Physical activity assessments for health-related research.* Champaign, IL: Human Kinetics; 2002:179–195.

15. McIver KL, Brown WH, Pfeiffer KA, et al. Assessing children's physical activity in their homes: the observational system for recording physical activity in children-home. *J Appl Behav Anal.* 2009;42(1):1–16. doi:10.1901/jaba.2009.42-1

16. Evenson KR, Catellier DJ, Gill K, et al. Calibration of two objective measures of physical activity for children. *J Sport Sci.* 2008;26(14):1557–1565. doi:10.1080/02640410802334196

17. Freedson PS, Melanson E, Sirard J. Calibration of the Computer Science and Applications, Inc. accelerometer. *Med Sci Sports Exerc.* 1998;30(5):777–781. doi:10.1097/00005768-199805000-00021

18. Pate RR, Almeida MJ, McIver KL, et al. Validation and calibration of an accelerometer in preschool children. *Obesity.* 2006;14(11):2000–2006. doi:10.1038/oby.2006.234

19. Hildebrand M, Hansen HS, van Hees VT, et al. Evaluation of raw accelerations sedentary thresholds in children and adults. *Scand J Med Sci Sports.* 2017;27(12):1814–1823. doi:10.1111/sms.12795

20. Lyden K, Keadle SK, Staudenmayer J, et al. The activPAL™ accurately classifies activity intensity categories in healthy adults. *Med Sci Sports Exerc.* 2017;49(5):1022–1028. doi:10.1249/MSS.0000000000001177

21. Ridley K, Ridgers ND, Salmon J. Criterion validity of the activPAL and ActiGraph for assessing children's sitting and standing time in a school classroom setting. *Int J Behav Nutr Phys Act.* 2016;13:75. doi:10.1186/s12966-016-0402-x

22. van Loo CM, Okely AD, Batterham MJ, et al. Validation of thigh-based accelerometer estimates of postural allocation in 5-12 year-olds. *J Sci Med Sport.* 2017;20(3):273–277. doi:10.1016/j.jsams.2016.08.008

23. Carlson JA, Jankowska MM, Meseck K, et al. Validity of PALMS GPS scoring of active and passive travel compared with SenseCam. *Med Sci Sports Exerc.* 2015;47(3):662–667. doi:10.1249/MSS.0000000000000446

24. Ellis K, Godbole S, Marshall S, et al. Identifying active travel behaviors in challenging environments using GPS, accelerometers, and machine learning algorithms. *Front Public Health.* 2014;2:36. doi:10.3389/fpubh.2014.00036

25. Oreskovic NM, Blossom J, Field AE, et al. Combining global positioning system and accelerometer data to determine the locations of physical activity in children. *Geospat Health*. 2012;6(2):263–272. doi:10.4081/gh.2012.144

26. Strath SJ, Kaminsky LA, Ainsworth BE, et al. Guide to the assessment of physical activity: clinical and research applications: a scientific statement from the American Heart Association. *Circulation*. 2013;128(20):2259–2279. doi:10.1161/01.cir.0000435708.67487.da

27. John D, Freedson P. ActiGraph and actical physical activity monitors: a peek under the hood. *Med Sci Sports Exerc*. 2012;44(suppl 1):S86–S89. doi:10.1249/MSS.0b013e3182399f5e

28. Wallace JP, McKenzie TL. Observed vs. recalled exercise behavior: a validation of a seven day exercise recall for boys 11 to 13 years old. *Res Q Exerc Sport*. 1985;56(2):161–165. doi:10.1080/02701367.1985.10608451

29. Jacobs DR, Ainsworth BE, Hartman TJ, et al. A simultaneous evaluation of 10 commonly used physical activity questionnaires. *Med Sci Sports Exerc*. 1993;25:81–91. doi:10.1249/00005768-199301000-00012

30. Hekler EB, Buman MP, Haskell WL, et al. Reliability and validity of CHAMPS self-reported sedentary-to-vigorous intensity physical activity in older adults. *J Phys Act Health*. 2012;9(2):225–236. doi:10.1123/jpah.9.2.225

31. Aaron DJ, Kriska AM, Dearwater SR, et al. The epidemiology of leisure physical activity in an adolescent population. *Med Sci Sports Exerc*. 1993;25(7):847–853. doi:10.1249/00005768-199307000-00014

32. Ainsworth BE, Leon AS, Richardson MT, et al. Accuracy of the college alumnus physical activity questionnaire. *J Clin Epidemiol*. 1993;46(12):1403–1411. doi:10.1016/0895-4356(93)90140-V

33. Kriska AM, Knowler WC, LaPorte RE, et al. Development of questionnaire to examine relationship of physical activity and diabetes in Pima Indians. *Diabetes Care*. 1990;13:401–411. doi:10.2337/diacare.13.4.401

34. Schulz LG, Harper IT, Smith CJ, et al. Energy intake and physical activity in Pima Indians: comparisons with energy expenditure measured by doubly-labeled water. *Obes Res*. 1994;2:541–548. doi:10.1002/j.1550-8528.1994.tb00103.x

35. Richardson MT, Ainsworth BE, Wu HC, et al. Ability of the atherosclerosis risk in communities (ARIC)/Baecke questionnaire to assess leisure-time physical activity. *Int J Epidemiol*. 1995;24(4):685–693. doi:10.1093/ije/24.4.685

36. Ekelund U, Sepp H, Brage S, et al. Criterion-related validity of the last 7-day, short form of the International Physical Activity Questionnaire in Swedish adults. *Public Health Nutr*. 2006;9(2):258–265. doi:10.1079/PHN2005840

37. Ball TJ, Joy EA, Gren LH, et al. Concurrent validity of a self-reported physical activity "vital sign" questionnaire with adult primary care patients. *Prev Chronic Dis*. 2016;13:E16. doi:10.5888/pcd13.150228

38. Sallis JF, Condon SA, Goggin KJ, et al. The development of self-administered physical activity surveys for 4th grade students. *Res Q Exerc Sport*. 1993;64(1):25–31. doi:10.1080/02701367.1993.10608775

39. Paffenbarger RS Jr, Wing AL, Hyde RT. Physical activity as an index of heart attack risk in college alumni. *Am J Epidemiol*. 1978;108(3):161–175. doi:10.1093/oxfordjournals.aje.a112608

40. Sallis JF. Seven-day physical activity recall. *Med Sci Sports Exerc*. 1997;29(6):S89–S103.

41. Sallis RE, Matuszak JM, Baggish AL, et al. Call to action on making physical activity assessment and prescription a medical standard of care. *Curr Sports Med Rep*. 2016;15(3):207–214. doi:10.1249/JSR.0000000000000249

42. Stewart AL, Mills KM, King AC, et al. CHAMPS physical activity questionnaire for older adults: outcomes for interventions. *Med Sci Sports Exerc*. 2001;33(7):1126–1141. doi:10.1097/00005768-200107000-00010

43. Godin G, Shephard RJ. A simple method to assess exercise behavior in the community. *Can J Appl Sport Sci*. 1985;10:141–146.

44. Crocker PR, Bailey DA, Faulkner RA, et al. Measuring general levels of physical activity: preliminary evidence for the physical activity questionnaire for older children. *Med Sci Sports Exerc*. 1997;29(10):1344–1349. doi:10.1097/00005768-199710000-00

45. Kowalski KC, Crocker PRE, Kowalski NP. Convergent validity of the physical activity questionnaire for adolescents. *Pediatr Exerc Sci.* 1997;9(4):342–352.
46. Kowalski KC, Crocker PRE, Faulkner RA. Validation of the physical activity questionnaire for older children. *Pediatr Exerc Sci.* 1997;9(2):174–186. doi:10.1123/pes.9.2.174
47. Pate RR, Ross R, Dowda M, et al. Validation of a 3-day physical activity recall instrument in female youth. *Pediatr Exerc Sci.* 2003;15(3):257–265. doi:10.1123/pes.15.3.257
48. Aaron DJ, Kriska AM. Modifiable activity questionnaire for adolescents. *Med Sci Sports Exerc.* 1997;29(6):S79–S82.
49. Bravata DM, Smith-Spangler C, Sundaram V, et al. Using pedometers to increase physical activity and improve health: a systematic review. *JAMA.* 2007;298(19):2296–2304. doi:10.1001/jama.298.19.2296
50. Tudor-Locke CE, Myers AM. Methodological considerations for researchers and practitioners using pedometers to measure physical (ambulatory) activity. *Res Q Exerc Sport.* 2001;72(1):1–12. doi:10.1080/02701367.2001.10608926
51. Bassett DR Jr, Ainsworth BE, Leggett SR. Accuracy of five electronic pedometers for measuring distance walked. *Med Sci Sports Exerc.* 1996;28(8):1071–1077. doi:10.1097/00005768-199608000-00019
52. Crouter SE, Schneider PL, Karabulut M, et al. Validity of 10 electronic pedometers for measuring steps, distance, and energy cost. *Med Sci Sports Exerc.* 2003;35(8):1455–1460. doi:10.1249/01.MSS.0000078932.61440.A2
53. Alsubheen SA, George AM, Baker A, et al. Accuracy of the vivofit activity tracker. *J Med Eng Technol.* 2016;40(6):298–306. doi:10.1080/03091902.2016.1193238
54. Lee JM, Kim Y, Welk GJ. Validity of consumer-based physical activity monitors. *Med Sci Sports Exerc.* 2014;46(9):1840–1848. doi:10.1249/MSS.0000000000000287
55. Murakami H, Kawakami R, Nakae S, et al. Accuracy of wearable devices for estimating total energy expenditure: comparison with metabolic chamber and doubly labeled water method. *JAMA Intern Med.* 2016;176(5):702–703. doi:10.1001/jamainternmed.2016.0152
56. Storm FA, Heller BW, Mazza C. Step detection and activity recognition accuracy of seven physical activity monitors. *PLOS ONE.* 2015;10(3):e0118723. doi:10.1371/journal.pone.0118723
57. Ferguson T, Rowlands AV, Olds T, et al. The validity of consumer-level, activity monitors in healthy adults worn in free-living conditions: a cross-sectional study. *Int J Behav Nutr Phys Act.* 2015;12:42. doi:10.1186/s12966-015-0201-9
58. Dannecker KL, Sazonova NA, Melanson EL, et al. A comparison of energy expenditure estimation of several physical activity monitors. *Med Sci Sports Exerc.* 2013;45(11):2105–2112. doi:10.1249/MSS.0b013e318299d2eb
59. Diaz KM, Krupka DJ, Chang MJ, et al. Fitbit(R): an accurate and reliable device for wireless physical activity tracking. *Int J Cardiol.* 2015;185:138–140. doi:10.1016/j.ijcard.2015.03.038
60. Diaz KM, Krupka DJ, Chang MJ, et al. Validation of the Fitbit One(R) for physical activity measurement at an upper torso attachment site. *BMC Res Notes.* 2016;9:213. doi:10.1186/s13104-016-2020-8
61. Dondzila C, Garner D. Comparative accuracy of fitness tracking modalities in quantifying energy expenditure. *J Med Eng Technol.* 2016;40(6):325–329. doi:10.1080/03091902.2016.1197978
62. Nelson MB, Kaminsky LA, Dickin DC, et al. Validity of consumer-based physical activity monitors for specific activity types. *Med Sci Sports Exerc.* 2016;48(8):1619–1628. doi:10.1249/MSS.0000000000000933
63. Evenson KR, Goto MM, Furberg RD. Systematic review of the validity and reliability of consumer-wearable activity trackers. *Int J Behav Nutr Phys Act.* 2015;12:159. doi:10.1186/s12966-015-0314-1
64. Mendoza AR. *A Comprehensive Validation of Activity Trackers for Estimating Physical Activity and Sedentary Behavior in Free-Living Settings* [dissertation]. Department of Kinesiology, University of Massachusetts Amherst; 2017.

IMPORTANT MILESTONES IN PHYSICAL ACTIVITY AND PUBLIC HEALTH

MORGAN N. CLENNIN | DANIEL B. BORNSTEIN

LEARNING OBJECTIVES

By the end of this chapter, the student should be able to

1. Differentiate between physical activity (PA) and exercise and provide examples of each.
2. Define and explain the difference between prevalence and incidence.
3. Distinguish among the different surveillance systems used in the United States to assess population levels of PA.
4. Explain how PA guidelines evolved over the 20th and 21st centuries to arrive at the most current PA guidelines in the United States.
5. Differentiate between federal PA guidelines and a national physical activity plan, and argue why both are important for increasing population levels of PA.

■ Introduction

This chapter will provide a brief history of the field of physical activity (PA) in public health and its relationship to the field of exercise science. Historical context is important as it helps to understand how the field emerged, where it is today, and where it is likely to go in the future. For example, as will be discussed later, our current PA guidelines evolved from the field of exercise science. As a result, confusion about the differences between PA and exercise remain. This confusion often leads to challenges when attempting to design, deliver, and evaluate interventions. Therefore, it is important to understand these differences as it may be incumbent upon you to clearly articulate the nuances of PA in public health when working with others in designing, delivering, and/or evaluating PA interventions.

■ The Difference Between PA and Exercise

The World Health Organization (WHO) defines **PA** as "any bodily movement produced by skeletal muscles that requires energy expenditure" (1). By the nature of this definition, PA includes a vast spectrum of activities.

BOX 3.1

Examples of PA

- Gardening
- Household chores
- Walking
- Playing with children
- Playing recreational sports
- Zumba class
- Bicycling or walking to work or to the grocery store
- Weight lifting
- Yoga

PA, physical activity.

As exemplified in Box 3.1, PA includes exercise. **Exercise** is defined by the American College of Sports Medicine (ACSM) as "a specific type of PA that is planned, repetitive, and done for a specific purpose of improving physical fitness" (2). Most people, when thinking about PA, do not distinguish it from exercise. Therefore, most people think of PA as something that is planned (e.g., I need to carve out a chunk of time during my day or I will need to bring a change of clothes), and is for the purpose of improving fitness (e.g., I am going to sweat and work hard). As you can imagine, carving out extra time, bringing a change of clothes, sweating, and working hard are things many people may want to avoid, rather than embrace as part of their daily routine. However, if people knew that PA could mean taking a meeting from the conference room to the park, or it included walking the ½ mile to lunch instead of driving, or that simply doing their household chores and gardening "count" as PA, it could be easier to get them engaged in a PA intervention. Therefore, when designing and delivering a PA intervention, it may be important for you to help your participants and colleagues understand the subtle, but important differences between PA and exercise, as they are importance differences.

■ Public Health Basics

When conducting PA interventions, either as a practitioner or researcher, you may or may not be working with other public health professionals. You may be the public health professional driving the intervention, and therefore will need to help others understand some basic public health concepts. If that is the case, this section will serve as a refresher and will help to contextualize those basic concepts in PA. If you are not currently a public health professional, this section will help provide you with some basic skills and understanding of public health so that you may better communicate and collaborate with others in conducting PA interventions, most of which are ultimately aimed at improving public health outcomes.

The WHO defines **public health** as "the art and science of preventing disease, prolonging life and promoting health through the organized efforts of society" (3). Notice WHO's emphasis on disease prevention and health promotion over disease treatment. As you read in Chapter 1, PA is one of the most important means for preventing disease. Therefore, increasing PA at the population level should lead to decline in the prevalence and/or incidence of disease. **Prevalence** refers to the total number of individuals within a population who have a particular outcome (e.g., diabetes, heart disease, or cancer). **Incidence** refers to the total number of *new* cases of a particular outcome. The terms *prevalence* and *incidence* are often associated with the subdiscipline of public health called **epidemiology**, defined as "the study of the distribution and determinants of health-related states or events in specified populations, and the application of this study to the control of health problems" (4). For example, the Centers for Disease Control and Prevention (CDC) estimates 30.3 million Americans have diabetes (5). This prevalence estimate is helpful because it provides clarity on the size of the problem, from which it becomes possible to estimate the total economic burden of diabetes. However, what this does not tell us is whether or not diabetes is a problem that is rising or declining. Knowing the incidence, or total number of new cases of diabetes, is the only way to know whether or not diabetes is growing or shrinking across the population.

Similarly, PA or physical inactivity, rather than a disease outcome such as diabetes, may be the epidemiological outcome of interest. As you will read later in this chapter, based on high prevalence of physical inactivity across the population, PA guidelines have been established in the United States and elsewhere. Before designing and delivering a PA intervention in a certain geographical area, it is important to know the prevalence of people who meet current PA guidelines in that area.

Measuring PA Prevalence

In 2014, the CDC published the *State Indicator Report on Physical Activity* (6), which helps provide important state-level information on the status of PA in each state. Knowing the status of PA in your state may help determine whether or not the intervention is even necessary, and if deemed necessary, can serve as the basis for evaluating the effectiveness of the intervention. For example, Figure 3.1 demonstrates that population prevalence of physical inactivity is higher among states located in the southern region of the United States. Based on this information, it may be concluded that conducting PA interventions in the south may be more of a priority than doing so on the west coast where physical inactivity prevalence is low. Additionally, as described by the CDC in Box 3.2 (7), there are a number of different national-level surveys in the United States that include measures of PA in order to estimate PA prevalence. Furthermore, Chapter 2 provides an in-depth look at different ways to measure PA.

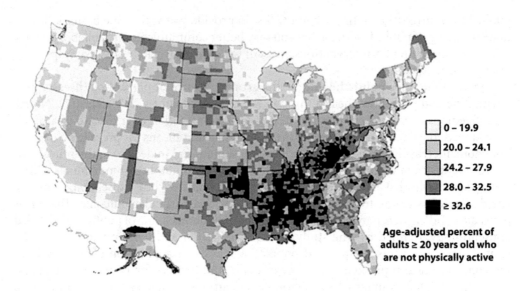

FIGURE 3.1 Physical inactivity prevalence among U.S. adults.

SOURCE: Centers for Disease Control and Prevention. *State Indicator Report on Physical Activity.* Atlanta, GA: U.S. Department of Health and Human Services; 2014.

BOX 3.2

U.S. National Surveys for Measuring PA

Currently, there are five separate nationally representative surveys that include questions about PA. Because of the manner in which PA data are collected in each survey, combining data from multiple surveys may provide the most complete understanding of trends in PA prevalence across the whole population, or within your state or region. For over 30 years, the United States has set national goals for improving the health of its residents, including PA, in a document called *Healthy People*. The goals and objectives of *Healthy People* are updated every 10 years, with the most current being *Healthy People 2020*. Some of the surveys listed in the following help provide data on whether or not the objectives in *Healthy People* are being met.

1. BRFSS: Beginning in 1984, BRFSS is a phone-based survey providing data on numerous health behaviors and health risks, including PA. BRFSS emphasizes state-level data across the 50 states. A sample BRFSS question aimed at assessing "leisure-time PA" as opposed to PA related to work or transportation is worded as follows:
   During the past month, other than your regular job, did you participate in any physical activities or exercises such as running, calisthenics, golf, gardening, or walking for exercise?

2. NHIS: Beginning in 1957, the NHIS uses household person interviews to collect data on a wide variety of heath topics. Data from NHIS are used to assess progress toward *Healthy People* goals.

3. NHANES: Beginning in the 1960s, NHANES couples information from direct physical examination and personal interview questions. In 2003, NHANES began using

(continued)

(continued)

accelerometers to measure PA. The greatest advantage to accelerometers over surveys is that they provide an objective assessment of PA. Subjective assessments such as phone interviews and surveys may be subject to "reporting bias," which is when individuals do not accurately recall their PA. Accelerometers, often attached at the waist or wrist, measure the frequency and intensity of movement in order to estimate their total PA over the period of hours, days, or weeks.

4. YRBSS: Beginning in 1990, the YRBSS monitors health risk behaviors that are known to be associated with leading causes of death, disability, and social problems among American adolescents. Specifically, PA data are collected every 2 years to help assess progress toward meeting the *Healthy People* goals.

5. NHTS: Conducted by the U.S. Department of Transportation, the NHTS is conducted every 5 years and provides data on the modes of travel, including active modes of travel. NHTS is also used to assess progress toward *Healthy People* goals.

SOURCE: Centers for Disease Control and Prevention. Physical activity. Surveillance systems. https://www.cdc.gov/physicalactivity/data/surveillance.htm. Published September 19, 2017. Accessed January 12, 2018.

BRFSS, Behavior Risk Factor Surveillance System; NHANES, National Health and Nutrition Examination Survey; NHIS, National Health Interview Survey; NHTS, National Household Travel Survey; PA, physical activity; YRBSS, Youth Risk Behavior Surveillance System.

Also worthy of note in the WHO's definition of public health provided earlier is the importance of society's efforts over any one individual's efforts. PA interventions are typically aimed at the population overall or certain subsegments of the population (e.g., middle-aged African American women living in rural areas). As you will read in later chapters of this book, successful PA interventions often consider the needs of society, or subsegments thereof, over those of any one individual. As a result, consideration must be given to environmental level correlates of PA (e.g., the physical or built environment, social environment, and/or the policy environment) as much as, if not more so than, individual level correlates (e.g., motivation or self-efficacy for PA). Exercise interventions, on the other hand, and much of the commercial fitness industry are often focused on individual-level behavior change (Box 3.3).

BOX 3.3

Examples of Environmental Correlates of PA

- Physical environment
  - Presence/absence of sidewalks, trails, and bicycle lanes
  - Location of stairs versus elevators
  - Presence/absence of standing workstations

(continued)

(continued)

- ■ Social environment
  - ● Infusing PA into traditional classrooms and lessons
  - ● Holding a "walking meeting" as opposed to a seated one
  - ● Having a "play street" where, once per week, the street is closed to vehicles and open to the community for PA
- ■ Policy environment
  - ● A corporation instituting a policy that allows workers to take three 10-minute PA breaks each day, in addition to a lunch break
  - ● A school system creating a policy that high-quality physical education will be offered 3 days per week for 60 minutes per day
  - ● A municipality legislating that sidewalks will connect residential areas to commercial areas and will be properly shaded with trees, will provide benches where people can rest, and will have easy access to water fountains

PA, physical activity.

■ Evolution of PA Guidelines

Our understanding of the relationship between PA and health has evolved. Across many ancient societies and civilizations, numerous scientists, philosophers, and physicians have acknowledged the importance of PA in promoting and maintaining an optimal level of health. However, only in recent decades has the body of knowledge regarding the relationship between PA and health begun to increase substantially. Many agencies and expert panels have utilized this emerging scientific evidence to develop recommendations for the public regarding the amount and types of PA needed to promote health. Over time, these PA recommendations have been revised to reflect new scientific evidence. The remainder of this section will document the seminal events leading to the development of first PA guidelines to promote population health and track their evolution.

> *Eating alone will not keep a man well, he must also take exercise. . . . And it is necessary, as it appears, to discern the power of various exercises, both natural exercises and artificial . . .*

- ■ Hippocrates, Regimen, ca. 400 BCE (8)

Groundwork

From the 1950s to 1970s, scientists began to systematically study the effects of exercise on health-related outcomes such as cardiovascular disease (e.g., London Bus Study, Early Harvard Alumni Study) (9, 10). As a result, the scientific knowledge about this relationship began to grow. During the 1960s, some of the first attempts to educate the public about the benefits of exercise and the amount and types required for good health emerged. One of the first publications was *Jogging*, a short paperback book written by Bill Bowerman (11). In his publication, Bowerman introduced a program that encouraged gradual and progressive increases in run duration and frequency. Some have credited Bowerman's *Jogging* with launching a fitness revolution. Another early publication that communicated with the public about the benefits of exercise and PA emerged in the late-1960s. In 1968, *Aerobics* was published by Dr. Kenneth Cooper, an Air Force physician (12). The book detailed a simple point system for exercises. Individuals could use this point system to determine the amount of exercise they should accumulate weekly. Cooper recommended that adults accumulate at least 30 points per week, with lower fit individuals starting at a level comparable with their current fitness level and then increasing gradually. Both of these early publications were some of the first attempts to communicate to the public about the importance and amounts of exercise needed to maintain good health and fitness.

Early Exercise Guidelines

During the same period, the field of exercise science began to examine the relationship between cardiorespiratory fitness and exercise. Box 3.4 defines cardiorespiratory fitness and how it is typically measured. Specifically, new studies exploring the effect of varying types, intensities, and volumes (frequency and duration) of exercise on fitness levels were emerging. With the abundance of new evidence, many organizations began to release exercise recommendations that identified the types and amount of exercise needed to promote fitness and health. This fitness-health paradigm emphasized steady-state aerobic exercise that lasted at least 60 continuous minutes. Notably, these early recommendations focused primarily on enhancing performance, especially cardiorespiratory fitness, by promoting increased intensity of endurance exercise. The rationale for this paradigm was that engaging in higher intensity endurance exercises would result in rapid increases in cardiorespiratory fitness, which in turn would reduce risk of cardiovascular disease.

BOX 3.4

Cardiorespiratory Fitness and VO_2

Cardiorespiratory fitness is commonly understood as the ability of the heart (cardio) and lungs (respiratory) to work together to provide oxygenated blood to the muscles of the body for the purpose of muscular contraction. The more efficiently the heart and lungs can provide oxygenated blood to the muscles of the body, through the body's vascular system, the greater one's level of cardiorespiratory fitness. The typical measure of cardiorespiratory fitness is VO_2 max, or the maximum volume of oxygenated blood that the heart and lungs are capable of producing. The unit of measure for VO_2 max is typically presented as milliliters of oxygen per kilogram of body weight per minute, or mL/kg/min. A person's VO_2 max is determined in part by some genetic factors, but is heavily influenced by the amount and intensity of PA they engage in regularly. For example, endurance athletes such as cross-country skiers have been shown to have high VO_2 max due to the demand of their sport (13).

PA, physical activity.

In 1975, the ACSM became one of the first organizations to formally produce exercise guidelines to promote health and fitness. The ACSM guidelines were first released in their exercise guidelines book (14). A few years later revised guidelines were released in a position statement (15). Concurrent with ACSM's release of their exercise guidelines, the American Heart Association (AHA) also published guidelines on "exercise prescription,"

TABLE 3.1. Early exercise recommendations and guidelines

ORGANIZATION	YEAR	QUALITY	QUANTITY
AHA's first guidelines	1975	Frequency	Three to four times per week
		Intensity	70%–85% maximal heart rate
		Duration	20–60 min
ACSM guidelines for exercise prescription	1975	Frequency	Three times per week
		Intensity	60%–90% VO$_2$ max
		Duration	20–30 min
ACSM position statement	1978	Frequency	3–5 d/wk
		Intensity	50%–85% VO$_2$ max (60%–90% maximal heart rate)
		Duration	15–60 min

NOTE: ACSM, American College of Sports Medicine; AHA, American Heart Association.

SOURCE: American College of Sports Medicine. *Guidelines for Graded Exercise Testing and Exercise Prescription, and Behavioral Objectives for Physicians.* Indianapolis, IN; 1976; American College of Sports Medicine. Position statement on the recommended quantity and quality of exercise for developing and maintaining fitness in healthy adults. *Med Sci Sports Exerc.* 1978;10; U.S. Department of Health and Human Services. *Physical Activity and Health: A Report of the Surgeon General.* Atlanta, GA: Centers for Disease Control and Prevention; 1996.

which were specific to patients with cardiovascular disease. The AHA's guidelines were based on emerging evidence of the immense benefits that exercise played in the rehabilitation of patients with poor cardiovascular function. These guidelines helped to communicate the importance of exercise, even among individuals with cardiovascular disease, in promoting significant health benefits. Table 3.1 summarizes these early exercise recommendations from the ACSM and AHA.

Evolution of Guidelines

Since the release of the first guidelines, the amounts and types of exercise deemed necessary to promote health and fitness have evolved to reflect new and emerging scientific evidence. During the 1980s and 1990s, PA recommendations shifted from an emphasis on higher intensity or vigorous *exercise* to the inclusion of moderate-intensity *PA*. This shift was the result of findings from several large-scale epidemiological studies, covered in detail in Chapter 1, that showed that the accumulation of moderate-intensity activities such as brisk walking and gardening were associated with health benefits. Specifically, new evidence showed that individuals that engaged in regular activity were less likely than sedentary individuals to develop or die from cardiovascular disease. More importantly, these same studies showed that the PA engaged in was predominantly from forms of moderate-intensity PAs such as walking. These epidemiological studies forced exercise scientists to reexamine the relationship between exercise intensity and health benefits. Findings from new exercise science studies also suggested that moderate-intensity PAs influenced fitness and health outcomes. Moderate-intensity PAs were found to increase fitness, but to a lesser extent than vigorous-intensity activity levels. Perhaps more surprisingly than changes in fitness, findings from these studies showed that moderate-intensity PA produced similar, or in some cases even better, health benefits.

This new evidence suggested that the amounts and types of exercise required to produce health-related benefits might differ from those necessary to improve fitness levels. More specifically, individuals did not have to engage in strenuous exercise of vigorous intensity to experience the health-enhancing benefits of PA. For example, one study noted that the largest decline in premature mortality was observed among individuals that engaged in enough PA to burn 1,500 calories per week, which equated to approximately 150 minutes of PA per week (9). This new evidence from the fields of epidemiology and exercise science sparked a shift in thinking. As such, the exercise guidelines began to shift from a more individual-level fitness paradigm to a more public health-focused paradigm that promoted engagement in moderate-intensity activities of daily living across the population. This more inclusive approach aimed to enhance population health and was thought to increase safety and acceptability among the public. A position statement released in 1990 from the American College of Sports Medicine highlights this shift toward a public health approach to the PA guidelines:

"Since 1978 an important distinction has been made between physical activity as it relates to health versus fitness. It has been pointed out that the quantity and quality of exercise needed to attain health-related benefits may differ from that recommended for fitness benefits. It is now clear that lower levels of physical activity than recommended by this position statement may reduce the risk of certain chronic degenerative diseases and yet may not be of sufficient quantity or quality to improve VO$_2$ max" (16).

The recognition of the importance of moderate-intensity PA is reflected in the gradual evolution of existing guidelines during the 1980s and 1990s. For example, the *ACSM's Guidelines for Exercise Testing and Prescription* was updated approximately every 5 years to reflect the evolving scientific knowledge about the relationship between PA, fitness, and health (2, 17). Table 3.2 compares the first ACSM exercise prescription guidelines to those endorsed 20 years later. While the components of the guidelines remained unchanged, we can see how the guidelines evolved to promote accumulated versus continuous physical activities at lower intensity levels.

During the mid-1990s, professional organizations and federal government entities released several publications supporting recommendations for PA to promote population health. A pivotal turning point was AHA's endorsement of physical inactivity as a risk factor for cardiovascular disease. In 1992, the AHA's *Statement on Exercise: Benefits and Recommendations for Physical Activity Programs for All Americans* position statement

TABLE 3.2. Comparison of ACSM guidelines for exercise prescription, 1975 versus 1995

	American College of Sport Medicine, 1975 (14)	American College of Sport Medicine, 1995 (2)
Frequency	3–4 times per week	3–5 d/wk
Intensity	70%–85% maximal heart rate	40%–85% VO$_2$ max
Duration	20–60 min	20–30 min

NOTE: ACSM, American College of Sport Medicine.

declared physical inactivity as a major and independent risk factor for development of cardiovascular disease (18). Additionally, AHA's position statement identified several recommendations for PA including that people of all ages could benefit from being more active. As you can see from the title of the position statement, however, the differentiation between exercise and PA may have remained unclear.

Despite numerous national organizations promoting the importance of PA and exercise, there was further confusion among the public regarding the amounts and types of activity necessary to promote health. While several organizations endorse recommendations that Americans should engage in more PA, many public health leaders acknowledged that increased clarity and messaging was needed. As a result, the U.S. CDC partnered with the ACSM to develop a public health statement about PA that could be used to effectively communicate with the public about the amounts and types of PA that should accumulate to maintain an optimal level of health. An expert panel was formed and charged with developing a statement based on strong scientific evidence that could be clearly and easily communicated to the public. The panel also aimed to develop a recommendation that was attainable by a majority of the public but still produced the desired benefits to health. Applying these criteria, the expert panel issued the following public health recommendation on PA in 1995:

> *Every U.S. adult should accumulate 30 minutes or more of moderate-intensity physical activity on most, preferably all, days of the week. (19) (p. 402)*

The recommendation, which was released in the *Journal of the American Medical Association (JAMA)*, introduced several novel approaches that differed from previous guidelines. For instance, the new statement highlighted the shift from vigorous and prolonged exercise to the endorsement of moderate-intensity activities that could be accumulated in bouts of 8 to 10 minutes in duration. This new statement aimed to provide the public with an attractive and attainable recommendation for PA. The expert panel noted that the greatest impact on public health would be the adoption of regular PA among sedentary individuals, which comprised a large segment of the American population.

While there was some controversy regarding the inconsistency of the new statement with previous guidelines, the new PA recommendation released by the CDC and the ACSM was quickly endorsed by the National Institutes of Health (NIH) and the WHO (20, 21). Following these endorsements was the landmark release of the *Physical Activity and Health: A Report of the Surgeon General* (22). To date, this report represented the strongest endorsement of the public health benefits of PA. The report examined extensive scientific evidence and summarized the health benefits of PA among adults and several special populations including adolescents, older adults, and persons with disabilities. In alignment with the CDC and ACSM recommendation, the Surgeon General's report on PA and public health also recommended that adults of all ages engage in at least 30 minutes of PA each day. A key message of the Surgeon General's report included that engaging in a moderate amount of PA on most days would result in significant health benefits and that additional benefits could be gained by accumulating a greater amount of PA. In the following years, these PA recommendations became widely accepted by many leading public health authorities. Over the next decade, the recommendation that adults accumulate 30 minutes of moderate or vigorous activity on most days gained validity as new research substantiating this recommendation emerged.

Despite widespread support for the latest PA recommendations, some individuals and public health authorities were skeptical of whether 30 minutes of daily PA was enough for individuals to accrue all of the desired health benefits associated with regular PA. One such organization was the U.S. Dietary Guidelines Advisory Committee. While language pertaining to a PA recommendation first appeared in the U.S. Dietary Guidelines for Americans in 1990, it included only a single sentence that acknowledged the role of PA for energy balance. Subsequent editions of the dietary guidelines did incorporate additional information with respect to the amounts and types of activity recommended. In 2004, the dietary guidelines expert panel reexamined existing evidence on the health benefits of PA and concluded that 30 minutes of moderate or vigorous PA on most days was associated with substantial health benefits. However, the panel also noted that additional PA beyond 30 minutes a day might be required to prevent excessive weight gain; and even greater amounts may be required to initiate and maintain weight loss among obese populations. These conclusions were included in the 2005 edition of the U.S. Dietary Guidelines for Americans.

2008 Physical Activity Guidelines for Americans

Unlike the U.S. Dietary Guidelines, the PA guidelines were still not federally mandated in the early to mid-2000s. Despite significant evidence of the health benefits, PA was still gaining momentum as a public health priority. In 2006, the Institute of Medicine (IOM), now known as the National Academy of Medicine, conducted a workshop to advise the Department of Health and Human Services (HHS) on the need for comprehensive PA guidelines. The conclusions drawn from the workshop included that the development of new PA guidelines would be feasible and was warranted given the substantial amount of recent high-quality evidence (23).

In response to the IOM workshop conclusions, the Secretary of HHS impaneled the PA Guidelines Advisory Committee. The advisory committee was tasked with conducting a detailed review of the scientific research on the relationship between PA and health and disease outcomes. The review of the scientific literature included an in-depth assessment of the dose–response relationship between PA and numerous chronic disease outcomes as well as examining this relationship among special populations (e.g., children and adolescents, persons with disability, minority subgroups) (24, 25). A detailed report offering an up-to-date summary of the scientific evidence regarding the PA and health relationship was produced by the PA Guidelines Advisory Committee (26). Guided by this report, the U.S. Department of HHS issued the 2008 *Physical Activity Guidelines for Americans (PAG)*. This document contained ***the first*** PA guidelines to be developed and endorsed by the U.S. federal government. It included a comprehensive set of guidelines that provided specific recommendations pertaining to the types and amounts of PA necessary for individuals across the life span (Box 3.5) (27).

National Physical Activity Plan

This seminal event marked an important turning point in which PA was formally elevated to a public health priority in the United States. In response to the 2008 PAG, a coalition of national organizations released the first U.S. National Physical Activity Plan (NPAP or the Plan) in 2010 (27,28, 29). The Plan was developed to complement and extend the impact of the 2008 PAG. It served as a strategic plan, or road map, aimed at decreasing chronic disease by having more Americans attain, or surpass, the 2008

PA guidelines. Understanding the important role that environments play in people's PA behavior, the Plan set out to enhance the environments where people live, work, play, and

---

BOX 3.5

2008 PA Guidelines for Americans

Children and adolescents (6–17 years) should participate in

- 60 minutes or more of daily moderate- or vigorous-intensity PA.
- Vigorous-intensity PA at least three times per week.
- Muscle- and bone-strengthening activities on 3 days per week.

Adults (18–64 years) should participate in

- At least 150 minutes of moderate-intensity PA per week or 75 minutes of vigorous-intensity PA per week (or a combination of the two).
- Muscle-strengthening activities on 2 or more days per week.
- Additional PA to gain greater health benefits.

Older adults[a] (65+ years) should participate in

- At least 150 minutes of moderate-intensity PA per week.
- Muscle-strengthening activities on 2 or more days per week.

NOTE: [a]Includes older adults who are generally fit and have no limiting health conditions.

SOURCE: U.S. Department of Health and Human Services. 2008 Physical Activity Guidelines for Americans. *Washington, DC: U.S. Department of Health and Human Services;*. 2008:6-17.

---

travel, rather than focusing on individual-level factors such as motivation, or self-efficacy for PA. The Plan was guided by a vision:

> *One day, all Americans will be physically active, and they will live, work and play in environments that encourage and support regular physical activity. (30)*

The NPAP includes a comprehensive set of evidence-based policies, programs, and initiatives designed to increase PA in all segments of the American population. Building on the NPAP, several states and municipalities across the United States have developed their own plans to increase PA, as detailed in Chapter 8. Since its inception, the NPAP has also evolved to reflect new scientific knowledge. In 2016, the original NPAP underwent revisions and was updated to reflect new evidence in the scientific literature. The revised NPAP was organized into nine societal sectors and overarching priorities to increase PA (Figure 3.2).

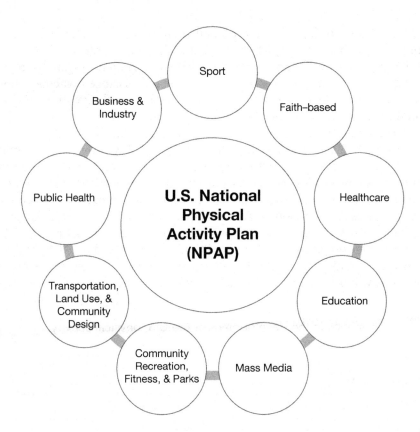

FIGURE 3.2 Nine societal sectors of the U.S.
NPAP. NPAP, National Physical Activity Plan.

The Future of the PA Guidelines

While the release of the 2008 PAG marked an important turning point for the field of PA in public health, new scientific evidence continues to emerge and refine our understanding of the PA and health relationship. As such, stakeholders from the multiple sectors, including the federal government, academia, and professional organizations, noted the importance of regularly updating the PAG to reflect new scientific knowledge. Since the release of the 2008 PAG, stakeholders and PA experts have reviewed new PA studies on several occasions to assess whether the guidelines should be updated or revised to reflect emerging evidence.

Approximately 4 years after the release of the 2008 PAG, a steering committee was formed to assess new findings from PA research. After reviewing evidence that had emerged following the release of the PAG, the committee concluded that the current recommendations would not change significantly if updated with new evidence. As a result, the steering committee recommended a Midcourse Report that would give experts the opportunity to review and highlight a specific topic of importance—the promotion of PA among youth. In 2013, the *Physical Activity Guidelines for Americans Midcourse Report: Strategies to Increase Physical Activity Among Youth* was released. The report informed public health practices with respect to youth and identified interventions across a variety of settings that showed promise in increasing PA levels among youth (31).

Chapters 13, 14, 15, and 16 all provide more detailed information about how to consider the needs of youth when designing, delivering, and evaluating PA interventions.

In 2014, PA experts from federal agencies and nongovernment organizations convened once again to examine the state of the science and discussed whether enough progress had been made in the field to warrant an update to the existing PAG. The consensus of the group was that sufficient scientific evidence had emerged; thus, the PAG would be updated to reflect the current state of the science. To initiate the update process, the Department of HHS solicited nominations for the 2018 PAG Advisory Committee. In 2016, 17 experts in PA and health were appointed to serve on the committee. The committee was convened to review the current scientific evidence examining the physical activity and health relationship. A scientific advisory report of evidence-based recommendations was then developed and circulated for public comment in early 2018 (32). Using the advisory committee's recommendations and comments received from the public, HHS then prepared the second edition of the PAG. The 2018 PAG were released in late 2018 and provide updated PA recommendations (33). These updated recommendations will help to inform the field of PA and public health for the years to come (Table 3.3).

TABLE 3.3. Key milestones in the development of the U.S. physical activity guidelines

DATE	MILESTONE
1975	ACSM and AHA independently release first PA recommendations
1990	PA statement included in U.S. Dietary Guidelines
1990	PA a focus area in Healthy People 2000
1992	AHA position statement
1995	JAMA article; CDC and ACSM's PA and public health recommendation
1996	NIH consensus statement released: Physical Activity and Cardiovascular Health
1996	Release of Physical Activity and Health, A Report of the Surgeon General
2006	IOM workshop: Adequacy of Evidence for Physical Activity Guidelines
2008	DHHS released U.S. Physical Activity Guidelines for Americans
2010	U.S. NPAP released
2012	PA established as APHA section
2013	Mid-course report: Strategies to increase PA among youth
2014	ACSM state of the science meeting
2016	U.S. NPAP updated and revised
2018	Anticipated release of the 2018 Physical Activity Guidelines for Americans

NOTE: ACSM, American College of Sport Medicine; AHA, American Heart Association; APHA, American Public Health Associatiojn; CDC, Centers for Disease Control and Prevention; DHHS, Department of Health and Human Services; IOM, Institute of Medicine; NIH, National Institutes of Health.

Current Issues

PA and Sedentary Behavior

While research has well established a relationship between moderate-to-vigorous PA and health, the potential detrimental effects of sedentary behaviors have been examined to a lesser extent. Some estimate that an average adult spends approximately 50% to 60% of the waking day in sedentary activities such as long periods of sitting or screen time (34). In the past decades, the opportunities for individuals to engage in sedentary activities have increased substantially. However, only in the past decade has research examining the adverse health effects of increased sedentary behaviors resurfaced. Recent reviews of the scientific literature have established a consistent relationship between sedentary behavior and numerous health outcomes including all-cause mortality, cardiovascular disease, diabetes, and some cancers (35–39). Existing scientific evidence suggests that there is a significant relationship between sedentary behavior and all-cause mortality, with risk of all-cause mortality increasing with time spent in sedentary behavior. Fortunately, recent studies also suggest that the increased health risks associated with sedentary behavior may be offset by high levels of moderate-to-vigorous PA (35, 40). Despite this evidence, additional research is needed to better understand the potential interactive effects of sedentary behavior and varying levels of PA on health-related outcomes. While more research is needed, existing evidence demonstrates the importance of engaging in moderate-to-vigorous PA to attenuate the health risk associated with increasingly sedentary lifestyles.

More Evidence on Dose–Response

Despite existing scientific literature, our current understanding of the dose–response relationship between PA level and health is still evolving. Existing scientific evidence strongly suggests an inverse relationship between moderate-to-vigorous PA level and mortality (all-cause and cardiovascular) (41–43). Notably, the greatest reduction in risk appears at the lower end of the dose–response relationship when sedentary individuals become PA. Among inactive individuals, relatively small increases in moderate-to-vigorous PA levels would have a significant impact on population health by reducing all-cause mortality and cardiovascular disease mortality. However, the risk of mortality appears to continually decline with increasing levels of moderate-to-vigorous PA levels. More research is needed to examine the dose–response relationship with respect to lower intensity physical activities and the possible increased risks associated with very high amounts of activity.

Summary

PA is a relative newcomer within the field of public health. Over the past 20 years, PA has become a subdiscipline within public health because of the many studies showing the relationship between PA and morbidity and mortality. The PA in public health field emerged largely out of the field of exercise science, which is why there may still be confusion about the subtle, but important differences between exercise and PA. As you work to design, deliver, and evaluate PA interventions, it will be important for you to understand and be able to articulate these subtle differences. It may also be important for you to use resources such as the 2018 Federal PA Guidelines for Americans, the U.S. NPAP, and Healthy People 2020 when designing, delivering, and evaluating PA interventions.

■ Things to Consider

- PA interventions often target policy, systems, and environmental changes, as well as individual-level change, while exercise interventions are more often focused on individual-level behavior change.
- For individuals, beginning and maintaining an exercise program often poses greater obstacles than becoming and staying more physically active.
- The 2018 Federal PA Guidelines for Americans, the U.S. NPAP, and Healthy People 2020 serve as useful resources when designing, delivering, and evaluating PA interventions.
- Existing evidence demonstrates the importance of engaging in moderate-to-vigorous PA to attenuate the health risk associated with increasingly sedentary lifestyles. However, more research is needed to examine the dose–response relationship between PA and health.
- As new scientific evidence emerges and continues to refine our understanding of the PA and health relationship, it is essential that the PAG are reviewed and updated on a periodic basis to reflect emerging evidence.
- When designing, delivering, and evaluating PA interventions, the 2018 Federal PA Guidelines for Americans can and should be used as a minimum benchmark for determining the effectiveness of the intervention, particularly among predominantly sedentary populations.

■ Resources

1. Physical Activity Surveillance:
   a. Behavior Risk Factor Surveillance System (BRFSS): https://www.cdc.gov/brfss
   b. National Health Interview Survey (NHIS): https://www.cdc.gov/nchs/nhis/physical_activity.htm
   c. National Health and Nutrition Examination Survey (NHANES): https://www.cdc.gov/nchs/nhanes/index.htm
   d. Youth Risk Behavior Surveillance System (YRBSS): https://www.cdc.gov/healthyyouth/data/yrbs/index.htm
   e. National Household Travel Survey (NHTS): http://nhts.ornl.gov
2. 2008 Federal Physical Activity Guidelines for Americans: https://health.gov/paguidelines/guidelines/summary.aspx
3. Healthy People 2020—Physical Activity: https://health.gov/paguidelines
4. U.S. National Physical Activity Plan: http://physicalactivityplan.org/index.html

References

1. World Health Organization. Physical activity. Available at: http://www.who.int/topics/ physical_activity/en/. Accessed January 16, 2018
2. American College of Sports Medicine. *Guidelines for Exercise Testing and Prescription.* Philadelphia, PA: Lea & Feibiger; 1995.
3. World Health Organization. Public Health Services. Available at: http://www.euro.who.int/ en/health-topics/Health-systems/public-health-services. Accessed January 15, 2018
4. Last JM. *A Dictionary of Epidemiology.* 4th ed. New York, NY: Oxford University Press; 2000.
5. Centers for Disease Control and Prevention. *National Diabetes Statistics Report, 2017.* Atlanta, GA: U.S. Department of Health and Human Services; 2017.
6. Centers for Disease Control and Prevention. *State Indicator Report on Physical Activity.* Atlanta, GA: U.S. Department of Health and Human Services; 2014.
7. Centers for Disease Control and Prevention. Physical Activity. Surveillance Systems. https://www.cdc.gov/physicalactivity/data/surveillance.htm Published September 19, 2017. Accessed January 12, 2018
8. Jones W, Wittington E. Works of Hippocrates. *Regimen in Health;* 1923.
9. Paffenbarger RS, Hyde R Jr, Wing AL, Jr. Physical activity, all-cause mortality, and longevity of college alumni. *N Engl J Med.* 1986;314(10):605–613. doi:10.1056/ NEJM198603063141003
10. Andrade J, Ignaszewski A. Exercise and the heart: a review of the early studies, in memory of Dr RS Paffenbarger. *Br Columbia Med J.* 2007;49(10):540.
11. Bowerman WJ, Harris WE. *Jogging: A Physical Fitness Program for All Ages.* New York, NY: Grosset & Dunlap; 1967.
12. Cooper KH. *Aerobics.* New York, NY: M Evans & Company; 1968.
13. Caspersen CJ, Powell KE, Christenson GM. Physical activity, exercise, and physical fitness: definitions and distinctions for health-related research. *Public Health Rep.* 1985;100(2):126.
14. American College of Sports Medicine. *Guidelines for Graded Exercise Testing and Exercise Prescription, and Behavioral Objectives for Physicians.* Philadelphia, PA: Lea & Febiger; 1976.
15. American College of Sports Medicine. Position statement on the recommended quantity and quality of exercise for developing and maintaining fitness in healthy adults. *Med Sci Sports.* 1978;10.
16. Pollock ML, Froelicher VF. Position stand of the American College of Sports Medicine: the recommended quantity and quality of exercise for developing and maintaining cardiorespiratory and muscular fitness in healthy adults. *J Cardiopulm Rehabil Prev.* 1990;10(7):235–245. doi:10.1097/00008483-199007000-00001
17. American College of Sports Medicine. *Guidelines for Exercise Testing and Prescription.* Williams & Wilkins; 1991.
18. Fletcher GF, Blair SN, Blumenthal J, et al. Statement on exercise: benefits and recommendations for physical activity programs for all Americans. A statement for health professionals by the Committee on Exercise and Cardiac Rehabilitation of the Council on Clinical Cardiology, American Heart Association. *Circulation.* 1992;86(1):340. doi:10.1161/01.CIR. 86.1.340
19. Pate RR, Pratt M, Blair SN, et al. Physical activity and public health: a recommendation from the Centers for Disease Control and Prevention and the American College of Sports Medicine. *JAMA.* 1995;273(5):402–407. doi:10.1001/jama.1995.03520290054029
20. Physical Activity and Cardiovascular Health. NIH Consensus Development Panel on Physical Activity and Cardiovascular Health. *JAMA.* 1996;276(3):241–246. doi:10.1001/jama. 1996.03540030075036
21. Fletcher GF, Balady G, Blair SN, et al. Statement on exercise: benefits and recommendations for physical activity programs for all Americans. *Circulation.* 1996;94(4):857–862. doi:10. 1161/01.CIR.94.4.857
22. U.S. Department of Health and Human Services. *Physical Activity and Health: A Report of the Surgeon General.* Atlanta, GA: Centers for Disease Control and Prevention; 1996.

23. Institute of Medicine. Adequacy of Evidence for Physical Activity Guidelines Development: Workshop Summary; 2007. Available at: https://www.nap.edu/catalog/11819/adequacy-of-evidence-for-physical-activity-guidelines-development-workshop-summary. Accessed November 9, 2017.
24. Haskell WL, Lee I-M, Pate RR, et al. Physical activity and public health: updated recommendation for adults from the American College of Sports Medicine and the American Heart Association. *Circulation*. 2007;116(9):1081. doi:10.1161/CIRCULATIONAHA.107.185649
25. Nelson ME, Rejeski WJ, Blair SN, et al. Physical activity and public health in older adults: recommendation from the American College of Sports Medicine and the American Heart Association. *Circulation*. 2007;116(9):1094. doi:10.1161/CIRCULATIONAHA.107.185650
26. Physical Activities Guidelines Advisory Committee. *Physical Activity Guidelines Advisory Committee Report*. Washington, DC: U.S. Department of Health and Human Services; 2008.
27. U.S. Department of Health and Human Services. *2008 Physical Activity Guidelines for Americans*. Washington, DC: U.S. Department of Health and Human Services; 2008. 6–17.
28. Kraus WE, Bittner V, Appel L, et al. The national physical activity plan: a call to action from the American Heart Association. *Circulation*. 2015;131(21):1932–1940. doi:10.1161/CIR.0000000000000203
29. Pate RR. A national physical activity plan for the United States. *J Phys Act Health*. 2009;6(suppl 2):S157. doi:10.1123/jpah.6.s2.s157
30. National Physical Activity Plan Alliance. National Physical Activity Plan. Available at: http://physicalactivityplan.org/theplan/about.html. Published 2016. Accessed December 15, 2017.
31. U.S. Department of Health and Human Services. *Physical Activity Guidelines for Americans Midcourse Report: Strategies to Increase Physical Activity Among Youth*. Washington, DC: U.S. Department of Health and Human Services; 2012.
32. U.S. Department of Health and Human Services. *Physical Activity Guidelines Advisory Committee. 2018 Physical Activity Guidelines Advisory Committee Scientific Report*. Washington, DC: U.S. Department of Health and Human Services; 2018. Available at: https://health.gov/paguidelines/second-edition/report/pdf/PAG_Advisory_Committee_Report.pdf
33. Office of Disease Prevention and Health Promotion. Physical activity. Available at: https://health.gov/paguidelines/. Accessed April 26, 2018.
34. Healy GN, Matthews CE, Dunstan DW, et al. Sedentary time and cardio-metabolic biomarkers in US adults: NHANES 2003–06. *Eur Heart J*. 2011;32(5):590–597. doi:10.1093/eurheartj/ehq451
35. Biswas A, Oh PI, Faulkner GE, et al. Sedentary time and its association with risk for disease incidence, mortality, and hospitalization in adults: a systematic review and meta-analysis. *Ann Intern Med*. 2015;162(2):123–132. doi:10.7326/M14-1651
36. Chau JY, Grunseit A, Midthjell K, et al. Sedentary behaviour and risk of mortality from all-causes and cardiometabolic diseases in adults: evidence from the HUNT3 population cohort. *Br J Sports Med*. 2013;49(11):737–742. doi:10.1136/bjsports-2012-091974
37. Sun J-W, Zhao L-G, Yang Y, et al. Association between television viewing time and all-cause mortality: a meta-analysis of cohort studies. *Am J Epidemiol*. 2015;182(11):908–916. doi:10.1093/aje/kwv164
38. Grøntved A, Hu FB. Television viewing and risk of type 2 diabetes, cardiovascular disease, and all-cause mortality: a meta-analysis. *JAMA*. 2011;305(23):2448–2455. doi:10.1001/jama.2011.812
39. Wilmot EG, Edwardson CL, Achana FA, et al. Sedentary time in adults and the association with diabetes, cardiovascular disease and death: systematic review and meta-analysis. *Diabetologia*. 2012;55(11):2895–2905. doi:10.1007/s00125-012-2677-z
40. Ekelund U, Steene-Johannessen J, Brown WJ, et al. Does physical activity attenuate, or even eliminate, the detrimental association of sitting time with mortality? A harmonised meta-analysis of data from more than 1 million men and women. *Lancet*. 2016;388(10051):1302–1310. doi:10.1016/S0140-6736(16)30370-1

41. Moore SC, Patel AV, Matthews CE, et al. Leisure time physical activity of moderate to vigorous intensity and mortality: a large pooled cohort analysis. *PLOS Med.* 2012;9(11):e1001335. doi:10.1371/journal.pmed.1001335
42. Arem H, Moore SC, Patel A, et al. Leisure time physical activity and mortality: a detailed pooled analysis of the dose-response relationship. *JAMA Intern Med.* 2015;175(6):959–967. doi:10.1001/jamainternmed.2015.0533
43. Sattelmair J, Pertman J, Ding EL, et al. Dose response between physical activity and risk of coronary heart disease: a meta analysis. *Circulation.* 2011;124(7):789–795. doi:10.1161/CIRCULATIONAHA.110.010710

4

ESTABLISHING THE VALUE OF PHYSICAL ACTIVITY FOR DIFFERENT STAKEHOLDERS

DANIEL B. BORNSTEIN | MICHELLE M. SEGAR

LEARNING OBJECTIVES

By the end of this chapter, the student should be able to

1. Identify and provide examples of the different stakeholders often needing to be considered when designing a physical activity (PA) intervention.
2. Explain how PA has historically been framed, and demonstrate how the socio-ecological model has helped to reframe PA.
3. Design a PA intervention aimed at two or more layers of the socio-ecological model.
4. Argue for why valuing PA exclusively for its health benefits may be problematic.
5. Discuss what it means to "find the hook" for different stakeholders, and describe how you would implement a plan for finding the hook with individual- and community-level stakeholders.

Introduction

As an individual interested in physical activity (PA), public health, or both, you may think active living and health are the most important things in people's lives. However, you have probably encountered individual citizens who do not think PA is that important or think that it is just for marathoners and bodybuilders. What about in the community? How do principals, developers, city council members, and physicians think about PA? What value do they find in developing active living communities? This chapter will explore how the value of PA can be established for a variety of different stakeholders in your community.

© Springer Publishing Company DOI: 10.1891/9780826134592.0004

▪ Individual and Organizational Stakeholders in PA

Value is defined as worth, usefulness, or "the degree of importance given to something" (1). This last phrase demonstrates the need for our discussion about how to establish the value of PA *within the context of* stakeholders' other values. PA is always competing for time or attention with something else. Thus, in order to more effectively promote PA to individuals and other stakeholders, we must understand how we can help it better compete with and/or facilitate our stakeholders' values and goals (2, 3). *Furthermore, what makes PA valuable to one person, group, or organization may be vastly different from what makes it valuable to others.*

In PA and public health, there can be many different stakeholders. Stakeholders can either be citizens who are affected by a course of action, or individuals and organizations who have interest in affecting a course of action. Individuals in settings such as schools, communities, places of worship, or businesses can be stakeholders in PA efforts. These citizen stakeholders are directly affected by the barriers and enablers to PA within those settings. Additionally, organizations and individuals are often stakeholders in PA-related enterprises, such as coalitions, which are trying to affect accessibility to PA for citizens within a single setting or across a variety of settings. As discussed in Chapter 7, PA coalitions are often comprised of health-focused organizations, such as hospital systems, parks departments, or public health agencies, all of which seemingly have a logical stake in increasing PA levels, given the well-established research on PA and health. It is well noted, however, that having more diverse composition of coalitions (4–6), to include nonhealth-focused organizations such as a chamber of commerce, school system, transportation department, law enforcement agency, or elected officials, is important for coalition success. However, if organizations do not actually perceive value in creating a more physically active population, then they are not likely to engage in helping improve environments that support active living. Similarly, most citizens have heard that they should be more physically active because it can improve their health. But what if health, as an outcome of PA, is actually not sufficiently valued by most citizens? As discussed throughout this chapter, making the assumption that health should be the targeted outcome we promote for PA may, in fact, be an erroneous assumption for many stakeholders.

This chapter focuses on understanding why our traditional approach to valuing and framing PA predominantly as "health promoting" is not an optimal motivator for many and discusses new ideas to increase the value of PA for different stakeholders as a key strategy to improving PA interventions. First, however, it is important to understand how the promotion of PA in our country has evolved.

▪ Contextualizing How PA Has Been Valued Historically

As PA professionals who want to increase the value of PA to our stakeholders, it is important to understand that PA has primarily been framed throughout our history as an individual and public health issue. For example, the American College of Sports Medicine, in collaboration with the American Medical Association, developed a program called Exercise is Medicine (EIM). The purpose of EIM is to "make the scientifically proven benefits of physical activity the standard in the U.S. healthcare system" (7). It seems logical that given the overwhelming evidence on the importance of PA for health, the release of PA guidelines, the adoption of national PA plans by countries, and the availability of programs like EIM (7), we should have substantially higher population levels of PA both nationally and globally. Yet, the lack of impact from efforts such as these can be understood once we recognize that our traditional approach to framing and promoting PA may be flawed. Our traditional approach is rooted in a health paradigm that is heavily influenced by individual-level behavior change theories. Health-based, individual-level behavior change theories emphasize the importance of personal responsibility. These theories often place the responsibility for becoming and staying active, and therefore healthy, primarily upon the individual. This individual-level approach operates under an assumption that the individual's context does not hold great influence on the choice to be active, and therefore assumes that individuals actually have control over becoming healthier or not.

Newer work in PA demonstrates the need for PA practitioners, advocates, and researchers to not solely focus on the individual as the primary or sole point of intervention (8–10). Specifically, the socio-ecological model has expanded our understanding by illuminating different contextual levels that influence PA behavior (11). As such, the socio-ecological model has been used to explain why an individual is challenged to become and/or stay physically active in the absence of environments and policies that support PA. As depicted in Figure 4.1 (11), the socio-ecological model identifies individual-, interpersonal-, organizational-, community-, and policy-level factors. Combined, these layers have been repeatedly shown to have significant influence over any individual's PA behavior.

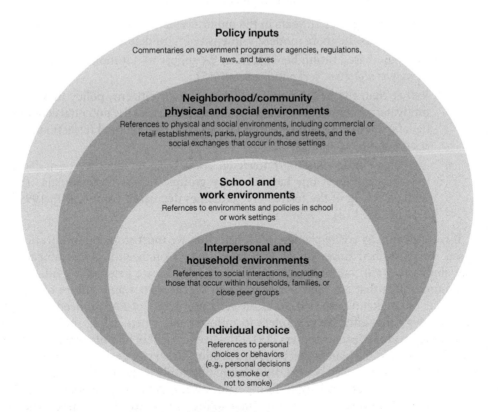

FIGURE 4.1   The social-ecological model of health behavior.

SOURCE: Sallis J, Cervero R, Ascher W, et al. An ecologic approach to creating active living communities. *Annu Rev Public Health.* 2006;27(14):1–14.

The socio-ecological model has unquestionably broadened our understanding of the contextual levels that influence PA behavior. It is now well recognized that to be highly effective in changing PA behavior at the individual and/or population levels, PA interventions should target different levels of the socio-ecological model. However, there is a lingering challenge with the application of the socio-ecological moodel and all of its layers. That challenge lies in sufficiently recognizing and engaging the many stakeholders that exist at each level of the model. The best way to engage key stakeholders at any level is to first understand why and/or how PA could be of value to them, *not us*. Since its inception, the field of PA in public health has generally assumed that since *we* value the health benefits of PA, our stakeholders will as well—therefore being motivated to take action. These assumptions appear to have undermined the uptake of PA by individuals and our population. These assumptions include

1. The health benefits of PA are sufficiently compelling to *get the attention* of policy makers.
2. Stakeholders will sufficiently *understand* our field's primary promotional strategy of PA: our PA guidelines, as seen in the Introduction to this book
3. PA guidelines' emphasis on the health benefits of PA will actually *engage and motivate* individuals to be regularly physically active.

Yet, as highlighted in the following, research suggests that assuming that we can hook our stakeholders on PA by emphasizing its health value is not correct (13):

- Despite being over 10 years in the public eye, less than 1% of the population understands the more moderate-intensity PA guidelines (14).
- The logic-based health benefits from PA appear to not motivate individuals as well as affective "feel good" effects (15).
- Rather than the health benefits of PA for their citizens, policy makers are motivated to support active living policies because of the potential economic benefits they bring to their communities (and the potential reelection better economies tend to bring) (16).
- The rate of understanding/knowledge about the guidelines has been declining among one of our key advocacy groups: fitness professionals. Their understanding of the formal PA guidelines decreased from 43% in 1999 to 19% in 2007 (17).

If we truly aim to create change in PA behavior, we must stop communicating solely based on prescribed doses of PA and their impact on health. Communicating this way emphasizes **our** values for PA. Instead, we must create persuasive evidence-based communications that are built out of research on the values and culture of our target audience: our stakeholders (18). In essence, as promoters of PA, we need to adopt the same strategy that effective marketers in industry use when selling their products or services to create repeat customers (19). Effective marketers identify what is called "the hook." The hook is the benefit that users of a product or service desire. We need to identify the "hook," or the primary benefit, from being physically active for each stakeholder. As noted earlier, stakeholders have differing values. So, unless we have done our diligence and/or research to discover what our stakeholders value, we should never assume we know what the hook for PA is for any stakeholder. Let us say, for example, that the goal of an intervention is to improve diabetes and heart disease outcomes in a given community through increased walking in that community. However, due to the poor condition of the sidewalks in that neighborhood, simply letting people know the health benefits of walking (intervening at the individual level) likely would not be sufficient to increase PA.

Rather, capital investment in improving the sidewalks (intervening at the community and public policy levels) is likely required. In this example, the local mayor is likely a critical stakeholder. If a known priority of the mayor is to help local businesses, you could have a conversation with the mayor and present the evidence on how improved sidewalks have been shown to boost sales for local businesses (20). Similar to this example, the remainder of this chapter is focused on effective strategies for building the value of PA among stakeholders at different levels of the socio-ecological model.

Building Value for Individual-Level Stakeholders: Motivating People to Value and Adopt Physically Active Lives

Framing PA as Health Enhancing for the Individual

The main goal of the field of PA, and general health, has been to help individual patients and the population as a whole to avoid disease or to assist them in disease management. So, it is logical that our field has framed PA as a health enhancement strategy. Let us consider the reasons why health might be valuable. Health is valuable because it provides the energetic resources people need to live well. Without health, people lack energy to live their lives. In this perspective, health is not the end goal. Rather, its function is as the intermediary of the real driver of what matters most: vitality and energy. We propose that by emphasizing health outcomes as the reason for being physically active, we are acting from OUR perspective and OUR values, something that most likely will not engage the population (18). For example, when PA is promoted to improve health (e.g., weight or blood pressure), people have to wait to receive feedback that their PA is effective (if they receive feedback at all). Research on behavioral self-regulation (how people manage and negotiate a behavior in their lives) suggests that people only continue to strive toward their goals when they receive feedback that they are approaching those goals (21). However, when people do not receive feedback that they are progressing toward their behavioral goals (e.g., weight loss, improved cholesterol), they quit. Furthermore, insights from behavioral economics show that people are more motivated by rewards that they will immediately experience (i.e., feeling good) rather than wait for, such as most health outcomes (22). Indeed, there is mounting research that improved health does not motivate PA participation. Rather, research shows that benefits that are related to positive affect, such as well-being and feeling good, are more effective motivators for PA (23, 24).

Framing PA as Affect Enhancing for the Individual

Research shows that affect (e.g., feelings or emotions) drives people's daily choices. Positive affect refers to experiencing pleasant feelings, whereas negative affect refers to unpleasant feelings. Anticipated affect (e.g., a person's expectation about how he or she will feel from being physically active) is thought to strongly motivate behavioral choices (25, 26). People use their feelings as information for what choices to make (27); they approach what feels good and avoid what feels bad. Thus, the literature on affect offers key insights into how public health practitioners can better sell PA to individuals. Studies across the life span suggest that positive affective benefits from exercise (e.g., "feeling good," "lifted mood") are better motivators than logical benefits such as "good health." One study that used text messages (randomized) among teens reported that among sedentary teens, the messages targeting positive affect (e.g., enjoyment) predicted participation more so than the logic-based health messages (24). In another study of midlife working women, being active to enhance quality of life predicted between 20% and 32% more participation over a 1-year period than health- and weight-related reasons (19). Other research among older adults (65–90 years) reported that the affective, feel-good expectations from being active, but not health-related expectations, predicted exercise participation 6 and 12 months later (23). Thus, positive affective experiences that are immediate, such as enjoyment, well-being, vitality, and connection with important others, might be the best way to establish the value of PA among individuals; a compelling way to feel happier and boost their daily quality of life.

Just like businesses, however, the only way to identify what would make PA relevant and compelling to individuals is to use inductive methods similar to traditional market research. The following case study describes a study we conducted to achieve this aim.

Individual and Interpersonal Case Study: What Walking Means to Moms

We were part of a team to study the meaning of walking for low-income urban mothers (28). Our goal was to understand what walking means to this specific group as a first step toward understanding how to make walking more relevant and valuable to them. We conducted focus groups among ethnically diverse participants from seven cities. Participants were on average 35 years old, with two children in grade school. Among the questions asked were why they walked, what counts as valid walking, and where exercise fits in daily priorities. Findings showed that some participants said that when they walked, they did it for functional reasons such as aiming to achieve a specific outcome like getting to work. Others said they liked to walk for more immediate benefits such as clearing their minds (individual level) or having time to share with friends (interpersonal level). However, many reported that they did not like walking in their neighborhood because they felt unsafe due to roaming dogs, shootings, or drug sales. These findings suggested that PA advocates can help low-income mothers place a higher value on walking by framing it as a way they can connect with others during leisure time or use walking as a way to revitalize themselves. Box 4.1 provides some helpful hints on how to identify value for stakeholders at the individual and interpersonal levels.

This study also sheds light on the limitations of focusing solely on the individual and interpersonal levels in PA interventions. Despite having identified new ways to help make PA valuable and culturally aligned among ethnically diverse women, women from this example were unlikely to walk without safer, more walkable environments. This emphasizes the need for the socio-ecological framework, and therefore identifying the values of different stakeholders across multiple layers of the framework.

BOX 4.1

How to Find "The Hook" For Stakeholders at the Individual and Interpersonal Levels

   I. Get to know your stakeholder(s):
      A. What matters most to the person or people you are promoting PA to?
      B. What priorities, goals, and experiences do they have?
         1. Use interviews, focus groups, or surveys to identify the priorities, goals, and experiences they value.

(continued)

(*continued*)

> C. What does science suggest, if anything, about how PA aligns with these valued priorities, goals, and desired experiences?
>
> D. Identify what beliefs people have about PA that make it hard to fit in or demotivating.
>
> E. Develop new messaging strategies that help people overcome the beliefs that are getting in their way of being active, as well as illuminating the real connections between PA and what matters most to them.
>
> PA, physical activity.

Building Value for Stakeholders at the Organizational, Community, and Public Policy Levels

As you will read in the following chapter, the environments and systems in which people work and learn (organizational level), play and pray (community level), and commute (public policy level) are largely determined by policies. Therefore, when attempting to design, deliver, and evaluate a PA intervention at these levels, the most important stakeholders are often policy makers who control those environments. Additionally, the stakeholders could be individuals or organizations seeking to advocate for active living policies among policy makers. For example, the National Coalition for Promoting Physical Activity (NCPPA) is an organization solely focused on advocating for PA policies and programs at federal and state levels.

Occasionally, stakeholders already value PA and its many benefits. For example, health-based organizations that join PA coalitions like the NCPPA often fully understand the myriad benefits associated with PA. Similarly, there are some individual policy makers who are regularly physically active individuals and may therefore be willing to support efforts to design, implement, and measure PA interventions. As stated previously in this chapter, however, this is not the norm. Many key stakeholders do not fully understand PA and its benefits. Nevertheless, opportunities still exist for getting buy in for PA interventions from key stakeholders. Getting key stakeholders bought in will come largely as the result of finding "the hook" for each stakeholder in the intervention. Similar to the case study presented earlier, which focused on the individual and interpersonal levels, an inductive approach must be used to identify value for key stakeholders at the organizational, community, and public policy levels. Box 4.2 provides guidance on that process.

BOX 4.2

How to Find "The Hook" For Stakeholders at the Organizational, Community, and Public Policy Levels

> I. Get to know your stakeholder:
>
> A. Lawmakers
> 1. Go to their website to know what committees they serve on.
> 2. From their website try to get information on their policy and political positions.

(*continued*)

(continued)

    3. See what their voting record has been on bills.

    4. Search their name on the Internet to see what they have been talking about or how they are being portrayed in the media.

    5. Search their name on the Internet to learn about their personal interests or background (e.g., they are a former athlete or are an avid hiker).

B. Nonelected policy makers (e.g., appointed officials, business owners, school principals)

    1. Know what organization or entity they represent and how long they have been there.

    2. Search their name on the Internet to see what they have been talking about or how they are being portrayed in the media.

    3. Search their name on the Internet to learn about their personal interests or background.

C. Organizations (e.g., corporations, nonprofits, coalitions)

    1. Use the Internet to

       a. Know what they do, what they build, or how they serve.

       b. Identify their mission and vision.

       c. Identify their strategic objectives or strategic plan.

       d. Know who their key people are (executives, directors).

          i. Identify whether or not one of the key people might already be a supporter/champion for a PA-related cause.

D. Communities (neighborhoods, towns, villages, places of worship)

    1. Try to identify a website for the community

       a. Learn about what the community values by exploring the content of their website.

          i. See if the community has a vision, mission, goals, and/or a strategic plan.

    2. Talk to community members

       a. Either through interviews or focus groups, ask community members what they value.

       b. Gather as much data as possible from different community members and try to identify common themes.

II. After learning about your stakeholders' key values, goals, and interests, determine whether or not there is evidence to show how increasing PA would positively impact those values, goals, or interests.

A. If the case can be made for how PA would be positively impactful, compile evidence and stories, and develop a one- to two-page brief that summarizes the evidence and how it will benefit them.

    1. The organization *Active Living Research* has excellent "brief" examples that you could use yourself or as a template for developing your own brief.

B. If the case cannot be made, move on to the next stakeholder.

PA, physical activity.

Case Study: Lessons Learned From Tobacco Control

The PA in the public health field is not alone in believing that having a health-based focus would prove to be sufficiently valuable to their stakeholders to initiate change. In tobacco control, for example, the evidence for the detrimental effects of smoking on health was indisputable. This evidence led to public health messaging campaigns that provided information about the harmful effects of smoking. Scientists believed that conveying this information would change individuals' smoking behavior. As it turned out, just providing information on the harmful effects of smoking did little to change individuals' smoking behavior. Similarly, it did little to change the policies and environments that could limit access to tobacco. However, when evidence on the ill effects of secondhand smoke became available, many policy makers understood the value in protecting nonsmokers from the harmful effects of secondhand smoke. As a result, policies such as taxes on cigarettes and rules on when and where people could smoke were adopted, and population-level usage of cigarettes declined (29).

However, getting buy in from policy makers was not always easy, and still remains a challenge. For lawmakers in particular, there was most definitely "competition" in the value proposition to implement tobacco control policies. Perhaps most notably, there was an entire tobacco industry lobbying against any tobacco control policies, which influenced the value proposition for politicians' willingness to enact policy change. For example, if a lawmaker's campaign was heavily subsidized by the tobacco industry, voting "yes" on tobacco control policies could be a political death sentence. More recent evidence demonstrating the economic impact of tobacco usage is being leveraged to further persuade lawmakers and other key stakeholders to further develop and implement policies that would limit tobacco usage, and ultimately improve health (30). Is there a secondhand smoke equivalent for PA policy?

Case Study: Physical Inactivity and National Security

One need not look much farther than the front page of most newspapers or listen to the first few minutes of a news broadcast to hear about national security. If national security is so prominent in the news, it must be because their consumers value it greatly. If our aim is to align PA interventions with what others perceive to be of value, why then is nobody using the impact of physical inactivity on national security as "the hook" for PA interventions? As it turns out, some organizations and scientists are talking about the importance of PA for national security. One such organization is called Mission Readiness. Mission Readiness, part of the Council for a Strong America, is an advocacy group of retired military leaders with the goal of "strengthening national security by ensuring kids stay in school, stay fit, and stay out of trouble." In the effort to help kids stay fit, Mission Readiness has produced a series of state-level reports called "Unfit to Fight." With Unfit to Fight reports for the states of Illinois, Colorado, Minnesota, and Texas, Mission Readiness proposes state-level policy and environmental solutions for how to improve the physical fitness levels of children within those states. For the state of Illinois, for example, two of the three solutions offered for improving the health and fitness of children are directly aimed at policy and environment and include (a) building PA back into communities and (b) keeping and improving PA in the school day (31).

The efforts being taken on by groups like Mission Readiness are due, in part, to mounting evidence on the impact of training-related injuries among military recruits. Through a series of epidemiological studies over the past two decades, the U.S. Department of Defense has become increasingly more aware of the economic and tactical problems associated with injuries that occur during basic training across the different branches of the military. Collectively, these studies have shown that after accounting for gender, physical fitness is the strongest predictor of injuries. Some studies have also shown that PA levels prior to entering the military are associated with injuries in basic training. As a result, many basic training stations across different military branches have instituted remedial physical fitness and injury prevention programs aimed at stemming the rising tide of injuries. However, the issue of training-related injuries persists because the real solution to the problem lies in creating a better candidate pool of applicants for military service. A recently conducted study investigated the physical fitness levels and injury rates of U.S. Army recruits on a state-by-state basis (32). Results from this study showed that a cluster of states located in the Deep South produced recruits who were significantly less physically fit and/or significantly more likely to become injured (see Figure 4.2) (32). Perhaps not so ironically, many of the states identified in this recent study are also well recognized for their high rates of heart disease, diabetes, obesity, and physical inactivity. Given how inherently interested the news media, lawmakers, organizations, and individual citizens are in national security, national security could provide a new "hook" for the importance of PA among lawmakers and other policy makers who value national security.

Identifying and Building Value for Other Key Stakeholders

Similar to identifying the hook for individual citizens and stakeholders such as politicians, we need to also understand what would motivate organizations and/or their leadership to support interventions aimed at establishing PA-friendly policies, systems, and environments. From worksites and healthcare settings to faith-based settings, and community parks and recreation, Section III of this book provides numerous examples of successful PA interventions at the community, organizational, and policy levels. Similarly, Section IV identifies successful PA interventions across the individual and interpersonal levels. As you read those chapters, pay attention to how the content therein can be applied to the content from this chapter in finding value for stakeholders at any or all levels of the socio-ecological model that may be critical to the success or failure of a PA intervention.

▆ Summary: Emphasizing Values to Go Beyond Building Knowledge to Changing Behavior

In order to increase the value proposition of PA such that it is truly important for individuals to do, organizations to invest in, and policy makers to change systems and environments for, our interventions and communications must aim to go beyond *building* knowledge to actually *influencing* behavior (13). The good news is that PA professionals are in great company at this time with this need because many other scientific communities have been struggling with the same challenges related to changing behavior rather than increasing knowledge. Across fields as diverse as politics to environmental sustainability, there is growing recognition of the need for more strategic communication and framing strategies that emphasize the value proposition for stakeholders, not us.

In fact, a scientific leader in promoting green behavior and sustainability says the following: "There are many reasons why the quality of the debate over climate change . . . is so distorted. One of them is that most academics don't see it as their job to communicate

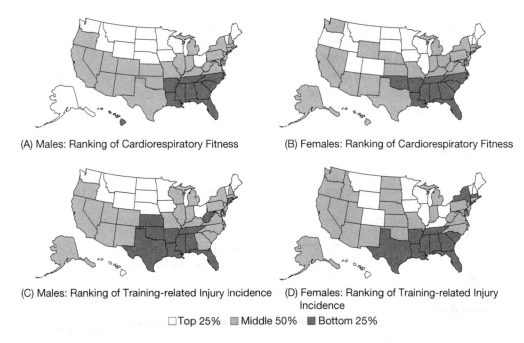

(A) Males: Ranking of Cardiorespiratory Fitness   (B) Females: Ranking of Cardiorespiratory Fitness

(C) Males: Ranking of Training-related Injury Incidence   (D) Females: Ranking of Training-related Injury Incidence

☐Top 25%   ■ Middle 50%   ■ Bottom 25%

FIGURE 4.2 States ranked by quartiles of cardiorespiratory fitness of males (A) and females (B). U.S. Army recruits and training-related injury incidence of males (C) and females (D). U.S. Army recruits entering basic training from 2010 to 2013.

SOURCE: Bornstein DB, Grieve GL, Clennin MN, et al. Which US states pose the greatest threats to military readiness and public health? Public health policy implications for a cross-sectional investigation of cardiorespiratory fitness, body mass index, and injuries among US Army recruits. *J Public Health Manag Pract.* 2018.

their science to the public. That is dangerous to the future of the academy—to become irrelevant in these debates." He further suggests creating training and incentives "to teach health behavior advocates how to more effectively communicate to boost the value of their behavior of interest" (13).

The past 30 years of science about exercise and PA has heavily invested in understanding the medical and physiological benefits of PA. If we are to effectively utilize the evidence from this science, the next generation of PA research and practice needs to prioritize the investigation of how to identify what our stakeholders might value about PA in order to foster the actual changes we aim to create in policies, environments, practices, and communities, as well as the daily decisions of individuals (33, 34).

▨ Things to Consider

- ■ Although improvements in health are a logical outcome for a PA intervention, stakeholders from outside the health or public health sectors may not consider improvements in health to be a compelling or valuable outcome.
- ■ When working with different stakeholders, it is incumbent upon you to identify the outcomes that are of relevance to them, and then be prepared to demonstrate how PA could positively impact the outcomes that are of value to them.

■ If there is no evidence for, or logical connection between, PA and the outcome(s) of interest to a stakeholder, then that person or organization is likely not a viable stakeholder.

■ When trying to identify what is valuable for a stakeholder, it is crucial to never make assumptions. Formative inquiry or research is essential to understand the perspective of the stakeholder you are targeting.

■ References

1. Value. Wiktionary website. https://en.wiktionary.org/wiki/value. Reproduced under the Creative Commons Attribution-ShareAlike 3.0 Unported License. Accessed December 1, 2018.
2. Segar M. *No Sweat: How the Simple Science of Motivation Can Bring You a Lifetime of Fitness.* New York, NY: AMACOM; 2015.
3. Bornstein DB, Carnoske C, Tabak R, et al. Factors related to partner involvement in development of the US National Physical Activity Plan. *J Public Health Manag Pract.* 2013;19:S8–S16. doi:10.1097/PHH.0b013e318284047d
4. Butterfoss FD. *Coalitions and Partnerships in Community Health.* San Francisco, CA: Jossey-Bass; 2007.
5. Butterfoss FD, Kegler MC. The community coalition action theory. In: DiClemente RJ, Crosby RA, Kegler MC, eds. *Health Promotion Practice and Research.* 2nd ed. San Francisco, CA: John Wiley & Sons; 2009.
6. U.S. Centers for Disease Control and Prevention. *Evaluation Technical Assistance Document: Partnership Evaluation Guidebook and Resources.* Atlanta, GA: Centers for Disease Control and Prevention, Division of Nutrition, Physical Activity, and Obesity; 2011.
7. American College of Sports Medicine. Cost effectiveness. Exercise Is Medicine website. Available at: http://www.exerciseismedicine.org/support_page.php/cost-effectiveness/. Accessed March 19, 2018.
8. Sallis J, Hovell M, Hofstetter C. Predictors of adoption and maintenance of vigorous physical activity in men and women. *Prev Med.* 1992;21:237–251. doi:10.1016/0091-7435(92)90022-A
9. Sallis JF, Floyd MF, Rodríguez DA, et al. Role of built environments in physical activity, obesity, and cardiovascular disease. *Circulation.* 2012;125(5):729–737. doi:10.1161/CIRCULATIONAHA.110.969022
10. Sallis JF, Glanz K. Physical activity and food environments: solutions to the obesity epidemic. *Milbank Q.* 2009;87(1):123–154. doi:10.1111/j.1468-0009.2009.00550.x
11. Sallis J, Cervero R, Ascher W, et al. An ecologic approach to creating active living communities. *Annu Rev Public Health.* 2006;27(14):1–14.
12. FitzGerald EA, Frasso R, Dean LT, et al. Community-generated recommendations regarding the urban nutrition and tobacco environments: a photo-elicitation study in Philadelphia. *Prev Chronic Dis.* 2013;10:E98. doi:10.5888/pcd10.120204
13. Segar M. How can the Physical Activity Guidelines go beyond building knowledge to influencing behavior? Public comment made on the 2018 Physical Activity Guidelines website. Available at: https://health.gov/paguidelines/pcd/. Published March 14, 2017. Accessed January 12, 2018.
14. Kay M, Carroll D, Carlson S, et al. Awareness and knowledge of the 2008 Physical Activity Guidelines for Americans. *J Phys Act Health.* 2014;11(4):693–698. doi:10.1123/jpah.2012-0171
15. Segar ML, Eccles JS, Peck SC, et al. Midlife women's physical activity goals: sociocultural influences and effects on behavioral regulation. *Sex Roles.* 2007;57(11/12):837–850. doi:10.1007/s11199-007-9322-1
16. Zwald ML, Eyler AA, Goins KV, et al. Understanding municipal officials' involvement in transportation policies supportive of walking and bicycling. *J Public Health Manag Pract.* 2014;23(4):348–355. doi:10.1097/PHH.0000000000000152

17. Ferney S, Moorheadb G, Baumanc A, et al. Awareness of and changing perceptions of physical activity guidelines among delegates at the Australian conference of science and medicine in sport. *J Sci Med Sport*. 2009;12:642–646. doi:10.1016/j.jsams.2008.09.014
18. Segar ML, Guerin A, Phillips E, et al. From a vital sign to vitality: selling exercise so patients want to buy it. *Curr Sports Med Rep*. 2016;15(4):276–281.
19. Segar M, Eccles J, Richardson C. Rebranding exercise: closing the gap between values and behavior. *Int J Behav Nutr Phys Act*. 2011;8:94. doi:10.1186/1479-5868-8-94
20. Hack G. Business Performance in Walkable Shopping Areas. Robert Wood Johnson Foundation, Active Living Research website. Available at: https://activelivingresearch.org/business-performance-walkable-shopping-areas. Published November 2013. Accessed March 19, 2018.
21. Carver C, Scheier M, Boekaerts M, et al. On the structure of behavioral self-regulation. In: Boekaerts M, Pintrich P, Zeidner M, eds. *Handbook of Self-Regulation*. San Diego, CA: Academic Press; 2000:41–84.
22. Hariri AR, Brown SM, Williamson DE, et al. Preference for immediate over delayed rewards is associated with magnitude of ventral striatal activity. *J Neurosci*. 2006;26(51):13213–13217. doi:10.1523/JNEUROSCI.3446-06.2006
23. Gellert P, Ziegelmann JP, Schwarzer R. Affective and health-related outcome expectancies for physical activity in older adults. *Psychol Health*. 2012;27(7):816–828. doi:10.1080/08870446.2011.607236
24. Sirriyeh R, Lawton R, Ward J. Physical activity and adolescents: an exploratory randomized controlled trial investigating the influence of affective and instrumental text messages. *Br J Health Psychol*. 2010;15:825–840. doi:10.1348/135910710X486889
25. Bagozzi R, Dholakia U, Basuroy S. How effortful decisions get enacted: the motivating role of decision processes, desires, and anticipated emotions. *J Behav Decis Mak*. 2003;16(4):273–295. doi:10.1002/bdm.446
26. Baumeister RF, Vohs KD, DeWall CN, et al. How emotion shapes behavior: feedback, anticipation, and reflection, rather than direct causation. *Pers Soc Psychol Rev*. 2007;11(2):167–203. doi:10.1177/1088868307301033
27. Chang HH, Pham MT. Affect as a decision-making system of the present. *J Consum Res*. 2013;40(1):42–63. doi:10.1086/668644
28. Segar ML, Heinrich KA, Zieff S, et al. What walking means to moms: insights from a national sample to frame walking in compelling ways to low-income urban mothers. *J Transp Health*. 2017;5:5–15. doi:10.1016/j.jth.2016.06.004
29. Wang TW, Falvey K, Gammon DG, et al. Sales trends in price-discounted cigarettes, large cigars, little cigars, and cigarillos—United States, 2011–2016. *Nicotine Tob Res*. 2017.
30. U.S. National Cancer Institute and World Health Organization. *The Economics of Tobacco and Tobacco Control*. Bethesda, MD; 2016.
31. Mission: Readiness. *Illinois: Unfit to Fight*. Available at: https://strongnation.s3.amazonaws.com/documents/275/05cfd356-3a67-47b3-b98a-1b1204a91096.pdf?1493998128&inline;%20filename=%22Unfit%20to%20Fight_MR_IL.pdf%22. Published 2016. Accessed March 4, 2018.
32. Bornstein DB, Grieve GL, Clennin MN, et al. Which US states pose the greatest threats to military readiness and public health? Public health policy implications for a cross-sectional investigation of cardiorespiratory fitness, body mass index, and injuries among US Army recruits. *J Public Health Manag Pract*. 2018. doi:10.1097/PHH.0000000000000778
33. Segar M, Taber J, Patrick H, et al. Rethinking physical activity communication: using qualitative methods to understand women's goals, values, and beliefs to improve public health. *BMC Public Health*. 2017;17:462. doi:10.1186/s12889-017-4361-1
34. Segar ML, Richardson C. Prescribing pleasure and meaning: cultivating walking motivation and maintenance. *Am J Prev Med*. 2014;47(6):838–841. doi:10.1016/j.amepre.2014.07.001

II

PLANNING YOUR PHYSICAL ACTIVITY INTERVENTION

DEVELOPING POLICY AND ENVIRONMENTAL INTERVENTIONS

AMY A. EYLER

LEARNING OBJECTIVES

By the end of this chapter, students should be able to

1. Understand the advantages of policy interventions for promoting physical activity (PA).
2. Apply the levels of the PA policy research framework to at least one policy-related issue.
3. Apply the five interrelated steps of policy development to at least one policy-related issue.
4. Explain the importance of the multiple-streams framework for promoting PA policies.
5. Synthesize the reasons for policy evaluation.

Introduction

Defining the word "policy" is no easy task. The concept is broad and convoluted, yet is important to understand because it affects many aspects of our lives. We actually live, eat, drink, and breathe policy every day! Policies affect community planning and housing, the way our food is produced and sold, water purity, and air pollution. Policies have tremendous impact on our health, but what exactly is a "policy"? Although there are many different types of policies, they are mainly grouped into two categories. **Public policy** is usually defined as formal laws, rules, or regulations enacted by elected officials intended to direct or influence the actions, behaviors, and decisions of others (1). These public policies are often referred to as "**BIG P policies.**" Less formal policies such as organizational rules or practices, and at times normative behaviors in

© Springer Publishing Company DOI: 10.1891/9780826134592.0005

specific settings, are often referred to as "**LITTLE p policies.**" While federal, state, and local laws can affect PA behavior, so can policies within, for example, workplaces. The laws would be considered BIG P or public policies, and the workplace rules are LITTLE P policies (Box 5.1).

BOX 5.1

Examples of BIG P and LITTLE p Policies

BIG P

- State law requiring daily PE in public elementary schools
- County law outlining complete street mandates
- City ordinance related to required funding for park and trail maintenance

LITTLE p

- Organizational policy to keep stairwells open during work hours for employees to use instead of elevator
- School-level decision to require training for teachers on incorporating active learning lessons into curriculum

PE, physical education.

History shows that policies can be a successful part of interventions to improve population health. Every one of the top 10 public health achievements in the past century was facilitated by policy action to influence practice and prioritize resources (2) (see Table 5.1 for examples of these policies and health achievements). Even though many of these achievements are related to past health priorities such as infectious disease rates or improved quality of life, they attest that policies can be effective for broad reaching and sustainable population health improvements.

Policies and rules implemented through governments and organizations affect health and well-being in a variety of ways. First, these policies and rules can outline how money is collected (e.g., taxes) and spent (e.g., services, subsidies). For example, a policy can be enacted to tax city residents so the money can be spent on building or improving a public transit system or a park. Policies can also outline specific spending details related to budgets. Governmental and organizational budgets need to be developed, adjusted, and improved on a regular basis. Programs and initiatives related to health can be reprioritized, increased, or decreased, so budget allocation amounts vary annually. Governments also regulate behaviors and practices of groups and individuals. Safety belt mandates or motorcycle helmet laws are examples of this. Additionally, governments outline citizens' private rights and help ensure those rights are not violated. These policies may create ethical controversy among different groups and ideologies because of the conflict between individual rights versus the health and safety of the population. For example, clean indoor air policies have been the subject of such controversy and those who smoke may feel as if these policies violate their right to use tobacco. Government and organizational rules can foster economic growth, too. Cities can implement policies to create environments that could attract and incentivize business development. Lastly, policies can be used to promote an informed and educated population. Restaurant menu labeling and food packaging label requirements are examples of ways that policies can educate, inform, and increase population awareness.

■ History of PA and Policy

As mentioned in Chapter 4, being physically active is often thought of as an individual choice. You can *choose* to be physically active if, when, and where you want to; or conversely, you can *choose* to not be physically active. However, research over the past decade has shed light on the importance of factors related to PA beyond personal choice, such as the environment and policy. Evidence exists to show that "choice" is impacted by what is available and accessible. Effective intervention strategies should include policy and environmental changes designed to provide opportunities, support, and cues to help people become more physically active (3, 4). Public policies can create and enhance environments that make being physically active the healthy, easy choice. Policies can also help reduce barriers that inhibit PA and those that encourage sedentary behavior.

Policies related to PA have a significant historical background. One of the earliest examples is school physical education (PE). Policies requiring PE in schools have been around since the mid-1800s. In 1823, the Round Hill School, a private school in Northampton, Massachusetts, was the first to integrate PE into their curriculum. In 1866, California was the first state to pass a law that required twice a day exercise in public schools (5). Schools were also implementing policies related to PA beyond just PE. As early as 1947, the New York State Legislature enacted a statute requiring outdoor playgrounds for all New York City public schools. While school policies have historically been supportive of PA for students, there are several examples of the way past community policies have negatively impacted PA of residents. The 19th and early

TABLE 5.1. Examples of policies related to public health achievements of the past century

PUBLIC HEALTH ACHIEVEMENT	RELATED POLICIES
Vaccinations	■ School-entry vaccine requirements ■ Healthcare worker mandates ■ Funding for development
Motor vehicle safety	■ Speed limits ■ Safety belt mandates ■ Drunk and impaired driving laws
Safer and healthier foods	■ Improvements in food labels ■ Better industry accountability ■ Mandated food safety testing
Control of infectious disease	■ Sanitation mandates ■ Required water testing ■ Funding research on disease transmission and control

20th century brought the industrial era where cities grew to accommodate the masses of new workers. Land use policies were almost nonexistent, and the result was overcrowded and unsanitary communities with little green space. Postwar development created more distant neighborhoods in suburbs and widespread car ownership, and roads designed for these cars decreased active travel. Today, schools and communities are seen as places where policies can make a positive impact on active lifestyles. Chapters in Section III provide several detailed examples.

Current Focus on Policy and Environmental Change

The PA Policy Research Framework

Given the national attention on the importance of policy to PA, an organizational framework was developed by Schmid et al. (6) (see Box 5.2). This conceptual framework illustrates the different sectors and settings in which policies can be developed and applied; see Figure 5.1. The framework has guided PA policy research and continues to be used to show the intersectionality and breadth of the topic.

As indicated by Figure 5.1, this PA policy framework shows that policies can occur at multiple levels: federal, state, regional, local. Sometimes policies at one level work in concert with all other levels. For example, federal policy dictates the amount and specifications of federal transportation funds to be distributed to states for nonmotorized transportation. States then have rules and regulations for disseminating the funds for projects in regions or localities, which in turn have rules and regulations for prioritizing and implementing funded projects. Other times, the levels may conflict. There may be a state law allowing **joint use agreements** between schools and communities, but the schools can restrict this use to the extent that they wish. As described in Chapter 4, the ability to implement a joint use agreement may hinge upon the ability to identify how the school benefits, or derives value, from such an agreement.

The framework also shows the main sectors where policies and environmental changes to impact PA are likely to occur. While schools, worksites, parks, transportation, and health sectors are important venues for PA promotion through policy and environmental change, other sectors such as faith-based settings and housing have been suggested additions to the framework. All sectors can complement one another, making the total environment most conducive to PA.Schools with robust PE programs,

---

BOX 5.2

What is Joint Use?

A joint use agreement is a formal agreement between two separate government entities—often a school and a city or county—setting forth the terms and conditions for shared use of public properties or facilities (7). A common example of joint use is opening outdoor school facilities such as playgrounds or tracks for use during nonschool hours.

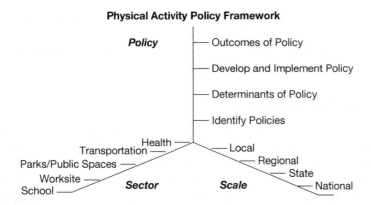

FIGURE 5.1   Schmid et al. (6) developed PA policy research framework.

PA, physical activity.

worksites that promote activity among employees, communities with safe and accessible parks, a healthcare system that integrates PA promotion to patients for prevention and treatment of disease, and a transportation system that allows for safe walking, cycling, and transit characterize best practices to positively impact population PA.

Policy and Environmental National Recommendations

With the current growth of PA policy research, the evidence on effective interventions is emerging. The *Guide to Community Preventive Services* identified three evidence-based environmental and policy strategies to improve population PA. Enhancing PE and PA within schools, designing streets and communities that support PA, and creating or enhancing access to safe places for PA are all recommended based on the evidence of their effectiveness in increasing population PA (8). The Institute of Medicine had also published documents with support for improving school (9) and community environments (10, 11) to increase PA and reduce obesity.

The National Physical Activity Plan (NPAP) also includes many policy-related recommendations (12). For example, the sector *Community Recreation, Fitness, and Parks* includes five recommended strategies, all of which are based on policy or environmental change. Improving opportunities, access, safety, leadership, and collaboration for PA in communities are priorities. Within the *Public Health* sector, strategies include engaging in collaborative partnerships to advocate for and develop PA policies, and to expand the monitoring of policy and environmental determinants of PA in communities. The NPAP also contains some overarching recommendations that have federal policy implications. Federal legislation to require and fund plan updates, as well as legislation to update the PA guidelines for Americans on a regular basis, are two large-scale, federal recommendations.

Policy Development and Implementation

Otto von Bismarck, a Prussian Statesman in the 1860s, is often credited with saying "Laws are like sausages. You should never watch either one being made." More than a century later, the policy process remains complex, messy, and sometimes unappetizing—but nonetheless extremely important. Anyone working to increase population PA and decrease sedentary behavior should know the basics of the policy process.

Federal, state, or local policies are all developed within an interactive, recurring process that typically involves five interrelated steps.

Step 1: Problem Prioritization

In this first step, the issue or problem is made known and the targeted solution includes some type of policy. Let us say a bicycle advocacy group has identified an increase in car–bicycle crashes in several areas of the community. They are proposing policies that would increase the safety of cyclists in the community. As discussed in Chapter 4, making the assumption that poor health outcomes are a problem or priority for many policy makers may not be a good assumption to make. As discussed in the following, PA-related policies often solve problems not necessarily related to health outcomes.

Step 2: Policy Formulation

There are usually many different policy solutions to the issue at hand. In this step, various policy solutions are conceptualized and vetted for feasibility, acceptance, and effectiveness. This is where examples from other communities, outcome evaluations, or best practices can be helpful. In the case of safety for cyclists, a good policy option would be to propose a requirement that all streets have highly visible, dedicated bicycle lanes. Support for safe bicycling can not only be seen as a PA issue, but the policies can also be formulated and supported by environmental advocates to reduce automobile emissions or by city planners who may be interested in reducing road congestion. The broader the support base, the more likely the rest of the policy process will be successful.

Step 3: Policy Enactment

In this step, the policy is formally adopted. This can happen through many different mechanisms including the legislative process, public vote, regulatory approval, executive order, or administrative law. This step can be arduous because of the barriers and limits within each of these systems. For example, states have limited time in their legislative sessions; usually about 6 months. It is only during this time when bills can be proposed, amended (likely more than once), and passed by both houses. At the local level, the barriers are often prioritization and competing demands. A proposal for requiring bicycle lanes might not take precedence when sewer systems or infrastructure are falling apart.

An often-cited policy theory that can help frame enactment is Jon Kingdon's multiple-streams framework; see Figure 5.2. Kingdon uses an analogy of "three streams converging to illustrate how policy change occurs" (13). In this model, the *problem* stream symbolizes the issue to be addressed. In our example, it would be increasing bicycle safety. The *politics* stream is about the mood, campaigns, or other legislative changes that might affect the success of the proposal. In the bicycle safety example, community residents may be more motivated to support pothole repair on roads or other infrastructure improvements over requiring bike lanes. This "mood" can impact policy enactment. The *policy* stream represents the different policy solutions to the problem. When these streams converge, a "window of opportunity" opens for policy success.

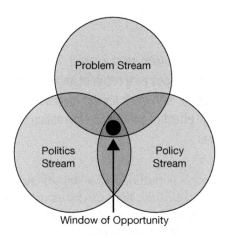

FIGURE 5.2 Multiple-streams framework.

Step 4: Policy Implementation

Enactment of a policy is not the end of the policy process. Once in place, the policies need to be implemented. Implementation involves taking what was approved, developing formal actions, and operationalizing the policy components. Typically, policies are implemented successfully if they are appropriately resourced and funded, have explicitly outlined responsible parties, and have provisions for enforcement. If the bicycle safety proposal was enacted, it would need to be implemented with resources for planning and prioritizing the development of bike lanes, the specific entities (e.g., streets division) who will mark the lanes, and some type of monitoring to ensure the lanes are being built to the specifications of the law.

Step 5: Policy Evaluation

Just like with interventions, evaluation is critical in determining success. Identifying effectiveness of an implemented policy can help tailor the policy for improvement or, if successful, be a tool to gain broader support for expansion of the policy effort. Policy evaluation is not just about outcome. Box 5.3 outlines several important purposes of policy evaluation. In the case of requiring bicycle lanes, evaluation might include changes in crash rates, cyclist prevalence, cost of lane development and maintenance, and driver and bicyclist perceptions.

BOX 5.3

Why Policy Evaluation?

- To understand the process of implementation
- To identify barriers and enablers of implementation
- To identify key players of support and opposition
- To compare what was planned with actual implementation

(*continued*)

(*continued*)

- To measure changes in the outcomes of interest
- To measure unintended changes as a result of implementation
- To compare policy outcome with other similar policies
- To identify any "dosing" effect of policy implementation
- To inform future actions

Although the policy process is outlined in a step-by-step framework, rarely does it follow a linear, sequential course. These steps can be interrelated, nonsequential, cyclical, intermittent, and not at all as well ordered as depicted. In spite of this, the basics and nuances of this process are important to know because to positively impact and sustain improvements in PA, policies will play a role.

LITTLE p Policies

Up until this point, the policy discussion was framed around BIG P or public policies. However, there are many venues for organizational or LITTLE p that can impact PA. Worksites (also discussed in Chapter 11) are a good example of this. Policies promoting PA in worksites can be formal such as health insurance incentives for those who are physically active or corporate discounts on gym memberships, but they can also be less formal such as acceptance of a casual dress code that allows for employees to comfortably engage in walking meetings or take walking breaks throughout the day.

Worksites can also facilitate policies and environmental changes to foster PA. Allowing for standing workstations, providing locker rooms and showers, or supporting active transportation options can create an environment that facilitates the "choice" to be physically active at work.

These organizational policies or environmental opportunities may not fit with the policy process outlined earlier, but still warrant evaluation. There is a need for more evidence on the outcomes of these policies in order to create and gain support for best practices.

■ Summary

Policies have played an important role in improving population health throughout history. Policies can create changes for broad populations and be sustained over time in ways that individual strategies and interventions cannot. Given the significant role that PA plays in health promotion and disease prevention, policies and environmental changes have emerged as recommended strategies to increase PA and decrease sedentary behavior.

The outline of the policy process can serve as a guide to understanding how and when researchers, practitioners, and advocates can become involved. The process, although complex, is vital to making lasting changes in the way we live, learn, work, and play and the places we do so.

Things to Consider

- Although there are frameworks and guides, the policy process is complex and often does not follow a linear path.
- Policy evaluation is an extremely important part of using policies and environmental changes to promote PA.
- Policies and environmental changes often work together to create the best opportunities to impact population PA.

References

1. Longest BB. *Health Policymaking in the United States*. 5th ed. Chicago, IL: Health Administration Press; 2010.
2. Centers for Disease Control and Prevention. Ten great public health achievements—United States, 1900–1999. *Morb Mortal Wkly Rep*. 1999;48(12):241–243.
3. Brownson RC, Haire-Joshu D, Luke DA. Shaping the context of health: a review of environmental and policy approaches in the prevention of chronic diseases. *Ann Rev Public Health*. 2006;27:341–370. doi:10.1146/annurev.publhealth.27.021405.102137
4. Brownson RC, Kelly CM, Eyler AA, et al. Environmental and policy approaches for promoting physical activity in the United States: a research agenda. *J Phys Act Health*. 2008;5(4):488–503. doi:10.1123/jpah.5.4.488
5. SPARK: Sports Play, and Active Recreation for Kids. The Evolution of Physical Education. Published October 15, 2015. Available at: https://sparkpe.org/blog/the-evolution-of-physical-education/. Accessed February 27, 2018.
6. Schmid T, Pratt M, Witmer L. A framework for physical activity policy research. *J Phys Act Health*. 2006;3(suppl 1):S20–S29. doi:10.1123/jpah.3.s1.s20
7. ChangeLab Solutions. What is a joint use agreement? Available at: https://www.changelabsolutions.org/publications/what-is-JUA. Published March 2009. Accessed February 27, 2018.
8. Centers for Disease Control and Prevention. Guide to community preventive services: Physical activity: built environment approaches combining transportation system interventions with land use and environmental design. Available at: https://www.thecommunityguide.org/findings/physical-activity-built-environment-approaches. Accessed February 27, 2018.
9. Institute of Medicine. *Educating the Student Body: Taking Physical Education and Physical Activity to School*. Washington, DC: The National Academies Press; 2013.
10. Institute of Medicine. *Accelerating Progress in Obesity Prevention*. Washington, DC: The National Academies Press; 2012.
11. Institute of Medicine. Advancing obesity solutions through investments in the built environment. In: *Proceedings of a Workshop—In Brief*. Washington, DC: The National Academies Press website. 2017. Available at: http://nationalacademies.org/hmd/reports/2017/advancing-obesity-solutions-through-investments-in-the-built-environment-proceedings-in-brief.aspx. Accessed February 28, 2018.
12. National Physical Activity Plan Alliance. The National Physical Activity Plan. Available at: http://www.physicalactivityplan.org/index.html. Accessed February 27, 2018.
13. Kingdon JW. *Agendas Alternatives Public Policies*. New York, NY: Addison-Wesley; 2003.

EFFECTIVE STRATEGIES FOR BUILDING AND MAINTAINING COALITIONS

DANIEL B. BORNSTEIN | JAY E. MADDOCK

LEARNING OBJECTIVES

By the end of this chapter, the student should be able to

1. Give examples of what coalitions can achieve.
2. Construct a vision and mission statement.
3. Explain the roles of members of the core team.
4. Generate SMART goals.
5. Illustrate the process of developing a community coalition.

Introduction

Physical activity (PA) coalitions have the power and potential to address important health issues from the local level on up through the regional, national, and global level. PA coalitions are usually comprised of private citizens and individuals who represent organizations that may be private, public, or a government agency. Traditionally, these individuals and organizations join PA coalitions because they are interested in increasing access to safe places for PA, supportive policies, or community design, or to promote PA generally throughout the community. A well-functioning coalition can be one of the most valuable tools in promoting PA and reaching goals that individual organizations could not achieve alone. However, a poorly functioning coalition can be an energy-draining disaster, which causes people to not want to work together and even lose interest in PA altogether. The goal of this chapter is to provide insights into what works well, and pitfalls to avoid, in developing and maintaining coalitions (Box 6.1).

BOX 6.1

Examples of Coalitions

There are a variety of types of PA coalitions. The following are some examples of PA coalitions in the United States, some local, some national. By investigating these coalitions a bit further through the Internet, you can learn a lot more about what they are focused on, who their members are, how they were established, and how they operate.

    National Alliance for Nutrition and Activity
    National Coalition for Promoting Physical Activity—National, not-for-profit coalition
    NPAP Alliance
    Get Fit Kauai—Public, county-level coalition run by a 501c3
    Get Active San Antonio

NPAP, National Physical Activity Plan; PA, physical activity.

◼ Steps to Developing an Effective Coalition

Developing Your Core Team

One of the most important first steps in developing a coalition is to bring together a small group of core members. This is a time to think small and get three to five individuals representing organizations that you already have a good working relationship with and would benefit from being part of the coalition. These individuals should already be champions of PA, but do not necessarily need to be in the health sector. They could be urban planners interested in active transportation or environmentalists who want to reduce our carbon footprint. One mistake often made is trying to get too big, too fast. If and when this happens, the first meetings of coalitions are often disorganized and unfocused, which can quickly lead members to question their membership and disengage from the coalition. Conversely, early meetings with a small group of known individuals often leads to initial planning meetings where brainstorming and free thinking are fun and quite productive in charting a course for the coalition in preparation for growth (Box 6.2).

BOX 6.2

Experience From Developing a Coalition in Hawaii

When we developed the Hawaii NPAC, we started with a core planning group that included the State Health Department, the University of Hawaii, and a few key advisors from local nonprofits (1). This group met for several months to figure out what we wanted to achieve and who should be involved. Our main tasks included examining the proposed structure of the coalition, developing sectors based on the state's PA and nutrition plan, and recruiting coalition and sector leadership.

NPAC, Nutrition and Physical Activity Coalition; PA, physical activity.

Developing Coalition Vision and Mission

After you have identified the three to five key individuals for your core team, work with this team to develop the coalition's vision and mission. This is the time for big-picture thinking and planning. The vision should reflect the ultimate dream of the coalition: what things would look like or be like if all the barriers were removed. The vision should then be concisely represented in a vision statement (Box 6.3).

BOX 6.3

Examples of Vision Statements

"Active living made easy"
"Better bike lanes, better communities"
"Safer streets, safer kids"
"Active community, healthy community"
"Better sidewalks, better home values"
"Active communities, lower healthcare costs"

The mission statement is similar to the vision statement in that it represents the big picture and is relatively concise. Where the mission statement differs from the vision statement is that it is more oriented toward action, is likely not as concise, and possibly describes what and why the coalition is going to achieve what it plans to achieve. Chapter 4 provides an in-depth look at strategies for identifying what achievements will provide value for the coalition members and for the populations being served by the coalition (Box 6.4).

BOX 6.4

Examples of Mission Statements

"Building safer streets through effective policy advocacy."
"Creating healthier, more active lives through systemic change."
"Improving home values and sense of community through robust systems for active travel."
"To help underserved youth establish lifelong habits for PA."

PA, physical activity.

Developing proper vision and mission statements often requires asking some key questions. Examples of questions you might want to ask your core team could include:

- What do you want to achieve?
- Is this going to be an obesity coalition, chronic disease coalition, a sustainability coalition, or one just focused on PA?
- Is the coalition trying to improve PA for everyone or is it focused on certain subpopulations (e.g., youth, older adults, disadvantaged groups)?

- What is the coalition's geographic scope (e.g., state, county, neighborhood, school district)?
- What type of strategies is the coalition focused on (e.g., legislative policy, school or workplace policy, community involvement, PA messaging campaigns)?
- Will the coalition be involved in lobbying or partnering with groups that lobby?
- What levels of commitment are you expecting from members and leaders?

These questions are essential questions to ask before you begin developing a larger group. People's time is valuable and you want to make sure that the right people are invited to the coalition meeting. For example, inviting the local Boys and Girls Club to a coalition that ends up being focused on older adults may be perceived as a waste of time. It is not that an organization such as the Boys and Girls Club might not have some interest in the coalition's activities down the line, but at this stage the coalition and the population being addressed may not fit with that organization's strategic interests and you might burn bridges for future collaborations. Research on effective PA coalitions has shown that organizations join coalitions when the mission, vision, and goals of the coalition align with the organizations' strategic interests (2, 3). As was discussed in Chapter 4, it is incumbent upon the coalition's core team to demonstrate to prospective coalition members how joining the coalition will provide value to them.

It is also okay to think small. If there is a specific issue in the community like creating a safe place for children to go biking, that can be a great place to start a coalition. Many groups start around these single-issue ideas and when they are achieved move to additional areas that help support the original mission. Starting with a small, single project is a perfectly acceptable way to develop your coalition.

Building Your Coalition Membership

Once your core group has figured out what you want to do (vision and mission), it is time to think about growing the coalition membership. This is still a time to be judicious and strategic, as this larger group will help determine the coalition's goals. It is entirely possible to have a very effective planning meeting with 50 people in the room, but these tend to be after a smaller group has been working together for a year or more. For the first coalition meeting, we think it works best to have 12 to 20 people who are excited and engaged in the topic. The earlier stages of building a coalition is not the time to bring in the nonbelievers.

Depending on the results of your discussion about vision and mission, the membership can vary dramatically, but should include individuals whom you know are PA supporters. If your coalition is focused on broad PA policies, you might want to engage a friendly elected official. For example, if your mayor regularly runs in road races, or maybe even rides her bike to work, she would be a great person to have on the coalition. Similarly, if part of your governor's platform is to improve quality of life in your state, and your coalition will be working on state-level policy change, then you can relate how your coalition's vision and mission will help him achieve his goals for improved quality of life. In fact, the governor of West Virginia played an instrumental role in establishing West Virginia's State Physical Activity Plan, which was developed by a coalition (4).

As mentioned previously, your coalition may be narrowly focused. For example, if the coalition wants to focus on Safe Routes to School, you might want someone from the local department of transportation and a school official, as well as parents, Parent-Teacher Association (PTA), and other concerned groups and individuals, while having the governor of your state likely is not necessary. If you do not know the name of the individual you want to invite, it is okay to think about both organizational titles (e.g., school principal) as well as names (e.g., influential leader in the community). The key point is that when approaching potential coalition members, you should demonstrate how the mission and vision of the coalition will *help them achieve what they believe is important* (5) (Box 6.5).

BOX 6.5

Coalition Membership Tool

Goal: Implement Safe Routes to School at all schools in our district
Skills needed: Someone who understands public works, someone with knowledge of school policies and procedures, parent representation, someone who can tell us if it actually works, champions
Possible invitees: Local public works department director, superintendent's office, school-level community liaison, PTA liaison, local bike/pedestrian advocacy group

PTA, Parent-Teacher Association.

It may also be important to have a coalition member that is a "spark plug," a champion of PA who can be an influential member (6). As an example, when developing new coalitions in Hawaii, we usually looked for an influential champion in the community. For our state childhood obesity task force, we asked the president of the University of Hawaii system, who was a noted diabetes researcher, and the vice president of a large healthcare organization, who had previously served as deputy director of health at the state health department, to serve as cochairs. Both were highly respected in the state and it helped us to recruit presidents, CEOs, directors, and legislators to the task force.

It is important to think about who is making the invitations to the coalition. The person or organization making the invitation can often influence if the person being asked agrees to serve. If a single agency is inviting everyone, this can be construed as an advisory board for the agency rather that a true participatory coalition. Another approach is to have the members of the core committee cosign the invitation letters. This is how the coalition for a Tobacco Free Hawaii started. At the beginning, it was an interagency group between the American Cancer Society, American Heart Association, Cancer Research Center, and Department of Health. Organizations were excited to join a coalition that already had influential members in the community onboard. Research has identified this as "organizational alignment." Organizational alignment is when different organizations see the value in joining with other organizational members of a coalition (7). Often times this value is in the power of multiple organizations or agencies working collaboratively toward a single goal. Part of the purpose of a coalition is to break down silos between groups or organizations so that people can come together in solving a problem and not duplicate efforts, or even worse, compete for resources.

Finally, consideration should be given to how you ask people to serve on the coalition. These days there is a tendency to send invitations via email or other social media. However, in this context, a more personal and professional approach will likely yield better results. A personal phone call to individuals you have identified as being possible key members of your coalition can be a much more persuasive way to recruit them. It lets them know that they were important enough for you to pick up the phone and call them. A bulk email on the other hand tells them they are not worth the time and that this meeting can be skipped. After the initial phone call, following up with an official hard copy letter of invitation, along with the details of the first meeting and thanking them for their participation, demonstrates both a personal and professional approach that will be welcomed. You may also want to consider limiting the time served on a coalition so individuals are able to consider their ability to serve. Often 2 to 3 year appointments are good places to start.

Steps to Maintaining an Effective Coalition

Goal Setting

Once you have identified your team of committed coalition members, the next step is to establish some short- and long-term goals for your coalition. Without clearly identified SMART goals and an ability to demonstrate success toward achieving those goals, your coalition may quickly lose momentum (Box 6.6).

BOX 6.6

SMART goals

Developing SMART goals is recognized as a key step in the strategic planning process for organizations and for individuals. SMART goals are specifically recommended by the CDC when developing PA coalitions and implementing PA programs. SMART stands for:
  Specific
  Measurable
  Attainable
  Realistic
  Time bound

CDC, Centers for Disease Control and Prevention; PA, physical activity.

Going for "easy wins," or goals that you are very confident can be achieved easily and early, can be critical to instilling confidence in your coalition's members and maintaining momentum. For example, an ambitious 1-year goal of your coalition could be to develop a PA plan for your community, city, or state. Given the many steps required to develop a PA plan (see Chapter 7), it may prove too challenging for your first year, and if not achieved could lead to member dissatisfaction with the coalition. A more modest 1-year goal might be to get more children walking and/or biking to school. In order to make that goal SMART, it might look like this: By August 1, the school task force will identify one element from the national organization Safe Routes to School that can be implemented in our community. This goal is now *specific* (you have identified that you will identify a strategy from a reputable source), **measurable** (you can easily measure whether or not you have identified one strategy from Safe Routes to School), **attainable** (it should not be difficult to identify a single strategy), **realistic** (given how accessible Safe Routes to School's information is, it is very realistic that your coalition could adopt one of its strategies), and **time bound** (you identified August 1 as your deadline). This goal should provide an easy win for your coalition.

A long-term goal, related to the short-term goal just provided, would be to implement the element of Safe Routes to School that you have identified. In order to make that goal SMART, it might look like this: By January 15, the school task force will have identified and trained a team of six teachers and parents prepared to implement a walking school bus on Monday and Friday mornings throughout the Spring semester (Insert photo of walking school bus). This goal is now **specific** (you have identified the specific strategy from Safe Routes to School, the number of people you will need to train, and the days on which your walking school bus will happen), **measurable** (you can measure the number of team members trained, and the number of days on which the walking schools actually happened), **attainable** (you should be able to identify and train a team of six individuals), **realistic** (it is realistic to think that you could train your team and then have the walking school bus occur two mornings per week, not necessarily every morning and every afternoon), and **time bound** (you have identified January 15 and the Spring semester as your time frame for achieving your goal).

In summary, having SMART, short- and long-term goals are the key steps in building and maintaining an effective coalition. One or more of your short-term goals should be easy wins for the coalition in order to build and maintain momentum by demonstrating that the coalition is experiencing success. It is okay to have short-term and long-term goals that are not necessarily easy, but they should still be SMART.

Establishing Leadership Roles

Coalitions often have bylaws that spell out the leadership structure and operational structure for the organization. Having bylaws when first establishing a coalition is not critical; however, it is important to identify key leadership positions within the coalition. Identifying leadership positions could be one of those "easy win" short-term goals that were just discussed. Establishing bylaws could still be a short-term goal, but is by no means an easy win. At a minimum, the leadership positions within a coalition should include a slate of officers, including: president or chair, vice president or vice chair, secretary, and treasurer. In the early stages, it can be implied as to what the roles of each officer are, but eventually, the roles of each officer should be explicitly stated in the coalition's bylaws or some similar document like a policies and procedures manual.

In addition to the key leadership positions identified earlier, depending upon the size of your coalition, it may also have a steering committee. The steering committee is typically comprised of a small group of coalition members (typically between three and 15 people) with the purpose of ensuring that the coalition stays true to its vision, mission, and goals.

Establishing Subcommittees

It is often the initial members of the coalition (e.g., the steering committee) that will work as a group to set up the coalition's vision, mission, and goals, as was discussed previously. However, as goals are determined and specific projects are identified, it is often important to establish subcommittees to manage specific projects of the coalition. Typically, a member of the steering committee will volunteer to lead or "chair" that subcommittee. For example, if the coalition agrees that one of its SMART goals is to start a walking school bus, it will be important to establish a subcommittee for that goal, with a chairperson who will be responsible for leading that subcommittee. The chair can then begin identifying key stakeholders in the community who can be approached to join that subcommittee, also sometimes called a task force. For the walking school bus example, it will be important to have the local elementary school principal and/or physical education teacher, member of the PTA, and possibly the local police chief as subcommittee/task force members.

Running Meetings

Running an effective and efficient meeting is critical to keeping coalition members engaged and excited. Here are some basic, but essential steps to consider when running coalition meetings:

- Establishing meeting frequency and times
  As simple as this sounds, actually finding a time when all members of your coalition can be present may pose a challenge. Using online meeting schedulers can be very helpful in setting an initial meeting, as well as follow-up meetings. Depending upon your coalition, you may need to meet more or less frequently. However, only meet as frequently as is necessary. Standing monthly meetings (e.g., meetings that occur on the first Thursday of each month at 2 p.m.) are quite common and effective. Your steering committee, if you have one, may choose to meet at additional times. Similarly, your subcommittees may also need to meet regularly; however, their meeting frequency and meeting times should be determined by the chair and members of the committee.

- Establishing a meeting place
  Where your coalition meets will largely depend upon whether or not it is local. Local coalitions will often meet at the office of one of the partner organizations. However, regional-, state-, or national-level coalitions will generally hold regular meetings via teleconference or web-based conference. Even if regular, monthly meetings are held via teleconference or web-based conferencing, it will be important to try and hold in-person meetings either annually or semiannually. Such in-person meetings are typically longer (e.g., 1–2 business days) than regular monthly meetings, which typically run 1 hour, as will be discussed in the following text on setting an agenda for meetings.

- Setting an agenda
  Typically, the coalition's president or chair is responsible for setting the agenda for each meeting. The agenda for your first meeting will look very different from that of future meetings. For your first meeting, which will be with your core group, the agenda may be as simple as

  - Member introductions
    Each member introduces him- or herself, states the organization he or she represents (if any), and maybe why he or she joined the coalition.

- Brainstorming
  - ◆ Discussion about the coalition's vision, mission, and goals
  - ◆ Thoughts about other key stakeholders that should be invited to join the coalition
- Setting up regular meeting schedule

Although this agenda is quite simple, it is still important to have prepared an agenda for the meeting that looks professional and that is emailed to all those coming to the meeting at least 24 to 48 hours prior to the meeting.

In the sample agenda from Box 6.7, there are some things that are worth noting as you develop your own meeting agenda. First, notice that the top of the agenda has the name of the coalition along with the meeting details (date, time, call-in number). This clearly is an example for a teleconference meeting. Were it an in-person meeting, the address for the meeting would be provided instead of a phone number. The agenda also delineates each agenda topic and the amount of time that will be spent on each topic. This is very helpful for keeping the group focused and efficient. Also notice that the agenda identifies the person responsible for each agenda item. Given that committee chairs may have a report to make, they should know that they are going to be on the agenda, which is also why the agenda should be sent well in advance of the meeting. Finally, note that the agenda states when the next meeting will take place. It is always a good idea to remind coalition members of when the next meeting, or next several meetings, will take place. Perhaps noticeably absent from the example earlier is the approval of minutes from the previous meeting. It is customary to have review and approval of minutes from the previous meeting among the first items on the agenda.

BOX 6.7

Sample Meeting Agenda

XYZ Coalition
Monthly Leadership Call Agenda
Date: December 2, 20XX
Time: 3:00 p.m. (Eastern Daylight Time)
Call in number: (XXX) XXX-XXXX
Passcode: XXXXX

  3:00–3:10—Welcome and introductions (Chair and all)
  3:10–3:15—Review and approval of minutes from previous meeting (All)
  3:15–3:40—The year ahead (Chair)
    Overall vision
      Committee structure
      Improve member retention
        Value in membership

(continued)

(continued)

Improve member recruitment
Fund raising
Making use of our recent policy success
Growing strategic partnerships
Vision for each committee

Discussion of vision (All)
New leadership positions (Chair)

Partnerships
Strategic planning
Treasurer

3:40–3:55—Committee updates and ideas (Committee Chairs)

Membership (Membership Committee Chair)
Student (Student Committee Chair)
Policy (Policy Committee Chair)
Communications (Communications Committee Chair)
Program Planning (Program Planning Committee Chair)

3:55–4:00—New business (All)
4:00—Adjourn
Next Meeting—Date: January 5, 20XX Time: 3:00 p.m. (Eastern Daylight Time)

■ Maintaining minutes
It is very important to accurately track the goings-on of each meeting in the form of meeting minutes. Typically, the person acting as the coalition's secretary will be responsible for taking notes during the call/meeting, and then formatting them and typing them up into a formal document that will be disseminated to all the coalition members. Your secretary should be a well-organized individual who can not only accurately record what happens during each meeting, but who can also somewhat quickly produce and disseminate the meeting minutes. The minutes should include what was discussed, any actions needed, and who is responsible for the actions by when.

■ Documenting successes and challenges
Progress toward, and/or challenges encountered in achieving, the coalition's goals and objectives should be documented regularly. Either during monthly meetings and/or in an annual report, the coalition's work should be well documented. When progress has been made, celebrate that success. Everyone likes to win; being able to provide feedback on progress helps keep coalition members engaged and excited. In some cases, you need to necessarily wait for an annual or semiannual meeting to report success. Similarly, everyone likes to be recognized for a job well done. If there were certain members of the coalition who were instrumental in progress having been made, be sure to recognize them by name, informally (mentioning their name during a meeting) and/or formally (presenting them with a certificate of appreciation).

Coalition examples from Dr. Maddock

In Hawaii, I had experience with starting and maintaining several coalitions. Early in my time in Hawaii, I was on the steering committee and eventually the chair of the Coalition for Tobacco Free Hawaii (CTFH). During my time as chair, the state legislature passed a comprehensive clean indoor air law, the major goal of our coalition. After that time, I served as the principal investigator and lead agency for the state nutrition and physical activity coalition (NPAC) as well as coalitions in Maui, Kauai, and Hawaii counties. My experience was decidedly mixed. Some of these coalitions folded with little success and others thrived. In 2015, our Get Fit Kauai Coalition was recognized with the Champions Award from the National Physical Activity Plan (NPAP) as one of the nation's best PA coalitions. Over these experiences, I was able to see what worked and what did not work in coalitions and how we can make these efforts more effective in meeting our goals.

One of the most important things that helped the coalition move forward was having a limited set of priorities. On the CTFH, our goal was very clear: influence the state to pass a policy to ban smoking in all indoor areas. While there were lots of other smoking-related policies that were important including increasing taxes and reducing youth possession, we knew that we could not focus on everything. By picking one major priority, we were able to focus all of our efforts to make sure that our voice was heard consistently and that we had the research and all other materials developed that eventually led to our success. In contrast, NPAC tried to adopt the first Hawaii state Nutrition and Physical Activity Plan for our goals. This plan had dozens of objectives which made coalescing around any particular focus hard and we saw limited success as a result.

A coalition example from Dr. Bornstein

I had the pleasure of working on the development, launch, and implementation of the NPAP over the course of 5 years. The NPAP was a national-level coalition comprised of "Organizational Partners" from government (e.g., CDC, U.S. Department of Agriculture), and a number of nonprofit organizations (e.g., American Heart Association, American Cancer Society, American College of Sports Medicine). Each organization selected an individual to represent its interests on the NPAP's "Coordinating Committee." Much like was discussed earlier in this chapter, the Coordinating Committee was a smaller, core group of committed individuals who really charted the course for the NPAP by mapping out its mission, vision, and goals. One thing that made the NPAP unique was that each Organizational Partner contributed money to the NPAP coalition in order to be represented on the Coordinating Committee. This "pay to play" scenario as it is often called was instrumental in providing the NPAP with resources necessary to carry out its mission. It is important to note, however, that these Organizational Partners also contributed capacity in other ways that were instrumental in developing and launching the NPAP. Typically, this is how coalitions work. They leverage the collective capacity of each other in order to move the goals of the coalition forward.

As the NPAP project grew, multiple committees and subcommittees were formed to help develop and advance the NPAP's more specific strategies and tactics. These committees and this process were open to any individuals or organizations interested in participating. Often it was members of the Coordinating Committee who knew certain individuals or organizations that they felt could contribute in meaningful ways to the NPAP coalition. For example, though not Organizational Partners, numerous small, medium, and large organizations, and even individuals with a passion for PA, joined the

NPAP's committees and subcommittees and provided tremendous capacity that would not have otherwise been possible.

One area where I believe the NPAP could have improved was in having an even more diverse set of organizations involved in the process. All of the NPAP's Organizational Partners, and many of the other organizations involved, were health- or PA-based organizations. This speaks to what was mentioned earlier in this chapter about having strategic alignment between the coalition and its members. However, given how strongly individuals' PA behavior is impacted by the environments in which they live, work, play, commute, learn, and pray, the NPAP could have benefitted from even greater representation from key organizations in areas such as education, the faith-based community, media, and industry. To the NPAP's credit, the revised version of the NPAP, released in 2015, included an entirely new faith-based section, thus including organizations and individuals who were not represented in the first iteration of the NPAP, released in 2010. The take-home message for a coalition you may be working with is to identify the organizations that could be positively impacted by your PA coalition. Once you have identified those organizations, health-based or not, work to demonstrate to them how joining your coalition will be of benefit to them.

Summary

Just as in other public health domains, successfully designing, implementing, and evaluating PA interventions is not easy. However, there is a long history of how coalition building can bring people, organizations, and resources together in such a way that achieving success becomes far easier than going it alone. Building and maintaining healthy, successful coalitions is not always easy, but by following the strategies from within this chapter and the resources provided at the conclusion of this chapter, you should be well on your way to bringing the requisite people together to overcome many of the obstacles standing in the way of increasing PA levels for all members of the population.

Things to Consider

- Achieving sustainable change often requires a team of organizations and/or individuals committed to the vision. Building a coalition is the most efficient way to formally organize such an effort. When looking for coalition members, identify organizations and/or individuals that have missions, goals, or strategic plans that would be positively impacted by the vision of the coalition.

- The vision for your coalition should reflect the ultimate dream of the coalition; what things would look like or be like if all the barriers were removed.

- In addition to having coalition members that are committed to the vision of the coalition, having a subset, or core team, of *highly* committed coalition members is essential to forming a coalition and moving its agenda forward.

- If involvement in the coalition can be part of a coalition member's existing job responsibilities, it will be that much easier to keep her/him engaged. For example, having an organization's Community Outreach Coordinator serve on your coalition will allow that person to devote existing work hours to the coalition as part of her/his regular work duties.

■ SMART goals are specific, measurable, attainable, realistic, and time bound, and will help you make progress toward your vision. When developing your goals, consider having some "easy wins," or goals that you know could be accomplished relatively easily and/or quickly. Being able to achieve some goals early on allows the coalition to demonstrate progress toward the vision, which is important for keeping coalition members engaged.

Resources

■ Butterfoss FD. Building and sustaining coalitions. In: Bensley RJ, Brookins-Fisher J, eds. *Community Health Education Methods: A Practical Guide.* Sudbury, MA: Jones & Bartlett; 2009.

■ Community Tool Box. Available at: http://ctb.ku.edu/en

■ National Center for Safe Routes to School. Available at: http://www.saferoutesinfo.org/

■ National Association of Counties. Available at: http://www.naco.org/sites/default/files/documents/Right-Way-to-Run-a-Meeting.pdf

■ American Federation of State, County, and Municipal Employees. Available at: https://www.afscme.org/news-publications/publications/afscme-governance/pdf/How_to_Chair.pdf

References

1. Maddock J, Aki NN, Irvin L, et al. Using coalitions to address childhood obesity: the Hawai'i Nutrition and Physical Activity Coalition. *Hawaii Med J.* 2011;70(7):48.
2. Bornstein D, Pate R, Beets M, et al. New perspective on factors related to coalition success: novel findings from an investigation of physical activity coalitions across the United States. *J Public Health Manag Pract.* 2015;21(6):E23–E30. doi:10.1097/PHH.0000000000000190
3. Bornstein D, Carnoske C, Evenson K, et al. Factors related to partner involvement in the U.S. National Physical Activity Plan. *J Public Health Manag Pract.* 2013;19(suppl 3):S8–S16. doi:10.1097/PHH.0b013e318284047d
4. Elliott E, Jones E, Bulger S. ActiveWV: a systematic approach to developing a physical activity plan for West Virginia. *J Phys Act Health.* 2014;11:478–486. doi:10.1123/jpah.2013-0083
5. Nelson JD, Moore JB, Blake C, et al. Characteristics of successful community partnerships to promote physical activity among young people, North Carolina, 2010–2012. *Prev Chronic Dis.* 2013;10:E208. doi:10.5888/pcd10.130110
6. Yancey AK. The meta-volition model: organizational leadership is the key ingredient in getting society moving, literally. *Prev Med.* 2009;49:342–351. doi:10.1016/j.ypmed.2009.09.004
7. Bornstein D, Pate R, Beets M, et al. New perspective on factors related to coalition success. Novel findings from an investigation of physical activity coalitions across the United States. *J Public Health Manag Pract.* 2015;21(6):E23–E30. doi:10.1097/PHH.0000000000000190

DEVELOPING PHYSICAL ACTIVITY PLANS

JAY E. MADDOCK | LAURA A. ESPARZA

LEARNING OBJECTIVES

By the end of this chapter, the student should be able to

1. Develop a community health profile.
2. Describe the steps to create a physical activity (PA) plan.
3. Analyze the organizations that would be invited to participate in the planning process.
4. Categorize strategies by feasibility and impact.
5. Discuss methods and channels for disseminating a PA plan.

▨ Introduction

The creation of active communities takes a variety of coordinated activities. As has been discussed in this book, interventions at the school, worksite, park, transportation, mass media, physician, and individual levels are all important in helping people meet their physical activity (PA) guidelines. While this can be exciting, it can also be overwhelming. Whether working to improve PA in a local community, a state, or even across the whole population, choosing what to do, how to do it, who will do it, and how progress can be measured can be a daunting task. This is where a PA plan comes in. A PA plan is like a road map. It helps identify where you are going and how you are going to get there. It is important to help guide not only what you are going to do but also what you are **not** going to do. This chapter will help guide you, step by step, in how to create a PA plan. We will share some of our experiences creating PA plans in hopes that they will be useful in creating your own plan.

© Springer Publishing Company DOI: 10.1891/9780826134592.0007

◼ The Planning Process

Getting Started

The first step to developing a plan is to develop a working group (1). This is usually a small group of people who can do the major writing of the plan and track its progress over time. While the plan will be collaborative, it is best to have a lead agency. This might be local government, a university, or a nonprofit in your community. The role of the lead agency is as a convener. The best lead agencies have a space to meet, some staff time to put the plan together and monitor its progress, and a little bit of resources. While it is not expensive to develop a plan, there are things like a website page and providing lunch that make the planning process more effective. The most important thing to remember is that the lead agency is a partner in the planning process. This is not *their* plan. Once a lead agency has been selected, the conveners can pull together the working group. This group should include people from different sectors. For instance, the National Physical Activity Plan (NPAP) has nine sectors:

- Business and industry
- Community, recreation, fitness, and parks
- Education
- Faith-based settings
- Healthcare
- Mass media
- Public health
- Sport
- Transportation, land use, and community design

These sectors may or may not be appropriate for your situation, so think through what sectors you want to include. It is good to have someone from each sector on your working group so that each of the sectors is represented by someone who is knowledgeable in the area. The current chapter takes a sector-based approach, as that has been the prevailing approach used in the United States. However, other approaches could be considered, such as a plan organized around specific subsegments of the population (e.g., older adults, children, persons with disabilities) (2).

One of the best places to get started is by reading other plans. This is not an exact science and is learned by trial and error. Reading a few plans before getting started is a good way to see what elements of a plan the group likes and what the group does not like about the way certain plans are written. This can help the working group think about how to structure the plan. Here are some sample plans at the national, state, and local level (Box 7.1).

BOX 7.1

Example PA plans

The National Physical Activity Plan: www.physicalactivityplan.org/index.html
    Be Active Western Australia: www.beactive.wa.gov.au/index.php?id=515

(continued)

(continued)

Active Texas 2020: sph.uth.edu/content/uploads/2012/06/Active-Texas-2020-full.pdf
West Virginia Physical Activity Plan: wvphysicalactivity.org/activewv2020
United kingdom: www.gov.uk/government/publications/health-matters-getting-every-adult
-active-every-day/health-matters-getting-every-adult-active-every-day#active-society

PA, physical activity.

Once the working group has a chance to look through a few plans, it is time to convene and start making some initial decisions. First, the focus of the plan is important. For large areas, like the United States and Texas, stand-alone PA plans have been developed. For smaller areas, these plans are often combined with nutrition, obesity, and/or chronic disease prevention (3). In Hawaii, the plan combined PA, nutrition, and obesity because many of the participants had these three areas in their job description and it would have been redundant to bring them together multiple times (3). The next decision is the time frame for the plan. In general, you can go as long as 10 years with a plan and as short as 5. The first plan in Hawaii was 5 years long. The steering committee (SC) decided after the first plan that a 7-year time frame worked better since the planning process took almost a year. Factors that should be considered include: length of time of the planning process, milestone dates (e.g., 2025), length of funding (if available), and any legislative or other mandates to create the plan.

Next, the working group needs to discuss the time to create the plan and a timeline. It can certainly take 6 to 12 months to develop a plan, especially if this is the first time. If this is the group's first attempt at a plan, then a year is realistic. The working group should also decide who is writing the plan. Some groups use an outside consultant or someone who is paid specifically to complete the plan. In other places, the working group divides sections of the plan. If people are writing the plan in their spare time, it will take longer to complete.

Developing a Community Health Profile

Once you have made some initial decisions about what you want to achieve and where you want to go, it is time to do some background work. Just like a road map, you need to know where you are starting from to find out where you want to go. The next step is to develop a community health profile. There are a lot of places to start putting together a picture of your community. First, you want to know about the level of PA in your community. The Behavioral Risk Factor Surveillance Survey (www.cdc.gov/brfss/index.html) has data on adult behavior for all 50 states and many metropolitan areas. Some states oversample to get county-level numbers. You can contact your state coordinator to find out what data your state collects (www.cdc.gov/brfss/state_info/coordinators.htm). For high school and some middle school students, there is the Youth Risk Behavior Survey (www.cdc.gov/healthyyouth/data/yrbs/index.htm), which provides similar information to the adult survey. The County Health Rankings (www.countyhealthrankings.org) also provide a variety of data about all counties in the United States and have lots of useful data in putting together a community health profile.

Once you have the outcome data, you want to create a policy scan. This can be done by sector and is one of the reasons why it is important to have a knowledgeable person for each sector. For instance, in education, what are the policies around recess, physical education, commuting to school, and other policies that affect PA? When someone is familiar or works in the school district, these policies will be easily accessible. This will be similar for parks and recreation, transportation, zoning, and other areas that you are interested in. In addition to policies, it is also important to assess what free and low-cost programming is occurring in the community. What classes do parks and recreation or the senior center offer? Many times, these classes are underenrolled and an item at the planning session is to develop new classes instead of linking people to existing ones.

The third part of the community data profile is to listen to community voices. This is essential so that you know what issues are facing your particular community. Are you interested in increasing PA in older adults, children, or certain ethnic groups? Each of these has different barriers. Focus groups are a great way to get input from a variety of stakeholders. Intercept surveys are another way to get quick data on different ideas. Observational methods also let you see how people are using the space. Are parks crowded at different times of the week? Do people use one feature heavily (e.g., basketball courts) while other features are empty (e.g., baseball fields)? At this point, you are trying to get big picture ideas. Later on when there are specific projects, then you will want to listen to community voices again to get ideas around solutions to particular issues (Box 7.2).

BOX 7.2

Steps in developing a community health profile

1. Collect or collate data on who, when, and where people are active in your community
2. Conduct a policy scan
3. Listen to community voices

Bringing Your Partners Together

Once you have completed your community profile, it is time to bring all of the partners together to develop objectives for the plan. So, who do you invite? The working group should know which sectors you want to include in the plan by now. If there is an existing coalition, you can start your guest list with them. If not, or if the group is small, have each sector leader start inviting people he or she knows. The goal should be to invite people who are knowledgeable about each sector and who are likely to implement pieces of the plan. This is the part of the plan to be as inclusive as possible. This is the plan for your state/community/region, so everyone who will be contributing to the plan should be invited. Oftentimes this can be done as a daylong meeting with an overall facilitator and table facilitators. There are several goals of this meeting. The first is to establish the vision and goals of the plan. This is discussed in more depth in Chapter 6 on coalitions. For these, it is best if the working group has a chance to draft some initial ideas. Putting out a few concepts and letting the group respond and add key words that they want included is a good way to stimulate the discussion. In the second goal, the group should review the community profile developed in the last section to get everyone on the same page, and the third goal is to brainstorm strategies to address each sector. If all of this is accomplished, the group has had a great meeting and has taken a significant step forward in creating the plan.

Sorting and Simplifying

Upon completion of this big group meeting, a series of ideas and strategies will have been identified. Next, it will be time to work with the group to reduce the overall number of ideas and strategies and to put these into similar formats that are clear and specific. Start by removing all duplicate items and items that are outside of your jurisdiction (i.e., federal and state policy changes if you are developing a local plan). Try to write each strategy clearly and specifically. For example, an unclear strategy might be, "Increase PE in all schools." A better strategy would be "Require quality, comprehensive PE in all Department of Education schools." The plan could even be more specific, requiring meeting specific guidelines around days and minutes a week. Once these strategies are reduced and written similarly, it is time to get input again. Some groups have done this online, but it could be done in group format also. Doing the survey by sector allows individuals to choose the sectors they want to complete, so people are not filling out areas where they have limited interest or expertise. For each sector, they had to indicate if it was a high-, medium-, or low-priority area and if they were willing to work on the area (Box 7.3).

BOX 7.3

Selecting priority strategies

The planning process tends to develop more strategies that can be addressed in the plan period. Deciding which strategies the group focuses on is an important task. One way to do this is to have each strategy ranked by (a) impact on PA and (b) feasibility. The items can then be plotted on a *x-y* axis with

a. High impact/high feasibility included in the plan

b. Low impact/low feasibility discarded

c. Low impact/high feasibility chosen only if they provide easy wins or are politically popular

d. High impact/low feasibility chosen only if it is very high impact and there are steps forward that can help it happen

---

The working group then reviews the data again and removes strategies that no one wants to work on or ones that are rated as low priority for most of the participants. The working group can contact a person/organization that was interested in working on a strategy and see if they are interested in taking the lead on moving this strategy forward. The working group takes on some of these positions and others are invited based on interest. One approach is matchup strategy, in which leadership within an organization has an issue as a priority and then has some resources (time, money, space, etc.) that it is able to put behind making it happen. For instance, in Hawaii, the AARP led efforts around reducing pedestrian deaths since it disproportionally affected their members and was also a national organizational priority.

The next step is to develop an evaluation plan. Evaluation is discussed more fully in Chapter 20 in this book. For PA plan evaluation, each strategy should have measures of success and data sources that correspond to them. For some items, no baseline data exists and these need to be developed. This needs to be considered in how many measures will need to be developed and if this is feasible. At this stage, the larger group should be brought back together by sector area, which will keep the total number in each group smaller. These groups should discuss the items that were selected and asked whether to add or delete items and if the rephrased items were understandable. Prioritization should also be done again with a 1-year time frame. For each sector group, tackling two to three issues was enough for the first year. The groups decide which items they wanted to start on, discuss what measures of success look like, and then move forward with implementation and evaluation.

Publishing and Disseminating the Plan

After prioritizing the items, developing an evaluation plan, and creating a 1-year action plan, you are almost ready to publish. The basics of the published plan include: who was involved in writing and developing the plan, a description of how the plan was written, the vision and goals of the plan, the community health assessment, the strategies for each sector, and the evaluation plan with data sources and baseline numbers. The working group should draft all of these elements of the plan and then send them out for public comment. Everyone who participated in the planning process should have a chance to see the document before it is published and make comments by a deadline that is provided. After an appropriate time for providing comments has passed (e.g., 6 weeks), the comments should be reviewed and incorporated into the document. You now have your plan and are ready to disseminate it. The plan can be disseminated in many ways. Some groups prefer hard copies, while others prefer web access. Most organizations today put the plan on the web and do a small amount of printing for elected officials, other VIPs, and planning committee members. One way to ensure use of the plan is to ask all of the organizations that participate in the planning process to formally endorse the plan. This helps to get organizations on board with the plan and keeps it an essential tool across the community. The group may also want to consider issuing a press release or press conference around the plan. Getting local media involved is another good method for spreading the word in the community.

■ The Plan is Written, Now What?

Once the plan is written and published, it feels like the work is done. But this is actually the start of the real work. How do you ensure the plan is usable and that you do not just have a pretty plan that sits on the shelves? One tool that is very effective is to develop a 1-year implementation plan. This plan should have one to two strategies per working group. These should be selected by the working group and be items that members are excited and ready to work on. This is also a good time to develop a SC. One of the most effective ways to do this is to elect a chair and vice-chair whose responsibility is to make sure the implementation is moving forward. The rest of the SC is usually comprised of the working group's leaders and the lead on the evaluation. This group should meet monthly to discuss progress and challenges to implementation. At the end of the year, it is important to bring the large group back together and celebrate the progress made over the year. The PA plan evaluation should be presented, and the next year's implementation plan developed.

While this process is more of an art than a science, if you follow these steps there will be a very good chance of developing a plan that is valuable to the community and help support progress in creating an active society. In the next section, we will describe specifically two of the PA plans that we are centrally involved in developing.

■ Examples of PA Plan Development

Developing the Active Living Plan for a Healthier San Antonio

The local health department of San Antonio, Texas, the City of San Antonio's Metropolitan Health District (SAMHD), was awarded $15.6 million in 2010 from the Centers for Disease Control and Prevention's (CDC) Communities Putting Prevention to Work (CPPW) program to implement a 2-year obesity prevention initiative. The overall goals of the initiative were to improve nutrition and PA behaviors by encouraging policy, environmental, and systems changes in school and community settings. Since the SAMHD's staff and program experience heavily favored nutrition, the addition of a PA focus was new territory for the department. The CPPW application called for the creation of a food policy council and, to create balance on the PA side, it also called for the creation of an active living council whose only defined deliverables were to develop a 3- to 5-year master plan and two policy recommendations.

To establish what would become the Active Living Council of San Antonio (ALCSA), SAMHD convened a SC composed of SAMHD staff and representatives of organizations involved in PA and/or health in the community. As the first active living initiative of its kind in San Antonio, the SC first defined "active living" for the group and set preliminary ALCSA goals:

- Provide forum to address active living issues
- Promote coordination across sectors
- Foster local PA and active living projects
- Promote access to PA places and programs
- Support PA-promoting policies

After brainstorming about ALCSA composition and agreeing that the group should be multisectoral, the SC established a membership structure that mirrored the defined sectors of the recently released *U.S. NPAP*, adding two additional membership categories (community, other) to ensure broad community participation:

- Business and industry
- Education, after school, and early childhood
- Healthcare
- Mass media
- Parks, recreation, fitness, and sports
- Public health
- Transportation, land use, and community design
- Volunteer and nonprofit
- Community
- Other

The SC developed an application process, SAMHD promoted the ALCSA to the community, and the SC selected 20 members (two members per sector), and scheduled ALCSA's inaugural meeting, a half-day retreat, and the first monthly meeting. Once the SC selected members and scheduled initial meetings, the SC dissolved and ALCSA's work began.

SAMHD engaged a facilitator to support ALCSA early on with team-building, development of mission and vision statements, and outlining a timeline to produce CPPW deliverables. Members soon developed a governance framework, elected officers, and established monthly plenary meetings in addition to ongoing individual and small-group work. ALCSA embarked on a months-long process of capacity-building about PA and active living based on current evidence and best practices, such as the 2008 PAGuidelines for Americans, the NPAP, and its accompanying *Make the Move* implementation guide. Members participated in teleconferences and webinars, attended a health policy development workshop organized by SAMHD to support CPPW activities, and conducted outreach to the San Antonio community to ensure that ALCSA understands local needs and priorities and that its work aligns with and supports other local initiatives. Though limited in number at the time, ALCSA studied existing PA plans to learn about how to develop a PA plan (see Table 7.1 for the challenges and lessons learned in the process of this development).

Following capacity building, the ALCSA established the following objectives to guide writing the plan:

> Articulate priorities
>
> Guide allocation of resources
>
> Establish measures of success
>
> Generate sense of urgency about PA and health

Developing the plan was a multistep, collaborative process that took 18 months to complete. The writing team, a subset of ALCSA members, drafted background material, overarching strategies, and target outcomes for the overall plan. ALCSA's sector partners drafted sector content. With input from sector constituents, sector partners identified two to three NPAP strategies and two tactics per strategy for the next 3 to 5 years, adapting the strategies and tactics to a local context. The writing team supported the work of sector partners by reviewing and revising the sections before seeking input on final drafts from sources outside the ALCSA, including local leaders and national content experts. The final document, the *Active Living Plan for a Healthier San Antonio*, represents the first local adaptation of the NPAP to a local setting. The 18-month process from the ALCSA's inaugural meeting to the plan's distribution resulted in an evidence-based plan that aligns with local priorities and initiatives.

Successes:

■ After producing the plan and separating from SAMHD, ALCSA continued functioning as an independent volunteer organization to advance the plan from the planning phase to adoption and implementation. ALCSA underwent a strategic planning process to establish goals and develop an action plan to guide this process.

■ CPPW funding allowed capacity building to occur within the local health department (LHD) and ALCSA with respect to the role of evidence-based

TABLE 7.1. Challenges and lessons learned in developing the ALCSA plan

CHALLENGES	LESSONS LEARNED
SAMHD provided little guidance to ALCSA about plan objectives and content. Despite SAMHD staff participation in all ALCSA meetings and inclusion of SAMHD leadership in ALCSA communications and ALCSA leadership meetings, SAMHD leadership was not directly engaged in the plan development process until the final editing stage. At this late stage, SAMHD prohibited ALCSA from including any instance of the word "advocate" or "advocacy" in the plan out of concern that it would be misconstrued with lobbying activities that could put federal grant funding at risk; SAMHD indicated it would withdraw support from the plan if these words remained. Although ALCSA disagreed with a mandate that changed the spirit of what was to have been a community-driven plan, ALCSA removed the objectionable words from the plan, considering it of benefit to the community to produce a plan with SAMHD support rather than to reject SAMHD's request and attempt to move forward in isolation. Once grant deliverables were fulfilled, ALCSA formally separated from SAMHD in order to continue its work as an independent volunteer organization.	Expectations about the process, product(s), and ownership should be clearly defined at the start of a planning process.
The CPPW deliverable of developing a 3- to 5-year master plan did not extend to implementation and evaluation. SAMHD plans did not include a role for ALCSA beyond the grant deliverables.	In addition to supporting plan development, funding should be available to support implementation, evaluation, and sustainability planning.
Separation from SAMHD brought an end to staff support and meals for lunch meetings.	While a group of committed volunteers is essential to drive the process, it is important to have staff who can facilitate meetings, guide communications, and coordinate logistics. Providing a meal (e.g., lunch) is helpful to members who take time out of their workday to attend meetings.
As city leadership changed, so did support for health-promoting initiatives. The mayor who established the MFC and oversaw a health department that drove multiple new obesity prevention initiatives left office. The subsequent mayor's priorities were quite different and resulted in weakened MFC and SAMHD focus on PA initiatives.	Successful plan implementation requires top-level leadership that prioritizes plan objectives.
While community leaders are not disinterested in promoting PA as a means to improving community health, policy makers are insufficiently motivated to take action (funding, policy) simply for the sake of benefitting community health.	Expanding the focus of PA promotion beyond health benefits to include environmental, safety, economic, and social benefits is likely to result in greater support among local decision makers.

NOTE: ALCSA, Active Living Council of San Antonio; CPPW, Communities Putting Prevention to Work; MFC, Mayor's Fitness Council; PA, physical activity; SAMHD, San Antonio's Metropolitan Health District.

strategies to promote PA. ALCSA used its new expertise to support local health promotion initiatives and promote plan implementation.

- The local Mayor's Fitness Council (MFC) adopted the plan in 2013, integrating ALCSA into its organizational structure as a permanent committee in order to prioritize implementation of strategies. MFC integration offered ALCSA the support of MFC (LHD) staff and funding as well as routine association with local health promotion efforts. ALCSA leaders served on MFC executive committee; ALCSA members served on MFC committees to promote plan implementation more broadly.

- SAMHD and MFC recognize the value of ALCSA member expertise and routinely invite ALCSA to participate in leadership roles in support of local initiatives. ALCSA have participated in many community health and policy initiatives, ensuring the integration of plan strategies in local initiatives:
  - Develop the SAMHD's legislative agenda
  - Serve on committees to draft the county's Community Health Improvement Plan
  - Serve on the SC to plan a local built environment and public health conference
  - Serve on committees to develop *SA Tomorrow*, a major comprehensive planning effort underway in San Antonio

- ALCSA members engaged in numerous education and outreach activities to promote plan strategies:
  - Delivered presentations at local, state, and national meetings
  - Developed sector-specific fact sheets for stakeholders and policy makers
  - Published manuscript in peer-reviewed scientific journal
  - Published editorials and articles in local media
  - Established presence on MFC website and social media
  - Organized *Speak Up for Healthy Living*, a town hall event to engage residents
  - Developed a *Speak Up for Healthy Living* tool kit to support implementation of a variety of community events
  - Established an awards program to recognize local businesses that support active living

The Hawaii Physical Activity and Nutrition Plan, 2013–2020

In March of 2012, we began the planning process for the Hawaii Physical Activity and Nutrition Plan, 2013–2020 (PAN Plan). We brought together an eight-person planning group from the Hawaii Department of Health, the University of Hawaii, and an outside consultant from the island of Kauai, with the Health Department serving as the lead agency. Several of the members of the planning group had worked on the development of the 2007–2012 PAN plan and were able to use that experience to help improve the process the second time. We agreed on three principles to base the objectives on:

1. Focus on policy, systems, and environmental change throughout the state
2. Use existing or impending tools for measuring outcomes

3. Be implementable given the capacity and resources in the state

From here, given the small size of the state, we decided to have only four sectors in the plan:

1. Community design and access
2. Worksite, industry, and business
3. Educational systems
4. Healthcare systems

For each of these areas, we recruited well respected, knowledgeable members of the community to serve as chairs and vice-chairs of each area with a goal of ensuring gender, ethnic, and island diversity in the group.

In August 2012, the planning committee met with the sector chairs and vice-chairs to present current data, outline evidence-based practices, discuss priority objectives, outline their roles and responsibilities as chairs/vice-chairs, and have them work with members of the planning committee to draft objectives for the plan. The chairs and vice-chairs outlined preliminary objectives and submitted them to the planning committee. Some of the chairs vetted the objectives among other colleagues/key informants. The planning committee further refined the objectives and incorporated priorities from a variety of resources including national guidance documents, other state task forces, and university experts.

In September 2012, the Department of Health reached out to a broad spectrum of stakeholders to seek volunteers in the community interested in participating in advisory workgroups to provide feedback to one or more specific sectors. One hundred and thirteen stakeholders expressed interest in working on one or more sectors. After obtaining the list of participants for each workgroup, the planning committee developed a survey in December 2012 to distribute to the sector workgroup members and chairs/vice-chairs to collect additional feedback on the initial plan objectives. Participants were asked if the objective was a priority or interest to their organization and if the wording needed revision. They were also asked to identify gaps or missing priorities and to add general comments or other recommendations. Responses were received providing comments, suggesting changes in language, and identifying gaps. These comments were incorporated into the next set of revisions and two more objectives were developed in January 2013. This draft list of 22 objectives was sent to approximately 1,000 stakeholders for final feedback in February 2013. One-hundred and seventy-two) people responded and feedback was incorporated into the final version of the objectives.

In May of 2013, the PAN Plan was officially launched at a PAN summit held in Honolulu. The summit included a breakout session for each of the sectors along with a release of the data and how the plan would be evaluated. This planning process provided the state with an excellent foundation to implement strategies to increase PA and supports for active living. It is still the foundation document that provided a road map for the state in these efforts.

See http://health.hawaii.gov/physical-activity-nutrition/files/2013/08/Hawaii-PAN -Plan-2013-2020.pdf for a complete description of the planning process.

Things to Consider

- A PA plan provides a road map for your community to keep on track with its efforts.
- A Community Health Profile contains data and information about the health of your community.
- Priority strategies can be sorted by feasibility and impact.
- While developing a plan is important, ensuring implementation, evaluation, and sustainability is also essential.
- A successful plan requires top-level leadership that prioritizes plan objectives.

Resources

- The Active Living Plan for a Healthier San Antonio is available at www.fitcitysa.com/wp-content/uploads/2017/05/Active_Living_Plan.pdf.
- Active Living Research website on building a plan: https://activelivingresearch.org/developing-active-living-plan-healthier-san-antonio-lessons-learned

References

1. Maddock JE, Bornstein D. Effective strategies for building and maintaining coalitions. In: Bornstein DB, Eyler AA, Maddock JE, et al, eds. *Physical Activity and Public Health Practice.* New York, NY: Springer Publishing; 2019:87–99.
2. Bornstein D, Pate R, Pratt M. A review of the national physical activity plans of six countries. *J Phys Act Health.* 2009;6(suppl 2):S245–S264. doi:10.1123/jpah.6.s2.s245
3. Hawaii Physical Activity and Nutrition Plan, 2013–2020. Honolulu, HI: Hawaii Department of Health;

PHYSICAL ACTIVITY POLICY TO PRACTICE

AMY A. EYLER | LAURIE WHITSEL

LEARNING OBJECTIVES

By the end of this chapter, the student should be able to

1. Describe the key components for successful policy to practice in improving population physical activity.
2. Differentiate the importance of each of the key components in policy to practice.
3. Argue the relevance of transdisciplinary involvement in moving physical activity policy to practice.
4. Examine recommendations for successfully moving policy to practice in improving population physical activity.
5. Compare and contrast examples of successful policy to practice.

■ Introduction

As discussed in Chapter 4, policies play an important role in improving and sustaining physical activity behavior at a population level. Evidence to demonstrate the impact of these policy strategies has been growing steadily over the past few decades (1, 2), but there is still a gap between knowing that policies are effective in improving physical activity and actually putting those policies into practice. To make matters even more complex, merely having a policy in place does not guarantee that this improvement in population physical activity is imminent. Policies must be implemented, adequately resourced, communicated, enforced, and evaluated to ensure that the policy results in its intended outcome. For example, the Community Guide recommends enhanced school-based physical education to increase physical activity. Enhanced school-based physical education involves changing the curriculum and coursework for k-12 students to increase the amount of time they spend engaged in moderate- or vigorous-intensity physical activity during physical education classes (3). In order to facilitate these improvements in physical education and subsequent physical activity, policies at the district or state level need to be developed, implemented, adequately resourced, communicated, and enforced (4). The case study outlined in Box 8.1 provides an example of not only lack of implementation, but also the subsequent consequences.

BOX 8.1

California State Physical Education Law and School District Compliance

Physical education is a main source of physical activity for schoolchildren (5). In 2005, the state of California passed a law that requires schools to provide students in grades one through six with a minimum of 200 minutes of physical education every 10 days (6). In a 2012 study, Sanchez and colleagues studied compliance—or failure to comply—with state physical education laws and the impact on children's fitness levels (7). They found that over half of the 55 districts studied failed to comply with the state physical education law, and that school districts with higher percentages of students eligible for free and reduced priced meals were more likely to be noncompliant districts compared with higher socioeconomic status districts. Of the fifth graders in the districts studied, only 58% were classified as being physically fit based on their performance on standard school fitness tests.

Researchers were not the only ones to realize the noncompliance of state laws. In 2013, parents and a physical education advocacy group (Cal200) sued 37 California school districts for not providing 200 minutes of physical education as outlined by state law (8). The movement began in 2009 when a parent realized that his third-grade son was not getting the state-required amount of physical education in his school. Upon further investigation, he found that noncompliance with the state physical education law was rampant, which resulted in a series of lawsuits against these districts. In 2015, the lawsuits were settled; elementary schools in California are now required to prove they are providing at least the minimum amount of physical education required by state law. Under the settlement agreement, teachers in the district must report the minutes they spend teaching physical education, provide the schedules to parents and school boards, and be subject to spot checks by principals. The settlement also requires that the 37 districts split the costs of the $1.2 million in attorney's fees.

In fall of 2015, lawsuits were filed against 89 more California school districts for not providing documentation of physical education or allegedly falsifying the documentation to show compliance with the physical education requirement. These lawsuits happened in spite of a new state law urgently enacted in October 2015 (CA AB 1391) prompting changes in state statutes designed to keep individuals or organizations from initiating a lawsuit, without first taking more local action via a district's uniform complaint procedure (9). Nevertheless, the years of legal action brought to light the need for schools to be more objectively accountable for implementing the state physical education requirements. Not only will children get equal amounts of physical education across districts, there will be records of this which will be helpful in assessing overall policy outcomes such as improved student fitness.

◾ Key Components for Policy to Practice

In order for physical activity policies to be successfully implemented and integrated into practice, there are several key components that must be addressed (Box 8.2). The first is **funding**. Implementing public policies requires money, and costs must be determined at the development and proposal phase. In order to gain support for policy efforts, policy makers need to know (or get an estimate) of how much it will cost to put the policy into practice and if there will be cost savings over time. At the federal level, much of this work is done by the Congressional Budget Office (CBO). The CBO supports the Congressional budget process, is strictly nonpartisan, and is required by law to produce formal cost estimates (often referred to as a CBO score) for nearly every bill that is approved by a full committee of the House or the Senate (10). These cost estimates are a key determinant of political support. In a challenging fiscal environment, legislation with a high CBO score will have a difficult road to passage if there are not potential revenue streams to offset the cost of implementation.

There are also often differences in funding between the authorization and appropriations processes. Authorizing laws establish, continue, or modify programs and are a prerequisite under House and Senate Rules for the Congress to appropriate budget authority for programs. Some authorization laws provide spending directly (often referred to as direct or mandatory spending) and other authorization laws require appropriations legislation (referred to as discretionary spending) for actual budgetary allocation. Very often, there is a difference in the amount of funding that is authorized versus what is actually appropriated.

Whereas bills with small budgets are more likely to be enacted, changes in practice will not occur without adequate funding. As was discussed in Chapter 4, framing the costs along with any savings or benefits is critical for stakeholder support and effective implementation (11). Just like what is done at the federal level, at the state and local level, broad economic effects or the revenue impact are written into fiscal notes that coexist with the policies. A fiscal note is a written estimate of the costs, savings, revenue gain, or revenue loss. Let us say that a city has identified four intersections with dangerous crosswalks. If evidence shows that requiring curb bump outs at these crosswalks will actually save money due to fewer injuries and damage from accidents, economic analyses of costs of construction and the estimated savings should be promoted through the fiscal note. However, since budgets and priorities are fluid, amounts identified in the fiscal note are not guaranteed in the appropriations process.

BOX 8.2

Summary of Key Components for Policies to Practice

- ◾ **Funding**
- ◾ **Effective regulatory process**
- ◾ **Communication and awareness building**
- ◾ **Capacity to execute policy actions**
- ◾ **Accountability**

Federal, state, and/or local budgets are funding sources for many policies related to physical activity. Sometimes a single-level source is used, but more often, a combination of the various funding levels is used. For example, the federal government has made funds available for active transportation in several successive federal transportation laws, with funds increasing significantly since the 1970s; however, there is competition with other multimodal transportation projects. It is worth noting that the lion's share of federal transportation funding, historically called the Surface Transportation Program (STP), *may* be used for pedestrian, bicycle, and transit infrastructure. So, one of the most promising ways to increase that infrastructure is to include it routinely, as part of all surface transportation projects at the state and local level. For example, the Nashville Metropolitan Planning Organization (MPO) has increased the importance of pedestrian, bicycle, and pedestrian accommodation in scoring their priority transportation projects (12). The result has been a dramatic increase in road and bridge projects that automatically include pedestrian, bicycle, and transit facilities. Increasingly, state and local governments will have to amplify funding coming from the federal level (13). There are several potential sources for that funding including sales tax measures, transportation impact fees, gas taxes, congestion pricing, user fees, tolls, project revenue streams, and financing (14–17). More and more, local governments are implementing taxes, issuing bonds, providing general fund allocations, seeking private/public partnerships, or levying impact fees on developers to shift financial burden from taxpayers to pay for the infrastructure that supports development (18–20). One focus of the funding should be to assure that resources are directed to vulnerable communities.

Funding allows for projects and programs to be implemented as outlined in the policies, as well as paying for enforcement and maintenance of the policy provisions. For instance, if a community creates a policy requiring sidewalks within all new developments, there must be money allocated to building and maintaining those sidewalks, in addition to staff who will enforce and follow-up with implementation of the policy. As demonstrated in the Case Study, policies should also include funds for evaluation and reporting if this is an expectation of the policy.

A second component for successful transference of policies into practice is an effective regulatory process where regulatory agencies with oversight are responsible for assuring legislation is put into practice and can be implemented effectively. For example, when a regulation is enacted requiring a certain amount of instructional minutes for physical education in public schools, there must be a process outlining oversight on how the regulation is being implemented. The public and physical activity advocates have an important opportunity to influence the regulatory process through public comment and relationship building with the agencies of jurisdiction to share best practices, case studies, experiential learning, and expertise to best inform how regulations are written. School districts, local governments, and community agencies can all share information on best practices for influencing this regulatory oversight.

Another component of successful implementation of policies is **communications and awareness building** such as regulatory agencies with oversight communicating to those who will be impacted by the law, advocacy organizations communicating to their grassroots networks or the media about legislation that has passed, or physical activity advocates communicating through their own social media channels. National advocacy organizations like the American Heart Association and SHAPE America, for example, communicated with educational leaders after passage of the Every Student Succeeds Act (ESSA) in 2015 to make sure that they knew school districts could prioritize physical education in Title IV funding applications. This communication creates awareness about the new law and sets the stage for implementation. Legislation that provides funding for local bike and pedestrian infrastructure must be communicated to local stakeholders so they know that they can apply for the funds. Many laws are ineffective because the general public or affected stakeholders simply are not aware of their passage or implications. This communication and awareness building, along with technical assistance and implementation resources, are especially important for vulnerable communities to assure policies are equitably implemented.

Another key component for successful transference of policies into practice is **capacity** to execute tasks as outlined in the policy. States, municipalities, schools, or organizations need people, training, and infrastructure to execute tasks effectively. In 2016, Colorado changed early childcare regulations to require 60 minutes of accumulated daily physical activity for preschool-age children, and imposed limits on screen time for all state-licensed early care facilities (21). Issues to consider related to capacity in this case include providing technical support to centers to interpret and comply with the new regulations, and also include staff and systems to assess, follow-up, and enforce the new rules.

Accountability for compliance is a final key component of implementation. Without proper accountability and enforcement, it is uncertain whether the activities outlined in the policy will occur, and expected outcomes may be negatively affected. As seen in the California physical education policy case study, the law was in place but clearly not being implemented as intended. If evaluation of the state law relied on changes in children's physical fitness levels, nonstandardized implementation of the requirements across districts may have resulted in inconsistent fitness improvements. Policy makers, upon seeing the inconsistent (or nonexistent) improvements, may view the policy as having little value and retract it.

Without accountability, those responsible for policy implementation may not prioritize efforts to comply. Accountability also encompasses strategies to address noncompliance with policies. Systems, infrastructure, and personnel are needed for technical assistance, inspection, notification, fines, and follow-up. Accountability provisions outline the context, frequency, and outcome of noncompliance. If a city has a law that requires all outdoor events to provide bicycle parking, personnel is needed to check if the event organizers consistently comply, and follow-up with noncompliance strategies outlined in the policy. Similarly, if a municipality is required to provide maintenance on a recreational trail, inspections must occur with reporting on physical conditions of the trail. It is important to note that governments can decide to offer waivers for entities that may not be able to comply with the required policy actions. Advocates need to be vigilant in the monitoring of waiver use to ensure accountability of policy implementation remains strong.

Physical Activity Policies Are Transdisciplinary

Policies play an important role in addressing many complex health issues. In 2010, the campaign for *Health in All Policies (HiAP)* began. HiAP is a collaborative approach to improving the health of all people by incorporating health considerations into decision making across sectors and policy areas (22). This collaboration promotes the inclusion of diverse governmental partners and stakeholders to work together to promote health, equity, and sustainability. In order to facilitate this, organizations such as the American Public Health Association (i.e., HiAP Guide for State and Local Governments) and the

National Association of County and City Health Officials (i.e., HiAP technical assistance) are providing assistance to practitioners in learning how to implement this collaborative framework. The *HiAP* approach fits well with physical activity policy efforts.

Public policy that influences physical activity is often driven from outside of public health and thus implementation requires transdisciplinary effort. Transportation, urban planning and design, parks and recreation, housing, emergency response, healthcare delivery, education accountability, public safety, and sustainability are all examples of transdisciplinary areas where physical activity policies may be developed and put into practice. Even though increased physical activity may be an outcome of these policies, it may have not been an original intent or priority. Consider the following examples:

- City development has resulted in a decreased number of downtown parking spaces. In order to encourage visitors to use public transportation or walk to destinations, the city officials institute a parking fee increase and a campaign to increase awareness of active transportation routes. This may encourage fewer vehicular trips and an increased active transportation of residents.

- With a concern for increasing rates of bicycle and pedestrian injuries, a city planning department implements a policy that requires safer bike lanes and crosswalks on city streets. These infrastructure improvements create actual and perceived safety of biking and walking, and rates of these activities may increase, while prevalence of injuries decrease.

- Representatives from a local school district apply for and receive funding for sidewalk improvements as part of their Safe Routes to School program. They work with city planning to develop the routes and engage public safety to train crossing guards. These improvements increase parents' confidence that their children will be safe and protected during their commute and this may result in more children using active transportation modes to get to and from school.

- Under the ESSA, the federal government provides new flexibility for states to develop school accountability, data reporting, and consolidated state plans that ensure every child gets a high-quality and well-rounded education. These new requirements for accountability around a well-rounded education allow for inclusion of physical education and physical activity measures within the state plans and other data reporting.

- The Affordable Care Act allowed employers the opportunity to vary health-care premiums for their employees within worksite health promotion programs with certain consumer protections in place. These outcomes-based incentive designs allow integration of physical activity and physical fitness assessment and programming for all employees with supportive leadership role modeling, worksite culture, and policies that promote physical activity before, during and after the workday.

In each of these scenarios, multiple stakeholders from different fields are involved in moving the policy to practice. Partnerships and collaboration among different disciplines can aggregate efforts and resources so that each group's priorities are recognized and outcomes are what were intended. Becoming part of coalitions that include many different types of community or organizational stakeholders is a way to become aware of potential partnerships and policy actions. It is also a good way to introduce health and physical activity outcomes as a by-product of policies that may have different, but complementary, outcome goals. Groups that are likely to help in efforts to increase physical activity are sometimes missing from these collaborations. A study of state physical activity plans revealed that few plan development teams included transportation or land use/community design partners (4). These groups should be highly involved in these plans as their work intersects with both physical activity policy and infrastructure.

Climate change and sustainability efforts are emerging as complementary to physical activity promotion and should be considered in transdisciplinary collaborations related to policy planning and implementation. Promotion of walking, rolling, and cycling for transportation, along with public transportation or any other active mode, presents a promising strategy to not only address problems of urban traffic strain, environmental pollution, and climate change, but also provide substantial health benefits with special emphasis on vulnerable communities and those with disabilities (23). Supporters of sustainable community development have the expertise and evidence to show that reducing motor vehicle travel has far-reaching benefits, which can also be used to promote physical activity policy. Active transportation modes such as bicycling, walking, and rolling can improve the local environment as well as have a positive impact on population health. Working together can create strong teams that can develop and implement strategies that resonate with a wide broad audience (i.e., both environment and health).

■ Recommendations for Better Policy to Practice

There are several other recommendations for successfully moving from physical activity policy to practice. Guidance and best practices exist for many topic areas such as Safe Routes to School, Complete Streets, and Physical Education. National advocacy agencies often provide venues for sharing of success stories, model policies, and implementation guidance. For example, the National Complete Streets Coalition within Smart Growth America provides resources on their website (smartgrowthamerica.org/program/national-complete-streets-coalition/) to facilitate policy implementation and give technical assistance for state and local agencies to "develop and implement effective policies and procedures." Shape America, The Society of Health and Physical Educators, developed guidance documents for physical education policy with recommended language, accountability measures, and rationale for policy components as well as implementation checklists. (www.shapeamerica.org/advocacy/upload/Guide-for-Physical-Education-Policy-9-23-14.pdf). These organizations are excellent resources and should be considered essential to those looking to develop, implement, and evaluate physical activity policies.

In addition to organizations, other states and communities can serve as examples of physical activity policy "lessons learned." States have been called "democratic laboratories" by policy diffusion experts because of the incremental way that many policies are developed and implemented (24). Exploring states and communities who may have been innovators in physical activity policy can provide insight into how best to replicate or modify implementation. Municipalities wanting to improve walkability and bikeability can look to Portland, Oregon, Denver, Colorado, and Washington DC to identify ways in which their policies to support active transportation have been implemented successfully. States such as Oregon (1971) and Florida (1984) were among the first to champion "routine accommodation" in which the needs of cyclists and pedestrians would be considered in all roadway projects; over the past 30 years, other states have followed this trend using information from the early innovative state policies (25).

The body of evidence on effective physical activity policies and environmental changes is growing. As more empirical studies are being conducted and subsequent results are being disseminated, the *Guide to Community Preventive Services* builds recommendations on evidence of effectiveness. Using these recommendations in development of policies can, in turn, increase the probability of effective translation to practice as well as positive physical activity outcomes (26). As of December 2016, built environment approaches combining transportation system interventions and land use and environmental design are recommended by the *Community Guide*. Enhanced school-based physical education is also recommended, as is creating or improving places for physical activity (3). The Community Guide should be used to align physical activity policy with national evidence-based recommendations (26).

Even though evidence supporting physical activity policy to practice is growing, gaps remain. These gaps are predicated on the fact that policy and environmental changes often happen quickly, without time for rigorous evaluation planning and baseline data collection. One way to fill these research gaps is to conduct "natural experiments" on changes related to physical activity policy and environmental change. Natural experiments provide ways to examine causal connections between the built environment, the social environment, and physical activity and can be alternatives to traditional randomized controlled trials (27, 28). One example of a natural experiment related to physical activity policy was conducted by Ogilvie and colleagues. The effect of a new bus network (segregated bus track) accompanied by a traffic-free path for pedestrians and cyclists on active travel was examined, and showed an increase in the proportion of commuting trips involving any active travel, a large decrease in the proportion of trips made entirely by car, and of an increase in weekly cycle commuting time. In order to build more evidence through natural experiments, stakeholders, researchers, and practitioners need to be aware of potential opportunities for these studies. Additionally, because rigorous studies require funding, funding agencies should recognize the challenges and inherent differences in natural experiments and make accommodations in requests for proposals. Natural experiments can provide unique insight into the effects and outcomes of physical activity policy and should be considered as a way to inform practice.

Summary

As noted in this chapter as well as Chapter 5, policies can be an effective and sustainable way to increase population physical activity. However, moving policy to practice is often difficult. Ways in which to encourage successful policy implementation include ensuring the policy is funded, has effective regulatory processes, includes components of communication and awareness building, and takes into account capacity and accountability. Policy development and implementation should be inclusive of all impacted stakeholders, making it a transdisciplinary effort. Evidence, either through best practices or empirical studies, should be considered when planning for successful movement of policy into practice.

Things to Consider

- Understand that impacting population physical activity means going beyond having a policy in place:

- Appropriate funding, regulatory processes, communication, capacity, and accountability all play a role in making policies related to physical activity more effective.
- Groups that develop and implement physical activity policies should represent diverse sectors and adhere to the *HiAP* framework.

References

1. Bauman AE, Reis RS, Sallis JF, et al. Correlates of physical activity: why are some people physically active and others not? *Lancet*. 2012;380(9838):258–271. doi:10.1016/S0140-6736(12)60735-1
2. Pratt M, Perez LG, Goenka S, et al. Can population levels of physical activity be increased? Global evidence and experience. *Prog Cardiovas Dis*. 2015;57(4):356–367. doi:10.1016/j.pcad.2014.09.002
3. Community Preventive Services Taskforce. Physical activity: enhanced school-based physical education. 2013. Available at: https://www.thecommunityguide.org/findings/physical-activity-enhanced-school-based-physical-education. Accessed September 9, 2017.
4. Chriqui JF, Eyler A, Carnoske C, et al. State and district policy influences on district-wide elementary and middle school physical education practices. *J Public Health Manag Pract*. 2013;19(3 suppl 1):S41–S48. doi:10.1097/PHH.0b013e31828a8bce
5. Institute of Medicine. *Educating the Student Body: Taking Physical Activity and Physical Education to School*. Washington, DC: The National Academies Press; 2013.
6. State of California. *California Education Code Sections 51210-51212 Article 2. Course of Study, Grades 1 to 6*. Sacramento, CA; 2005. https://leginfo.legislature.ca.gov/faces/codes_displaySection.xhtml?sectionNum=51210.&lawCode=EDC. Accessed September 9, 2018
7. Sanchez-Vaznaugh EV, Sanchez BN, Rosas LG, et al. Physical education policy compliance and children's physical fitness. *Am J Prev Med*. 2012;42(5):452–459. doi:10.1016/j.amepre.2012.01.008
8. Adams J. Lawsuit agreement to force schools to provide physical education. EDSource website. Available at: https://edsource.org/2015/lawsuit-agreement-to-force-schools-to-provide-physical-education/73544. Published February 1, 2015. Accessed September 15, 2017
9. Simmons S, Collins A, Ngo S. Fit to defend: a primer on the physical education instructional minutes litigations. Lozano Smith, Attorneys at Law website, News & Insights. Available at: http://www.lozanosmith.com/news-clientnewsbriefdetail.php?news_id=2471. Published January 29, 2016
10. Congressional Budget Office. *Introduction to Congressioal Budget Office*. 2017. https://www.cbo.gov/about/overview. Accessed September 15, 2017.
11. Howie EK. The "ins" and "outs" of physical activity policy implementation: inadequate capacity, inappropriate outcome measures, and insufficient funds. *J School Health*. 2014;84(9):581–585. doi:10.1111/josh.12182
12. Meehan L, Skipper M, Pate R, et al, eds. Incorporating physical activity and health outcomes in regional transportation planning. *Implementing Physical Activity Strategies*. Champaign, IL: Human Kinetics; 2014:337–347.
13. League of American Bicyclists. *States: Infrastructure and Funding*. 2015. https://bikeleague.org/content/states-infrastructure-funding. Accessed September 15, 2017.
14. Bergman P, Grjibovski AM, Hagstromer M, et al. Congestion road tax and physical activity. *Am J Prev Med*. 2010;38(2):171–177. doi:10.1016/j.amepre.2009.09.042
15. Deehr RC, Shumann A. Active Seattle: achieving walkability in diverse neighborhoods. *Am J Prev Med*. 2009;37(6 suppl 2):S403–S411. doi:10.1016/j.amepre.2009.09.026
16. McDade A. *Tools for Financing Local Bicycle and Pedestrian Improvements: Moving from Planning to Implementation in a Fiscally Constrained Environment*. San Luis Obispo, CA: City and Regional Planning, Cal Poly; 2014.
17. Samdahl D. Multi-modal impact fees. ITE 2008 Annual Meeting and Exhibit Compendium of Technical Papers. Anaheim, CA; 2008.

18. American Planning Association. *APA Policy Guide to Impact Fees.* 1997. https://www. planning.org/policy/guides/adopted/impactfees.htm. Accessed September 9, 2018.
19. Peters S. *Impact Fees for Complete Streets.* Los Angeles, CA: Urban Planning, University of California; 2012.
20. Riggs W, McDade E. Moving from planning to action: exploring best practice policy in the finance of local bicycling and pedestrian improvements. *Case Stud Trans Policy.* 2016;4(3):248–257. doi:10.1016/j.cstp.2016.06.004
21. Colorado Office of Early Childhood. *Colorado Child Care Regulations.* Denver, CO; 2016.
22. Rudolph L, Caplan J, Ben-Moshe K, et al. Health in all policies: improving health through intersectoral collaboration. 2013. http://www.phi.org/uploads/application/files/q79jnmxq5krx9qiu5j6gzdnl6g9s41l65co2ir1kz0lvmx67to.pdf, Accessed September 9, 2018.
23. de Hartog JJ, Boogaard H, Nijland H, et al. Do the health benefits of cycling outweigh the risks? *Environ Health Perspec.* 2010;118(8):1109–1116. doi:10.1289/ehp.0901747
24. Boushey G. *Policy Diffusion Dynamics in America.* New York, NY: Cambridge University Press; 2010.
25. New Jersey Bicycle and Pedestrian Resource Center. History of complete streets in the United States. New Jersey Bicycle & Pedestrian Resource Center website. http://njbikeped.org/services/history-of-complete-streets-in-the-united-states/. 2013. Accessed September 15, 2017
26. Community Preventive Services Taskforce. Develop evidence-based policies. The Community Guide website. Available at: https://www.thecommunityguide.org/about/policy-development. 2016. Accessed September 15, 2017
27. Ogilvie D, Griffin S, Jones A, et al. Commuting and health in Cambridge: a study of a 'natural experiment' in the provision of new transport infrastructure. *BMC Public Health.* 2010;10(1):703. doi:10.1186/1471-2458-10-703
28. Olsen JR, Mitchell R, Mackay DF, et al. Effects of new urban motorway infrastructure on road traffic accidents in the local area: a retrospective longitudinal study in Scotland. *J Epi Comm Health.* 2016;70:1088–1095. doi:10.1136/jech-2016-207378

III

IMPLEMENTING PHYSICAL ACTIVITY INTERVENTIONS IN SPECIFIC COMMUNITIES AND SETTINGS

PHYSICAL ACTIVITY AT THE WORKPLACE

NICOLAAS P. PRONK

▓ Introduction

Almost 63% of U.S. civilians aged 16 years and over participate in the labor force (1). On average, only slightly more than half receive "sufficient" leisure-time physical activity (LTPA), where LTPA is categorized as sufficiently active (moderate intensity, ≥150 minutes per week), insufficiently active (10–149 minutes per week), and inactive (<10 minutes per week) (2). Variation exists among industry groups, as it has been noted that professional and technical service-type jobs (~60%) may well have double the prevalence of sufficient activity compared to farming, fishing, and forestry groups (~30%) (3).

Employment appears to be good for physical activity levels as it has been noted that among men, full-time employment, even in sedentary occupations, is positively associated with physical activity compared to not working. For both men and women, job type has a major impact on daily activity levels (2, 3). Overall, a larger proportion of white-collar compared to blue-collar workers were engaged in sufficient LTPA. However, it has been reported that during the half century between 1960 and 2010, daily occupation-related energy expenditure has decreased by more than 100 calories (4). This reduction

© Springer Publishing Company DOI: 10.1891/9780826134592.0009

in energy expenditure accounts for a significant portion of the increase in mean U.S. body weights for both women and men. During that same period, obesity rates among workers have doubled, physical activity levels remain below par, and cardiorespiratory fitness levels often do not meet minimal job requirement standards (4, 5). Despite these sobering statistics, it appears that since 2004, based on National Health Interview Survey data, LTPA has significantly increased in most occupational and industry groups (3).

Given this situation, it is clear that the workplace represents an important setting for public health efforts. In order to effectively and efficiently increase the prevalence of sufficiently high levels of physical activity among workers, individual employers, business and industry as a sector, and other governmental and nongovernmental agencies need to find ways to collaborate based on principles of shared value. Those collaborations need to consider the evidence of effectiveness of available interventions, ensure activity patterns that avoid prolonged sitting or standing, integrate physical activity into comprehensive worksite health promotion program design, and adapt learnings from successful examples in the field to apply to the local situation.

■ Business Rationale for a Physically Active Workforce

Physical activity and exercise have a profound benefit on the body and the mind. The nervous system, including the neural connections in the brain; the immune, endocrine, and musculoskeletal systems; and the distribution of body fat, are all positively impacted by regular physical activity and exercise (6). Furthermore, when physical activity is a routine part of a person's daily set of activities, the benefits extend into improved management and prevention of major chronic conditions, such as diabetes, cardiovascular disease, and certain cancers, as well as improvements in mood states and mental health. These benefits have a direct influence on how people function, and function manifests itself in the workplace into factors such as productivity, interactions among team members, and relationships with customers (7, 8). In addition, less illness reduces medical care costs (9). Thus, increasing physical activity to levels associated with health benefits can create a healthier workforce, reduce incidence of new disease, enhance management of existing disease, reduce debilitating chronic conditions, reduce sick leave and injuries at work due to disease and ill-health, enhance worker and family earnings, enhance the social relationships among coworkers, and increase productivity (4–12).

Furthermore, when companies invest in the health and well-being of their workforce, including the promotion of physical activity, they need to consider programs in a broader context. As such, the workplace culture has been recognized as a central component of successful efforts to improve workforce health and well-being (13). When companies are recognized for building a successful culture of health and safety, they also tend to benefit from superior marketplace performance. In fact, such firms generate significantly higher profits and stock returns. In addition to 5% to 18% higher annualized returns on shareholder investment portfolios, these companies report a more engaged workforce, a more loyal and satisfied customer base, better relationships with stakeholders, greater transparency, a more collaborative community, and a better ability to innovate as some of the contributing factors to obtain this competitive advantage (14–18) (Table 9.1).

Finally, the business case closes the loop with public health as we recognize that companies with healthy workforces also play an important role in sustainability for environmental, social, and economic performance in society. Linking health and well-being of the workforce, the community, and the marketplace performance of the company provides an example of creating shared value in which benefits accrue to all stakeholders

TABLE 9.1. Benefits of an active and physically fit workforce.

EMPLOYEE BENEFITS	EMPLOYER BENEFITS
■ Prevention of illness and disease ■ Improved management of chronic conditions ■ Reduced pain ■ Improved mood states ■ Improved mental health ■ Improved overall function ■ Reduced healthcare need ■ Reduced healthcare-related expenses ■ Increased worker income ■ Increased overall family earnings ■ Lower debt ■ Lower long-term unemployment ■ Improved overall health and well-being ■ Higher job satisfaction	■ Lower healthcare costs ■ Lower disability costs ■ Higher productivity ■ Enhanced mood states ■ Improved coworker interactions ■ Enhanced customer interactions ■ Lower illness absence ■ Lower presenteeism ■ Reduced injury rates ■ Improved overall health and well-being of workers ■ Improved culture of health and well-being ■ Enhanced marketplace performance ■ Enhanced corporate image ■ Attractive option for recruitment of talent ■ Enhanced retention of talent ■ Higher job satisfaction

involved. A stronger economy, a vital community, and positive sustainable growth and prosperity for people involves multiple, interactive, and interdependent stakeholders and sectors to partner for success (19). Recognition of these macroeconomic considerations in the business case for building a healthy and functional workforce is important. Hence, considering the role of physical activity in the creation of a business case for investment in workforce health is connected to a much larger play than merely the impact of activity on illness prevention or management. Rather, it fits perfectly with the need to address noncommunicable disease prevention and sustainable development goals as major public health objectives (20, 21).

■ Current Issues

Physical Activity Prevalence Among Employees

Most adults do not engage in sufficient physical activity to enjoy the health and well-being benefits—in fact, less than 5% meet the threshold for a healthy level of physical activity based on accelerometer data (28). However, employment tends to be a beneficial factor in physical activity behavior. Based on data from the National Health Interview Survey (NHIS) collected between 1997 and 2004, 36% of male employees and 31% of female employees met the Healthy People 2010 guidelines for physical activity (29). Despite this, over the past five decades, the workplace has increasingly become an environment that promotes sedentary behavior. As a result, sedentary behavior and

physical inactivity have received increased attention from both researchers and practitioners to better understand the implications to health, functioning, and workplace
performance (30, 31).

Besides aerobic activity (e.g., walking, running, swimming), physical activity guidelines also recommend strengthening exercise because of its beneficial effects (32). Muscle
strengthening exercises are effective in building strength and muscular endurance.
Workplace-based strength training programs have shown results related to reductions
in neck, shoulder, upper extremity, and lower back pain, blood pressure reductions,
increases in flexibility, headache reductions, maintenance in the ability to perform work,
and reductions in absenteeism (32–37). In a cross-sectional analysis of 10,956 employees
who completed a health assessment (response rate of 75%), results indicated that 6,182
employees met the guideline for strength exercise (two or more days per week) as
opposed to 4,774 who did not. Hence, prevalence of strength training in this sample
was 56%. Results of this analysis showed that those who participated in strength training
exercises on two or more days per week experienced higher levels of function (physical
and emotional), self-perceived general health status, fewer health risk factors, and were
more productive as compared to their counterparts who reported participation in less
than 2 days per week of muscle strengthening exercises (38).

Fitness of the U.S. Workforce

In a review of the literature organized around a definition of "fitness" that was based on
three components, namely obesity, physical activity and exercise, and cardiorespiratory
fitness, the overall characterization of the fitness profile of the U.S. workforce was that
fitness levels were relatively low and appeared to have declined over the past five decades.
Obesity prevalence among workers has doubled over the past several decades, overall
occupational energy expenditure has reduced by more than 100 kcal per day since 1960,
sedentary behavior at the workplace has increased, and the workforce may be classified as
being in "fair" to "poor" levels of cardiorespiratory fitness (5). Significant variability exists
among various jobs and sectors; however, across all business and industry sectors, a need
exists to enhance movement; among specific sectors (e.g., police, military, firefighters,
among others), fitness levels need to be improved in order to ensure that all employees
meet the minimum standards for job performance.

What Works in Promoting Physical Activity at the Workplace?

In order to learn about what works in promoting physical activity in the workplace, we
need to review the literature on programs implemented in the context of the workplace
and find out if they indeed increased physical activity levels. A second question would
be to find if such programs also benefit health-related or other important factors such as
productivity or costs outcomes.

Systematic Review and Meta-Analytic Findings

A recent in-depth review notes that physical activity interventions can significantly
increase levels of physical activity, especially when such interventions include partnerships and coordinated efforts among several stakeholders such as schools, healthcare systems, or businesses (39). A recent meta-analysis on worksite physical activity
interventions reported on a set of substantially heterogeneous studies across 38,231

subjects and noted significant impacts on physical activity levels (40). This study also looked at additional health and worksite-relevant outcomes and noted other significant effects for fitness, lipids, anthropometric measures, work attendance, and job stress. These data indicate that some workplace interventions can increase physical activity among employees and improve important health and worksite outcomes. Unfortunately, due to the large heterogeneity among the interventions, this analysis was not able to elucidate what type of programmatic aspects are most important to generate the impact.

Another systematic review that addresses this topic was conducted by the Community Preventive Services Task Force and reported on the effectiveness of assessments of health risks with feedback (41). Eighteen studies reported physical activity changes with a median relative increase of 15.3% in the proportion of people being physically active from baseline to follow-up. However, when considering the program design, only those studies that added follow-up programs to the assessment of health risks with feedback were effective in improving physical activity. This study begins to answer the important question about what factors are important to include in program design in order to ensure successful outcomes—assessments by themselves are important but not sufficient. Additional programmatic services are needed in order to see significant impact on the outcomes of interest. In addition to the reported outcomes for physical activity, this review also documented evidence of positive economic impact based on eight studies that reported positive return on investment ratios.

Physical Activity Policies at the Workplace

Chapter 5 provides an in-depth analysis of the importance of policies, systems, and environments in influencing physical activity behavior across multiple contexts and settings. The workplace is a perfect example of this. The definition of health policy as introduced by the World Health Organization refers to

> decisions, plans, and actions that are undertaken to achieve specific health care goals within a society. An explicit health policy can achieve several things: 1) it defines a vision for the future which in turn helps to establish targets and points of reference for the short and medium term; 2) it outlines priorities and the expected roles of different groups; and 3) it builds consensus and informs people (42).

Based on this definition, it appears reasonable to expect that a policy application to physical activity interventions implemented at the workplace may be an effective means to stimulate and promote activity among workers. However, in practice, the definition of "workplace policy" is confusing and often includes programmatic aspects that should not fall under policy classifications (e.g., promotion of walking the stairs as an organizational policy as opposed to a programmatic tactic to promote activity). Specific to physical activity policy at the workplace, Schmid and Witmer (43) proposed three levels of policy: (a) formal written codes, regulations, or decisions bearing legal authority, such as legislation or zoning; (b) written standards that guide behaviors; and (c) unwritten social norms. Based on this framework, it is possible to organize various approaches to physical activity policy and consider the associated health and business outcomes. For example, the impact of employer subsidies for public transportation on overall physical activity or a tax-benefited reimbursement for bicycling to work as a result of the Bicycle Commuter Act may be considered and studied (44). More specifically, action principles that may support the implementation of employer-sponsored physical activity programs include (a) the organization of physical activity interventions within a framework that leverages the interrelationships between individuals and their work environment (8, 44, 45); (b) prioritizing the use of evidence-based and evidence-informed interventions (5, 8, 40, 41, 44); and (c) the alignment of selected physical activity programs with best practices for comprehensive worksite health promotion programs (5, 8, 46–48).

■ Application of Systems Science: the Interdependent, Interactive, and Reciprocal Nature of the Workplace, the Home, and the Community

The workplace may be described as a complex social system. Pronk and Narayan state (45, p. 124):

> The workplace might be viewed as a community of individuals sharing knowledge and expertise and collaborating toward the achievement of a common goal or mission. The work situation involves sociology as there are interpersonal relationships, social networks, task assignments, and flow dynamics related to interpersonal communications and experiences. Socialization, or belonging to a valued group, is another important spatiotemporal example of a complex set of interactions that is directly related to being or becoming an effective team member at work—it is also an important personal need as it ranks second highest on Maslow's five-level hierarchy. Collectively, this set of social interactions create a complex situation that is dynamic, interactive, interdependent, non-linear, stochastic, information limited and difficult to predict—all properties of complex systems.

Hence, interventions designed to increase a specific behavior, such as physical activity, need to be explicit in recognizing and optimizing the interactive, interdependent, and complex relationships at play within and outside the worksite setting.

There is widespread recognition and agreement among experts that in order to improve health outcomes, reduce disease incidence, and mitigate disease sequelae, programs, practices, and policies need to be multicomponent, multifaceted, comprehensive, and multilevel. Furthermore, while they need to include and engage the individual, the focus should be on environmental factors in the context of change among groups, institutions, and communities (22). Specifically, the creation of safe spaces to be active enables employees and their families to make healthy choices. Walkable neighborhoods, safe playgrounds, and public transportation make for good examples. Additionally, employment in itself, affordable housing, and the promotion of community development are important factors in building communities that flourish and address the underlying inequities that contribute to violence and disparities. In the context of addressing health equity, fostering social cohesion will help people feel included, provides individuals with a sense of ownership and belonging, and promotes social order and community participation (49). Social cohesion may be considered a highly valuable asset to communities as the underlying social networks increase mutual trust and support positive social norms. Addressing these types of factors is a complex task that calls for nonlinear approaches and longer term thinking. They also require us to look beyond the walls of the workplace and consider how physical activity patterns extend into the family and community context.

Business and Community

Connecting physical activity promotion efforts to the family and the available community resources is another important consideration. Supporting workers in adopting and maintaining physical activity behavior change should be specific aspects of the programs being implemented. Increasingly, companies see the importance of connecting to larger community health needs. However, once again, the context of decision making for any company to invest in such programs will need to be based on a set of criteria that is broader than physical activity alone. The reasons to invest in community health needs will include the potential to attract and retain top talent, and for the workforce to perform at high levels; and to reduce costs, increase safety, enhance job satisfaction, enhance the company's community image, and increase manufacturing reliability, to name a few (46).

Best-Practice Design Principles

The context in which physical activity programming happens matters. As a result, the design of the program needs to take context in consideration. Furthermore, the context needs to be engaged early on in the process so that decisions are made with buy in from all parties. Based on this, it makes sense to consider implementation of physical activity programs in the context of the broader workplace health strategy for any given company.

The broader workplace health strategy needs to consider design elements that make programs successful. When considering the scientific literature on this, only a handful of studies emerged that have looked at the underlying principles that make programs successful. A review of these studies and subsequent identification of best practices was published in the practice literature in 2014 (47). This analysis identified 44 best practices that were collapsed into nine best-practice program design principles. These principles are summarized in Table 9.2.

Field testing was conducted to test the nine best-practice program principles both in a retrospective and prospective manner. Based in part on these efforts, the American Heart Association reflected these principles in their workplace wellness recognition guidelines (48) and data-driven practice-based case studies were observed from a variety of companies. The Turck Corporation explained their status as an industry exemplar following a retrospective review covering the past 10 years of their program experience (50). In addition, Indiana University completed a successful redesign of their program based on the nine best-practice program design principles (51). The principles were also used in Finland to test how a corporate wellness provider was able to implement programs and generate successful outcomes (52). This particular approach suggests that improvements in program implementation can be made by using these principles in a systematic process and connecting the program design phase to the implementation phase. Finally, a formal assessment using the nine best-practice principles was conducted by HealthPartners for their Be Well program (53). The data was generated using a 2-hour dialogue session during which business unit leaders ($n = 98$) from across the organization rated their organization's degree of implementation with each of the best-practice design principles. Results were tabulated and subsequently associated with results of the employee health assessments by major business units and indicate that the higher the best-practice design principles score, the lower the number of health risks in the population (see Figure 9.1). The analysis showed that the best-practice assessment score explained approximately 30% of the variation in population health risks ($r = 0.54$; $p = .045$).

TABLE 9.2. Best practice program design principles.

DESIGN PRINCIPLES	EXPLANATION
Leadership	Elements that reflect program vision, organizational policy, resources, and implementation support
Relevance	Elements that address factors critical to program participation and connecting to the intrinsic motivations of workers
Partnership	Elements that relate to integration efforts with other groups or entities such as unions, other internal departments, external vendors, and community organizations, among others
Comprehensiveness	The five components as defined by *Healthy People 2010* that create a comprehensive program: health education, supportive physical and social environments, integration of the worksite program into the organization's structure, linkage to related programs, and worksite screening programs
Implementation	Elements that ensure a planned, coordinated, and fully executed work plan and process tracking system
Engagement	Elements that promote ongoing connections between employees and the program through activities and behaviors that build trust, respect, and an overall culture of health and well-being
Communications	Elements that reflect a strategic communications plan that maintains high program visibility and recognition
Being data-driven	Elements that ensure program measurement, reporting, evaluation, and continuous improvement
Compliance	Elements that ensure the program meets regulatory and ethical requirements and protect the personal information of employees and participants

SOURCE: Adapted from Pronk NP. Best practice design principles of worksite health promotion programs. *ACSM's Health & Fitness Journal.* 2014;18(1):42-46. doi:10.1249/FIT.0000000000000012.

■ Workplace Recognition Programs

As companies exert efforts to introduce, expand, or evolve their workplace health and well-being programs, a useful development has been the guidance provided by recognition programs. Over the years, various workplace recognition programs have been introduced that highlight and celebrate organizations that have implemented exemplary programs. Most, if not all, of these programs are based on current evidence of what works and best practices in the field. A recent review of such workplace recognition programs noted that the majority of the existing programs draw on the nine best-practices principles outlined in Table 9.2 (48). Notable recognition programs include the CEO Gold Standard for Cancer Prevention (American Cancer Association), the Corporate Health Achievement Award (American College of Occupational and Environmental Medicine), Fit Friendly Worksites/My Life Check (American Heart Association), Health-Lead (U.S. Healthiest), Best Employers for a Healthy Lifestyle (National Business Group on Health), or the Well Workplace Award (WELCOA). Typically, recognition programs

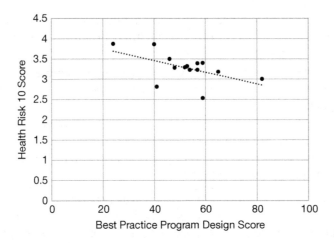

FIGURE 9.1 Best practice program design score by number of health risks.

involve a submission of the program activities, participation, and outcomes, and a review by an expert panel in order to generate a decision to recognize the program or not. In rare cases, the program may be audited with an on-site inspection, such as the American College of Occupational and Environmental Medicine's Corporate Health Achievement Award or the HealthLead program introduced by the U.S. Healthiest organization (48, 54). Regardless of which recognition program a company decides to apply for, the interest should be to celebrate milestones achieved, progress toward implementation of a successful program, and to identify areas for improvement. The best recognition programs provide useful feedback for the company that outlines areas for improvement and supports planning for the next phase of the program.

Cultural Considerations

A healthy workplace culture may be defined as

a workplace ecology in which the dynamic relationship between human beings and their work environment nurtures personal and organizational values that support the achievement of a person's best self while generating exceptional business performance (13, 55).

To achieve such a healthy culture, the organization needs to adopt inclusive paradigms that commit people to shared rules and standards around which to act, practice, behave, and work their trades. Such inclusive paradigms include participatory practices to encourage a sense of program ownership among workers, alignment of workplace health promotion objectives with business goals, a focus on interdisciplinary and multidepartmental teams, and multilevel program development (e.g., individual, team, and organizational levels). Furthermore, building cultures of health and well-being at the workplace is a longer term goal that needs the input of sustained energy and effort. At a high level, the following process steps in shaping a culture of health and well-being will prove important to consider (55)

- *Surfacing*: It refers to the approach by which an organization holds an ongoing dialogue with its people in order to identify the most important issues, concerns, and values that matter most.

- *Communicating*: It refers to the manner in which the company connects the values and issues identified with the processes and audiences that allow for the change to happen.

- *Aligning*: It refers to the process by which the organizational policies and practices are connected to the values and issues. This step is important in ensuring that everyone will feel heard and respected and has an opportunity to be actively engaged in shaping the culture.

Taken together, surfacing, communicating, and aligning will generate a process that leads to an organizational environment that is open, credible, and respectful; allows for learning, growth, and achievement; and builds toward exceptional business performance.

Case Studies—Insights From the Field

Regions Hospital Be Well Program

Regions Hospital, one of the largest HealthPartners business units with its team of 5,100 dedicated professionals, is a level one trauma center with one of the Twin Cities' busiest EDs (53). The stressors related to hospital care are ever-present and the jobs are physically, emotionally, and mentally challenging. In order to deliver great care, service, and experience for patients and families, the Regions leadership team knew they had to make the health and well-being of employees as much a priority as the care provided to patients—because "you cannot give to others what you do not have yourself." The Regions health and well-being journey started in earnest when leadership used data to identify relationships between healthcare costs and gaps in employee health. The Regions experience between 2009 and 2016 was evaluated formally and this case example highlights the key drivers and the population health impact over that period.

Over the course of 7 years, Regions Hospital was successful at improving the health and well-being of its employee population. Compared to an expected increase of 0.9 risks due to the natural decline associated with aging in the absence of access to a comprehensive health and well-being program, the population of approximately 5,100 employees reduced their risks by 0.28 risk units. This difference was associated with an estimated $28.5 million savings in medical and pharmacy claims costs and reduced productivity loss. Specific examples of changes in the risk factors for the Regions Hospital population include reductions in the proportion of employees with low physical activity of 1.4%, low fruits and vegetables intake of 18.3%, a change in tobacco user prevalence of 5.7% (from 8% in 2009 down to 2.3% in 2016), and a reduced proportion of employees reporting poor self-perceived general health status of 1.5%.

The learnings generated by the implementation of the Be Well program over the 7 years highlight the importance of three particular elements: (a) leadership awareness and commitment to making health and well-being a priority and leading a culture of change; (b) redesigning employee health benefits around individual needs and incenting healthy behaviors; and (c) providing access to great health and well-being resources at work. In the words of the Regions Hospital CEO, Megan Remark: "The big idea was to start small, listen with intent for expressed needs of people, engage employees from the beginning, and making them the power behind a healthy, productive, and high-performing workplace."

Quality Bicycle Products (QBP)

Quality Bicycle Products (QBP) is a medium-sized manufacturer and major distributor of bicycles and bicycle parts located in Minneapolis, MN. Founded in 1981, QBP has built a strong bicycle-friendly workplace culture and has closely aligned both its corporate health and well-being program and its corporate social responsibility efforts to its business goals and objectives (56). As a result, QBP has emphasized bicycling to work as a specific strategy to optimize worker health and well-being.

Between 2009 and 2013, QBP engaged in a variety of initiatives to stimulate bicycling to work along with other efforts to improve the health and well-being of its employees. These efforts included such traditional resources as medical and dental benefits, access to 401(k) savings programs, college savings accounts, employee assistance programs, referral bonus, profit-sharing bonus, mentorship program, and tuition reimbursement. In addition, novel workplace benefits were offered such as balance balls, massage service, yoga, and snow shoeing events, among others. Trip-end facilities were built within the company, including shower and locker facilities and a large indoor bicycle parking facility along with a specified area for bicycle repair (with complimentary tools to use). Furthermore, financial incentives were provided for every day the employee bicycled to work and free emergency rides home as well as access to a company-owned pool of bicycles was provided for short trips, errands, or recreations (e.g., short work break).

Results of the program included the observation that between 2009 and 2013, the annual number of bicycle commuters doubled from 210 out of 425 (50%) to 340 out of 623 (55%) employees. Based on a review of QBP's Human Resources Department records, the company reported an overall reduction of healthcare premiums of 4.4% between 2007 and 2011. This result compares favorably to the average increase of 24.6% in member-per-month costs for companies across the country during this same period.

Summary

Increasing the level of physical activity among employees is increasingly difficult to achieve due to the changing nature of work. Work is increasingly sedentary and approaches to address this need to be multilevel, multicomponent, and comprehensive. Physical activity programming and policy approaches need to be considered in context of a larger well-designed workplace health strategy; this may be accomplished by following best-practice program design principles that are based on evidence of effectiveness.

Things to Consider

How do you get started on building a successful physical activity program at the workplace? Here are a couple of things to consider when getting started.

- Fundamentally, it is a good idea to start with what we know works. So, begin by considering evidence-based recommendations for physical activity programs applied to the workplace setting (see the Resources section for some excellent examples).

- Next, consider the context of the workplace and how activity programming needs to fit into the workflows and the work processes.
- Additionally, consider how programs for physical activity promotion fit within the larger health and well-being program at the company. The best-practice program design principles outlined in Table 9.2 should be helpful in thinking about how best to put the pieces of the puzzle together.
- Finally, consider what types of measurement approaches make the most sense and how best to report on progress.

Resources

- American College of Sports Medicine (ACSM)
  http://www.exerciseismedicine.org/support_page.php/schools-and-workplaces
- American Council on Exercise (ACE)
  https://www.acefitness.org/acefit/fitness-fact-article/3120/fostering-a-workplace-culture-of
- Canadian Best Practices Portal
  http://cbpp-pcpe.phac-aspc.gc.ca/public-health-topics/physical-activity
- Centers for Disease Control and Prevention (CDC)
  https://www.cdc.gov/physicalactivity/worksite-pa/index.htm
  https://www.cdc.gov/workplacehealthpromotion/tools-resources/workplace-health/physical-activity.html
  https://www.workhealthresearchnetwork.org/wp-content/uploads/2016/05/CDC-WHRN-Physical-Activity_Employer-Guide-FINAL.pdf
  https://www.cdc.gov/workplacehealthpromotion/index.html
- The Community Preventive Services Task Force (CPSTF)
  https://www.thecommunityguide.org/stories/putting-community-guide-work-workplaces-partnering-reach-employers
  https://www.thecommunityguide.org/setting/workplaceworksite
- The International Association for Worksite Health Promotion (IAWHP)
  www.iawhp.org
- The National Institute for Health and Care Excellence (NICE)
  https://www.nice.org.uk/guidance/ph13
- The National Physical Activity Plan (NPAP)
  http://www.physicalactivityplan.org/index.html
- The World Health Organization (WHO)
  http://www.who.int/dietphysicalactivity/Quintiliani-workplace-as-setting.pdf

References

1. Labor Force Statistics. Bureau of Labor Statistics. United States Department of Labor; Available at: https://data.bls.gov/timeseries/LNS11300000. Accessed January 4, 2018.
2. Van Domelen DR, Koster A, Caserotti P, et al. Employment and physical activity in the U.S. *Am J Prev Med*. 2011;41(2):136–145. doi:10.1016/j.amepre.2011.03.019
3. Gu JK, Charles LE, Ma CC, et al. Prevalence and trends of leisure-time physical activity by occupation and industry in U.S. workers. The National Health Interview Survey 2004–2014. Ann Epidemiol. 2016;26(10):685–692. doi:10.1016/j.annepidem.2016.08.004
4. Church TS, Thomas DM, Tudor-Locke C, et al. Trends over 5 decades in U.S. occupation-related physical activity and their associations with obesity. *PLOS ONE*. 2011;6(5):e19657. doi:10.1371/journal.pone.0019657

5. Pronk NP. Fitness of the US workforce. *Ann Rev Public Health.* 2015;36:131–149. doi:10. 1146/annurev-publhealth-031914-122714

6. Bassuk SS, Church TS, Manson JE. Why exercise works magic.. *Sci Am.* 2013;309(2):74–79. doi:10.1038/scientificamerican0813-74.

7. Pronk NP, Martinson B, Kessler RC, et al. The association between work performance and physical activity, cardiorespiratory fitness, and obesity. *J Occup Environ Med.* 2004;46(1):19–25. doi:10.1097/01.jom.0000105910.69449.b7

8. Pronk NP. Physical activity promotion in business and industry: evidence, context, and recommendations for a national plan. *J Phys Act Health.* 2009;6(s2):S220–S235. doi:10.1123/jpah.6.s2.s220

9. Wang F, McDonald T, Champagne LJ, et al. Relationship of body mass index and physical activity to health care costs among employees. *J Occup Environ Med.* 2004;46:428–436.

10. U.S. Bureau of Labor Statistics. Economic news release: employer costs for employee compensation. Available at: https://www.bls.gov/news.release/ecec.nr0.htm. Accessed September 22, 2017

11. Fronstin P, Werntz R. The "business case" for investing in employee health: A review of the literature. EBRI Isuue Brief. Washington, DC: Employee Benefit Research Institute. 2004. Available at: https://www.ebri.org/content/the-business-case-for-investing-in-employee-health-a-review-of-the-literature-and-employer-self-assessments-495. Accessed September 22, 2017.

12. Walker TJ, Tullar JM, Diamond PM, et al. The longitudinal relation between self-reported physical activity and presenteeism. *Prev Med.* 2017;102:120–126. doi:10.1016/j.ypmed.2017.07.003

13. Pronk NP. Population health management and a healthy workplace culture: a primer. In: *Engaging Wellness. Corporate Health and Wellness Association.* 2012.

14. Fabius R, Thayer RD, Konicki DL, et al. The link between workforce health and safety and the health of the bottom line: tracking market performance of companies that nurture a "culture of health". *J Occup Environ Med.* 2013;55(9):993–1000. doi:10.1097/JOM.0b013e3182a6bb75

15. Grossmeier J, Fabius R, Flynn JP, et al. Linking workplace health promotion best practices and organizational financial performance: tracking market performance of companies with highest scores on the HERO scorecard. *J Occup Environ Med.* 2016;58(1):16–23. doi:10.1097/JOM.0000000000000631

16. Goetzel RZ, Fabius R, Fabius D, et al. The stock performance of C. Everett Koop award winners compared with the Standard & Poor's 500 index. *J Occup Environ Med.* 2016;58(1):9–15. doi:10.1097/JOM.0000000000000632

17. Conradie C, Smit E, Malan D. Corporate health and wellness and the financial bottom line: evidence from South Africa. *J Occup Environ Med.* 2016;58(2):45–53. doi:10.1097/JOM.0000000000000653

18. Eccles B, Ioannou I, Serafeim G. *The Impact of a Corporate Culture of Sustainability on Corporate Behavior and Performance.* Boston, MA: Harvard Business School; 2011. Working Paper 12-035.

19. Yach D. Health as a cornerstone of good business and sustainable development. *Am J Public Health.* 2016;106(10):1758–1759. doi:10.2105/AJPH.2016.303387

20. Von Schirnding Y. Health and sustainable development: can we rise to the challenge? *Lancet.* 2002;360:632–637.

21. Pronk NP, Malan D, Christie G, et al. Health and well-being metrics in business: the value of integrated reporting. *J Occup Environ Med.* 2018;60(1):19–22. doi:10.1097/JOM.0000000000001167

22. Pronk NP. Placing workplace wellness in proper context: value beyond money. *Prev Chronic Dis.* 2014;11. doi:10.5888/pcd11.140128

23. Berry LL, Mirabito AM, Baun WB. What's the hard return on employee wellness programs? *Harvard Bus Rev.* 2010;88:104–112.

24. Conley D, Glauber R. Gender, body mass, and socioeconomic status: new evidence from the PSID. *Adv Health Econ Health Serv Res.* 2007;17:253–275.

25. Kosteas VD. The effect of exercise on earnings: evidence from the NLSY. *J Labor Res.* 2012;33:225–250. doi:10.1007/s12122-011-9129-2

26. Münster E, Rüger H, Ochsmann E, et al. Over-indebtedness as a marker of socioeconomic status and its association with obesity: a cross-sectional study. *BMC Public Health.* 2009;9:286.

27. Crabtree S. Obesity linked to long-term unemployment in US. Gallup. June 18, 2014.

28. Troiano RP, Berrigan D, Dodd KW, et al. Physical activity in the United States measured by accelerometer. *Med Sci Sports Exerc.* 2008;40(1):181–188. doi:10.1249/mss. 0b013e31815a51b3

29. Caban-Martinez AJ, Lee DJ, Fleming LE, et al. Leisure time physical activity levels of the US workforce. *Prev Med.* 2007;44:432–436. doi:10.1016/j.ypmed.2006.12.017

30. Tremblay MS, Aubert S, Barnes JD, et al. Sedentary Behavior Research Network (SBRN)— Terminology Consensus Project process and outcome. *Int J Behav Nutr Phys Act.* 2017;14:75. doi:10.1186/s12966-017-0525-8

31. Pronk NP. Sedentary behavior and worksite interventions. In: Zhu W, Owen N, eds. *Sedentary Behavior and Health Concepts, Assessments, and Interventions.* Champaign, IL: Human Kinetics. 2017. 297–305.

32. U.S. Department of Health and Human Services, Office of Disease Prevention and Health Promotion. 2008 Physical Activity Guidelines for Americans. Available at: https://health. gov/paguidelines/guidelines/. Accessed September 22, 2017

33. Gram B, Andersen C, Zebis MK, et al. Effect of training supervision on effectiveness of strength training for reducing neck/shoulder pain and headache in office workers: cluster randomized controlled trial. *Biomed Res Int.* 2014;693013. doi:10.1155/2014/693013

34. Mortensen P, Larsen AI, Zebis MK, et al. Lasting effects of workplace strength training for neck/shoulder/arm pain among laboratory technicians: natural experiment with 3-year follow-up. *Biomed Res Int.* 2014;845851. doi:10.1155/2014/845851

35. Pedersen MT, Andersen CH, Zebis MK, et al. Implementation of specific strength training among industrial laboratory technicians: long-term effects on back, neck and upper extremity pain. *BMC Musculoskeletal Dis.* 2013;14:287. doi:10.1186/1471-2474-14-287

36. Sundstrup E, Jakobsen MD, Brandt M, et al. Workplace strength training prevents deterioration of work ability among workers with chronic pain and work disability: a randomized trial. *Scan J Work Environ Health.* 2014;40(3):244–251. doi:10.5271/sjweh.3419

37. Zavanela PM, Crewther BT, Lodo L, et al. Health and fitness benefits of a resistance training intervention performed in the workplace. *J Strength Cond Res.* 2012;26(3):811–817. doi:10. 1519/JSC.0b013e318225ff4d

38. Pronk NP, Bender EG, Katz AS. Health, function, and performance benefits of workplace strength training programs. *ACSM's Health Fitness J.* 2016;20(5):69–71. doi:10.1249/FIT. 0000000000000235

39. Heath GW, Parra DC, Sarmiento OI, et al. Evidence-based intervention in physical activity: lessons from around the world. *Lancet.* 2012;380:272–281. doi:10.1016/S0140-6736(12) 60816-2

40. Conn VS, Hafdahl AR, Cooper PS, et al. Meta-analysis of workplace physical activity interventions. *Am J Prev Med.* 2009;37(4):330–339. doi:10.1016/j.amepre.2009.06.008

41. Soler RE, Leeks KD, Razi S, et al. A systematic review of selected interventions for worksite health promotion. *Am J Prev Med.* 2010;38(2S):S237–S262. doi:10.1016/j.amepre.2009.10. 030

42. World Health Organization. Health Policy. Available at: http://www.who.int/topics/health_ policy/en/. Accessed September 22, 2017

43. Schmid T, Pratt M, Witmer L. A framework for physical activity policy research. *J Phys Act Health.* 2006;3:S20–S29. doi:10.1123/jpah.3.s1.s20

44. Pronk NP, Kottke TE. Physical activity promotion as a strategic corporate priority to improve worker health and business performance. *Prev Med.* 2009;49:316–321. doi:10.1016/j.ypmed. 2009.06.025

45. Pronk NP, Narayan KMV. The application of systems science to addressing obesity at the workplace: tapping into unexplored potential. *J Occup Environ Med.* 2016;58(2):123–126. doi:10.1097/JOM.0000000000000648

46. Pronk NP, Baase C, Noyce J, et al. Corporate America and community health: exploring the business case for investment. *J Occup Environ Med*. 2015;57(5):493–500. doi:10.1097/JOM. 0000000000000431

47. Pronk NP. Best practice design principles of worksite health and wellness programs. *ACSM's Health Fitness J*. 2014;18(1):42–46. doi:10.1249/FIT.0000000000000012

48. Fonarow GC, Calitz C, Arena R, et al. Workplace wellness recognition for optimizing workplace health: a presidential advisory from the American Heart Association. *Circulation*. 2015;131:e480–e497. doi:10.1161/CIR.0000000000000206

49. Centers for Disease Control and Prevention. *A Practitioner's Guide for Advancing Health Equity*. Atlanta, GA: US Department of Health and Human Services. 2013.

50. Pronk NP, Lagerstrom D, Haws J. LifeWorks@TURCK: a best practice case study on workplace well-being program design. *ACSM's Health Fitness J*. 2015;19(3):43–48. doi:10. 1249/FIT.0000000000000120

51. Hoffman L, Kennedy-Armbruster C. Case study using best practice design principles for worksite wellness programs. *ACSM's Health Fitness J*. 2015;19(3):30–35. doi:10.1249/FIT. 0000000000000125

52. Äikäs AH, Pronk NP, Hirvensalo MH, et al. Does implementation follow design? A case study of a workplace health promotion program using the 4-S program design and the PIPE Impact Metric evaluation models. *J Occup Environ Med*. 2017;59(8):752–760. doi:10.1097/ JOM.0000000000001067

53. Global CMO Network. Be Well at Regions Hospital in Saint Paul. Minnesota, USA. *Health: Our Business*. 2017;Vol. 2:66–73. Available at: https://www.bupa.com/~/media/files/site-specific-files/our%20purpose/workplaces/health%20our%20business%20ii.pdf. Accessed September 22, 2017.

54. Katz AS, Pronk NP, Chestnut K, et al. Congruence of organizational self-score and audit-based organizational assessments of workplace health capabilities: an analysis of the Health-Lead workplace accreditation. *J Occup Environ Med*. 2016;58(5):471–476. doi:10.1097/JOM. 0000000000000697

55. Pronk NP. *ACSM's Worksite Health Handbook*. 2nd ed. Champaign, IL: Human Kinetics; 2009.

56. Pronk NP. Bicycling to work at Quality Bicycle Products: a case example for active transportation in the business and industry sector. *ACSM's Health Fitness J*. 2014;18(5):49–52. doi:10.1249/FIT.0000000000000060

FAITH-BASED SETTINGS AND PHYSICAL ACTIVITY PROMOTION

BENJAMIN L. WEBB | BROOK E. HARMON | MELISSA BOPP

LEARNING OBJECTIVES

By the end of this chapter, the student should be able to

1. Describe the benefits of partnering with faith-based organizations (FBOs) to promote physical activity (PA).
2. Describe the connection between religion and health.
3. Discuss the role of FBOs in PA promotion.
4. Discuss the differences between faith-based versus faith-placed.
5. Create an effective plan for engaging stakeholders in FBOs to promote PA.

▓ Introduction

What Is a Faith-Based Setting?

There are many different ways that faith-based settings, hereon referred to as **faith-based organizations** (FBOs), can be defined. In general, an FBO is characterized as: (a) having direct ties with a faith (religious) community, (b) having a religiously oriented mission statement, and (c) receiving financial support from a religious institution (1). A typology of FBOs has also been proposed (2), where at one end of the continuum are FBOs that connect all aspects of the organization with their religious identification. These FBOs are typically places of worship, such as churches, synagogues, and mosques. At the other end of the continuum are FBOs historically linked with a religious tradition, but their services do not necessarily include a religious element. Examples of this type of FBO are charitable organizations such as the Salvation Army and the Y (formerly known as the

© Springer Publishing Company DOI: 10.1891/9780826134592.0010

YMCA). The former type of FBO (i.e., places of worship) is often sought out as a partner in delivering health-promotion interventions.

Why Partner With Faith-Based Organizations to Promote Physical Activity?

Connection Between Religion and Health

In ancient times, it was a commonly held belief that supernatural forces were the cause and remedy for all forms of illness (3). During the Middle Ages (5th–15th century), the care for the sick and dying in Europe was carried out largely by physicians that were also Christian clergy (e.g., monks) (4). In fact, most of the facilities used to care for the physically and mentally ill during the Middle Ages were hospitals and monasteries run by the Christian church (5). During the Enlightenment Period (1685 CE–1815 CE), there was decreased emphasis on the link between religion and health (6); however, the 20th century brought with it a renewed interest in the health effects of a religious life. In 1920, a physician named James Walsh wrote a seminal book entitled *Religion and Health*, in which he relied primarily on anecdotal evidence to assert the positive influence of religious practices on numerous health-related outcomes (e.g., longevity) (7). In it, he argued that religious practices, such as controlling the desire for excessive rest, would have a positive impact on the health and longevity of religious individuals. His thoughts on the importance of engaging in physical activity (PA) and avoiding sedentary behavior are as relevant today as they were nearly 100 years ago:

> *If mortification of the spirit were to be practiced by abstinence from overrest and by a definite amount of exercise every day, it would be an excellent thing for the religious as well as the physical life. This is one of the most frequent advices of those interested in the spiritual life as well as the bodily health for many generations. What people need is to keep busy. This is good for both their minds and their bodies (7).*

More recent literature reviews have relied on empirical evidence to examine the association between religion and health (8–11). These reviews often produce evidence for both religion's negative and positive influences on health, but they do highlight the continued relevance of religion in matters of health. In fact, a recent survey revealed that 90% of medical schools in the United States now include courses on spirituality and health in their curricula (12), indicating that the medical community recognizes the importance of religious beliefs and practices in healthcare.

Practicality

There are several practical reasons to consider partnering with FBOs to promote PA. First, there are an estimated 350,000 congregations in the United States (13). Approximately 77% of Americans claim a religious affiliation, with approximately 40% of U.S. adults reporting that they attend religious services at an FBO at least once per week (14). The percentage of individuals that consider religion important to their lives and that attend religious services on a weekly basis is greatest for subgroups often affected by health disparities (e.g., African Americans, females, and the elderly) (14).

Taken together, this indicates that FBOs

- Are present in most communities
- Provide physical space for health-promotion interventions
- Are frequented by millions of Americans on a weekly basis

- Are an important aspect of many Americans' lives, especially those affected by health disparities
- Can provide a resource from which to draw volunteers needed to support health-promotion interventions

Influential Leadership

Clergy (e.g., pastors, priests, rabbis, and imams) are the administrative and spiritual leaders of FBOs. Clergy are regularly cited as integral to health-promotion efforts involving FBOs due to their potential to influence the physical and social environment of FBOs (15, 16). Their importance and influence may be more pronounced in some subgroups of the population. For instance, African American churches are viewed as the most influential institution in the African American community, with African American clergy perceived as being vital to social change (17). The Catholic Church is central in the Latino community, with over 50% of all Latinos in the United States self-identifying as Catholic (18). It is argued that health-promotion efforts in the Latino community should include a religious element to enhance their effectiveness (19). There is also evidence that partnerships with Muslim clergy (imams) to promote health in the Muslim community have also been successful (20, 21). Imams recognize how important they are in promoting the health of their congregation, as well as helping their congregation make health decisions that are in line with the tenets of their faith (22, 23).

Role of Faith-Based Organizations in the Community

Although the role of FBOs in caring for the ill has been reduced, they have continued to play an important role in the community in other areas. David Moberg (24) describes FBOs as not only religious institutions, but also as social institutions due to their role in the socialization of individuals in a community, as well as their role in developing social relationships and unity among its members. Nationally, FBOs have served as a champion of social justice issues surrounding the civil rights of minorities (25), as well as borne a great deal of the humanitarian work carried out nationally and internationally (26). In local communities, FBOs have served in many social service roles, including providing food and clothing pantries (27), homeless shelters (28), and providing counseling services (29, 30). There are numerous examples of FBOs collaborating with public health researchers, or in some cases choosing to implement interventions on their own, to promote health-related outcomes such as cancer screening (31, 32), HIV/AIDS prevention (33), diabetes prevention and self-care (34–36), and healthy eating (37, 38).

Role of Faith-Based Organizations in Physical Activity Promotion

Although it is more common for PA to be included as a component rather than the primary focus of lifestyle interventions delivered in FBOs, there is precedence for partnering with FBOs to promote PA. A review examining PA interventions in FBOs identified 27 interventions that either focused on or included PA as an outcome of the study (39); 17 studies reported significant improvements in PA from baseline to follow-up. Since the publication of that review, there have been several more reports published on the development and/or efficacy of PA interventions delivered in FBOs (40–42), supporting the continued interest in partnering with FBOs to promote PA.

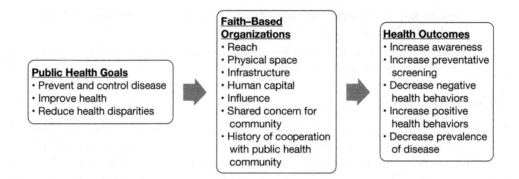

FIGURE 10.1 Model of the Mediating Role of Faith-Based Organizations in Attaining Public Health Goals.

FBO, faith-based organization.

Figure 10.1 summarizes how FBOs can serve as mediating structures in the community in pursuit of public health goals. Public health goals can be summarized as those that prevent and control disease, improve health, and reduce health disparities in the United States. The pursuit of these goals can be strengthened by developing partnerships with prominent community-based organizations, such as FBOs. FBOs serve as mediating structures to develop, deliver, and sustain interventions that align with public health goals. These partnerships can then help to bring about improvements in several health-related outcomes for the congregations of the FBOs, and also for the greater community for which they serve.

■ Current Issues

National-Level Support for Partnering With Faith-Based Organizations

There has been an emergence of interest at the national level in partnering with FBOs to deliver health-promotion interventions, including those related to PA.

The White House

The Personal Responsibility and Work Opportunity Reconciliation Act of 1996 (43) included in it a provision entitled, "Charitable Choice," which allows FBOs to receive federal funding to provide social services to Americans in need without requiring them to remove religious content from these services as long as the funds are not used for inherently religious activities (e.g., religious instruction), and the FBOs may not refuse services to anyone on the basis of their religious affiliation. In 2001, the White House Office of Faith-Based and Community Initiatives was created, which included the establishment of centers within various government agencies to help support faith-based and community initiatives (44). The name of the office was later changed to the Office of Faith-Based and Neighborhood Partnerships (45), but the overall mission of meeting the needs of Americans by partnering with FBOs and other community organizations remained the same.

The *Let's Move* initiative was started to address the issue of childhood obesity in America (46). In conjunction with this initiative, the *White House Taskforce on Childhood Obesity* (47) provided several recommendations on how to address childhood obesity through, among other things, increasing PA participation. Among their several recommendations, they encouraged federal and local agencies to work with nonprofits to increase access to recreation opportunities for youth. Many FBOs have gymnasiums and/or general-purpose rooms that could provide recreation opportunities for youth in the community. Funding these recommendations could prove difficult for some FBOs; however, the U.S. Supreme Court (48) recently issued an opinion that religious institutions should be eligible for public funds as long as the funds are used for secular purposes (e.g., making upgrades to a playground).

Healthy People 2020

Healthy People 2020 (*HP2020*) is a 10-year strategic plan to improve health outcomes among all Americans (49). Included in *HP2020*'s overarching goals is to "Create social and physical environments that promote good health for all." Having established that FBOs are part of the social and physical environment in many communities, it is feasible to conclude that FBOs would be a natural partner in pursuit of this goal, as well as *HP2020*'s subgoal to improve the health of Americans through participation in daily PA. The evidence-based recommendations for pursuing *HP2020*'s PA-related goals rely heavily on the recommendations of the Community Preventive Services Task Force (CPSTF).

The Community Preventive Services Task Force

The CPSTF is an independent panel of experts from the public health and medical sector that conducts extensive reviews of the scientific literature to make best-practice recommendations for promoting the health of the community. Their criteria for reviewing the evidence base includes factors such as the research design, the amount of available evidence, and the consistency of findings across studies. In regards to PA promotion, three of the CPSTF's (50) recommended strategies are highly applicable to FBOs:

1. Social support interventions in community settings
   - These interventions rely on new or existing social networks to provide supportive relationships for adopting and maintaining a physically active lifestyle.
   - Effective strategies include buddy systems, PA contracts, and group-based PA (e.g., walking groups).
   - FBOs provide existing social networks, communications infrastructure, and physical space that can be utilized to deliver PA interventions (e.g., support groups).
2. Community-wide campaigns
   - These interventions rely on the collaboration of multiple sectors within the community to deliver messages and interventions aimed at increasing PA awareness and participation.
   - Effective strategies include multiple components, such as delivering health messages via mass media, providing support groups and PA counseling, and offering health risk assessments and other PA-related events at various sites in the community.

■ FBOs provide communication infrastructure to increase awareness about community events and resources, provide a source for volunteers to assist with community events, and can provide the physical space to host community events and other PA-related services. The community ties of FBOs and their leadership have allowed them to collaborate with secular organizations for community-wide campaigns.

3. Creation of or enhanced access to places for PA combined with informational outreach activities

■ These interventions rely primarily on changing the environment to increase access and reduce barriers to opportunities to participate in PA.

■ Effective strategies include building walking trails, reducing facility usage fees, expanding facility hours, providing training in use of fitness/recreation equipment, and health education.

■ FBOs can make their facilities and recreational spaces available, either for free or for a nominal fee, to the community for the purpose of PA and other health education activities.

It is clear that FBOs fit well within the CPSTF's framework of "recommended" strategies for promoting PA participation. The preexisting social networks, communications infrastructure, and physical space offered by FBOs supports their suitability as a partner in PA promotion. However, it was not until the recently developed National Physical Activity Plan (NPAP) that specific strategies for partnering with FBOs to promote PA were recommended.

National Physical Activity Plan

When the National Physical Activity Plan was launched in 2010, FBOs were not represented among the sectors. After input from community practitioners, researchers, and public health professionals, the Plan was revised in 2016 to include a faith-based sector, with input from an expert panel. The addition of the faith-based sector expanded the reach of the original plan to some of the populations mentioned earlier and provided an avenue for culturally tailored approaches to promoting PA. The faith-based sector aimed to include diverse religious organizations, with a broad definition of FBOs to include houses of worship, organized religious denominations, faith-based social service agencies, and charities, but focusing more on religious congregations and denominations. The sector sought to build on the comprehensive, inclusive mission of many FBOs to address physical health along with spiritual and mental health among members. Within the sector, six strategies were identified for including PA in health ministries, encouraging partnerships with different organizations to promote PA, institutionalizing PA promotion for employees, and focusing on evidence-based practices (51):

■ Strategy 1 indicates that FBOs should work within their organizational structure to capitalize on health ministries, groups, missions, or other entities within the FBO to deliver health-related interventions, policies, and approaches. This strategy highlights the importance of having a "champion" within the congregation who is trained and skilled for leading and implementing these types of activities.

- Strategy 2 builds on the connection between religion, health, and the role of FBOs in communities, encouraging FBOs to partner with organizations from other sectors (e.g., education, healthcare) to promote PA in line with the values, beliefs, and practices of the FBO.

- Strategy 3 highlights the importance of creating a healthy workforce within the FBO, building on research that indicates that healthier clergy tend to have a healthier environment at their FBO.

- Strategy 4 focuses on how PA and health promotion can be institutionalized, working to deliver messages and strategies related to PA that are linked with scripture or ideas within the FBO's specific faith doctrine.

- Strategy 5 highlights the importance of working with other public health organizations to develop and deliver PA interventions that are accessible and tailored for many different population groups (e.g., women, older adults, teens).

- Strategy 6 is grounded in the dissemination of evidence-based strategies to FBOs, in line with the approach outlined in the CPSTF's *Community Guide* (52).

Case Example 1. Methodist Le Bonheur Healthcare's Congregational Health Network

In 2006, Methodist Le Bonheur Healthcare (Methodist) in Memphis, Tennessee, implemented a novel model that partners a traditional healthcare system with FBOs in the Mid-South region to improve health outcomes (53). Currently, approximately 500 FBOs have signed a covenant to participate in the Congregational Health Network (CHN). The model includes a director and nine navigators housed within Methodist's Faith and Health Division (FHD). Each FBO provides two volunteer liaisons and currently over 13,000 congregation members are CHN members. Through the partnership, which includes notification of a CHN pastor and liaison when a CHN member is admitted to the hospital and training FBO liaisons in chronic disease prevention and control, the healthcare system has shown a reduction in readmissions and mortality rates of CHN members compared to non-CHN members. The system has also seen a reduction in charges, particularly those related to chronic diseases such as diabetes and heart disease, among CHN members compared to non-CHN members (54).

Several PA initiatives for Latino communities have been made possible by the CHN and the FHD.

- Get Set: Created and implemented by a CHN navigator at Methodist, *Get Set* is a PA intervention that partners with FBOs to recruit participants and provide space for the intervention. The intervention targets Latino adults to improve both fitness and weight outcomes. The intervention includes a combination of high-intensity interval and cardiovascular endurance training, weight monitoring, and a run at the end of the intervention.

- Kids on the Move: A summer intervention for Latino children ages 5 to 12 that is offered in neighborhood parks, the CHN navigators at Methodist work with FBOs in the communities where the parks are located to recruit children to participate in the summer intervention. The intervention runs for 2 days in each park and is offered at multiple parks during the months of

June and July. The intervention focuses on engaging children in fun PA, as well as building skills related to being more active.

- Living Healthy Summer Camp: The FHD was instrumental in connecting representatives from 10 FBOs in the Memphis area to a team of public health researchers. With input from leaders of the FBOs, the camp expanded into a 4-month curriculum that included: weekly mailings of family-focused diet and PA education activities; a weeklong camp offering child-focused cooking and PA skill building; and four 2.5-hour sessions offered to parents that focused on diet, PA education, and skill building. Findings from the study have yet to be published, but preliminary analyses indicate the camp positively impacted children's perceptions of their cooking ability and time spent in moderate-to-vigorous physical activity.

Faith-Based Versus Faith-Placed

Partnering with FBOs to develop and/or deliver PA interventions does not necessarily mean that the intervention will include religious content. Generally, an intervention is considered to be faith-based if it includes religious content or themes in the intervention materials and/or the intervention was developed by an FBO. On the other hand, when FBOs are used only to recruit participants and/or as a site to deliver the PA intervention without any religious content or themes, then it is considered faith-placed. Understanding this distinction is important as it is argued that cultural competency is maximized when interventions are tailored at both the deep level (e.g., religious beliefs and values) and the surface level (e.g., delivered in an FBO) (55).

Several reviews have examined the effectiveness of both faith-based and faith-placed health interventions. In one review, 100% of faith-based interventions reported a significant effect on health outcomes compared to only 53% of faith-placed interventions (56). Another review that focused on interventions that reported on outcomes specifically related to PA found that approximately 63% of both faith-based and faith-placed interventions reported significant improvements in PA (39). A more recent review of obesity interventions in African American churches concluded that a greater percentage of faith-based interventions reported significant increases in PA compared to faith-placed interventions (45% vs. 20%, respectively) (57).

In addition to whether an intervention is faith-based or faith-placed, the following study design elements are also important to consider when weighing the evidence for PA interventions in FBOs:

- Research design: Studies do not always rely on rigorous research designs, such as randomized-controlled trials, when testing the effectiveness of an intervention. Some studies reporting significant effects use single-group designs, meaning there was no control group to compare with the intervention group. Those that do use a control group may use a quasi-experimental design where participants are not randomly assigned to the intervention and control group, which may limit the internal and external validity of the study. Also, some studies use small sample sizes and/or target-specific populations (e.g., Christians, African Americans), which may limit the generalizability of study results to other religious or racial/ethnic groups. Although single-group and quasi-experimental designs can provide important evidence to consider, preference should be given for randomized-controlled trials when possible.

- Measurement of PA: As you may have read in Chapter 2 of this book, measuring PA can take many different forms, depending upon the goals of the intervention. In FBOs, many studies use self-report measures to assess changes in PA because it is more affordable. Although there are valid questionnaires that have demonstrated acceptable accuracy and sensitivity to change (e.g., 7-day PA recall), self-report measures are inherently subject to biases compared to objective measures (e.g., accelerometers). For example, participants might under- or overreport their time spent in PA if they cannot accurately remember their previous PA behavior (recall bias), or overreport time spent in PA if they are aware that appearing to be active is socially desirable (social desirability bias). When possible, evidence based on objective measures of PA should be given more weight than evidence based on self-reported data alone.

- Intervention details: Although details of an intervention's components are sometimes published separately from the results of the intervention, many studies provide only a general description of the intervention rather than specific details on its various components, which prevents other researchers and practitioners from replicating the intervention. Details on intervention components such as the content of educational materials, structure of educational classes, and behavior change strategies used are necessary for translating effective interventions into practice. If the intervention is tailored at the deep level for FBOs (i.e., faith-based), it is also important to describe how religious beliefs and practices were incorporated into the intervention.

- Lack of a guiding theoretical framework: Some studies do not mention or thoroughly describe the theory used to guide the development of the intervention. Although interventions not based on a theoretical framework may result in significant improvements in PA participation, the lack of a theoretical framework to guide the development of the intervention makes it difficult to explain how and why PA increased (or not) as a result of the intervention. With a guiding theoretical framework, intervention content can be tailored to target specific psychosocial variables depending on the needs of the target population. These psychosocial variables can also be measured to determine whether they mediate changes in PA behavior as the theory proposes. Most faith-based PA interventions are informed by social cognitive theory (39), but it is likely that other theories and models would be appropriate for this setting. For example, the *Faith, Activity, and Nutrition* intervention used a social ecological framework to target multiple levels of influence on PA and eating behaviors (58).

Importance of Clergy in Physical Activity Interventions

Although the evidence on whether clergy support and participation in faith-based interventions leads to improvements in PA outcomes is equivocal (16, 59–62), cross-sectional studies have provided valuable information regarding the potential for the health and behaviors of clergy to influence the health environment in FBOs:

- Clergy who are more active and perceive themselves as healthy are more likely to offer health interventions in their FBO (63).

- Clergy who perceive themselves as healthy are more likely to provide health counseling to their congregants (64).
- Clergy who are more active are more likely to speak to their congregants about PA during sermons and during individual counseling (65).
- Clergy with healthier eating habits and identities are more likely to identify as role models to their congregation and offer health interventions (66).

These findings are promising; however, clergy in general are disproportionately affected by obesity and other chronic health conditions (65, 67–69). Despite the apparent need for health interventions for clergy, there are only a few published reports of interventions targeting the health and behaviors of clergy specifically (70, 71). At the very least, efforts to modify the health and behaviors of clergy may help to alleviate a potential barrier to partnering with FBOs to promote the health of the community.

Things to Consider When Partnering With Faith-Based Organizations

Background Research

Not only must the practitioner/researcher search for FBOs within the community, he or she will need to answer the following questions while searching for them:

- Where is the FBO located in relation to the target population for the intervention? Depending on the target population of the intervention, it may be important to consider whether proximity to the FBO could be a barrier to utilizing services and interventions at the FBO. It might also be important to consider the demographic composition of the FBO to ensure the target population will be reached through the FBO (see Box 3.10).

Box 10.1

Cultural Considerations

When conducting background research on FBOs, the researcher/practitioner should consider that religious beliefs and practices, and their relative importance to the target population, may vary by

- Religious tradition
- Denominational affiliation
- Region of the country
- FBO doctrine
- FBO leadership
- Demographics of the congregation

FBO, faith-based organization.

- What is the capacity of the FBO to engage in PA promotion? Answering this question will include reviewing what interventions the FBO offers, as well as what facilities they have available for PA interventions. It might also include consideration for the size of the church as evidence indicates larger FBOs have more infrastructure and capacity for funding interventions than smaller FBOs, but smaller FBOs often have stronger ties to the community (72).

- What is the mission of the FBO? The mission of the FBO may vary based on religious tradition, denominational affiliation, and leadership. In general, it would be advantageous to seek partnerships with FBOs that include in their mission a concern for the well-being of people in the community, and who are willing to collaborate with outside entities in pursuit of this mission.

Contacting the Faith-Based Organization

Practitioners/researchers should keep these things in mind when contacting FBOs:

- Use existing networks whenever possible. Members of the team should consider whether they know someone with personal ties to the FBO that can help establish initial contact with the leadership of the FBO. This may make scheduling an initial meeting with the leadership easier to accomplish.
- Meet face-to-face with leadership. Preference should be given for face-to-face meetings with FBO leadership. Not only does this put a face to the potential partner, but it also provides the researcher/practitioner an opportunity to demonstrate his or her commitment to the partnership and establish how the partnership aligns with the mission of the FBO.
- Meet face-to-face with the congregation. In order to gauge interest and support for the partnership, FBO leadership may invite the researcher/practitioner to speak to the congregation and/or other key stakeholders about the proposed partnership. This is a valuable opportunity for the researcher/practitioner to demonstrate a shared commitment between him- or herself and the leadership in pursuing the mission of the FBO.
- *Be patient.* Partnerships with FBOs may take time to materialize, especially considering the multiple barriers (e.g., perceived lack of time, resources, and motivation) that may be present at various times throughout the process. Researchers/practitioners can take advantage of this time to learn more about the FBO and to further demonstrate their commitment to partnering with the FBO in pursuit of their mission.

Involve Key Stakeholders

In line with the recommendations of community-based participatory research (CBPR) (73), the PA intervention should be developed in partnership between the researchers/practitioners, members and leadership of the FBO, and possibly with representatives from the community that might also benefit from the intervention. The CBPR approach allows partners to contribute their knowledge, expertise, and resources to the development of the intervention. In general, partnerships with FBOs should seek to include the following people:

- Leaders, who are respected in the FBO and surrounding community, have authority to make decisions about how resources are used in the FBO and the surrounding community, and have a track record of willingness to partner with other organizations.

- Members of the FBO that are respected in the FBO and surrounding community, and who have intimate knowledge of the issues facing individuals that attend the FBO and that live in the surrounding community.
- Other organizations in the community that could provide resources, experience, and infrastructure for components of the PA interventions.

Ensure the Intervention Is Sustainable

In this chapter, we have highlighted the potential for FBOs to provide space, resources, and a pool of volunteers for PA interventions. However, FBOs can often be stretched in terms of their resources and human capital. There is a risk of overburdening highly involved members of an FBO with an additional intervention to run and staff. To ensure that a PA intervention is sustainable, it is important that the responsibility for the intervention is shared among several individuals or groups in the FBO.

Case Example 2. The Faith, Activity, and Nutrition Intervention

One example of a sustainable faith-based intervention is the *Faith, Activity, and Nutrition (FAN)* intervention (58). The *FAN* intervention was a collaborative effort between several universities and the Seventh Episcopal District of the African Methodist Episcopal (AME) church in South Carolina. *FAN* was a culturally tailored intervention aimed at improving PA participation and healthy eating among individuals that attended one of the 74 AME churches that participated in the intervention. The research team worked with pastors, health directors (if available), *FAN* coordinators, and laypersons in the participating churches to identify strategies to increase availability and accessibility to opportunities to engage in PA (e.g., offer PA interventions at church, partner with local fitness clubs for discounted memberships, and offer education classes on how to be active). Churches had the flexibility of choosing which opportunities for PA to enhance or make available, depending on the needs and interests of the congregation. Churches submitted a formal plan to the research team for increasing opportunities for PA, as well as the budget needed to enact their plan. They were then provided with some financial support, all intervention materials, technical assistance, and participant incentives to help start and maintain the 15-month intervention. Congregants of AME churches that participated in the *FAN* intervention demonstrated small but significant improvements in PA participation compared to churches that were on the wait-list control group (74). A key feature of *FAN* was the decision by the research team to make sure the intervention would be sustainable after the study concluded by training church staff and members to deliver the intervention, as well as by ensuring the responsibility of maintaining the intervention was shared by numerous individuals within the church. Additionally, the *FAN* intervention was made available to all AME churches in South Carolina at the conclusion of the study. The materials and resources used for the *FAN* intervention are available online for any FBO to use free of charge (www.health-e-ame.com).

▓ Summary

- Historically, FBOs have been concerned with meeting both the spiritual *and* physical needs of the community.

- Many Americans report a religious affiliation and attend worship services at FBOs.
- FBOs can provide facilities, resources, and human capital necessary for the provision of PA interventions.
- Clergy are the spiritual and administrative leaders of FBOs. They are an important ally in the promotion of PA in FBOs. They may be more willing and effective in championing PA if they themselves are physically active.
- Many national agencies, such as the CPSTF and the NPAP Alliance, provide guidelines for working with community-based organizations such as FBOs to promote PA.
- Whether it is faith-based or faith-placed, the PA intervention should align with the mission and values of the FBO.
- There are several considerations to make prior to partnering with an FBO, as well when making initial contact with the FBO.
- The development and sustainability of the PA intervention will benefit greatly by involving key stakeholders from the FBO in all aspects of the planning and implementation process.

Things to Consider

- The primary mission of FBOs is to meet the spiritual needs of their congregants, with many FBOs also offering services to meet the practical, emotional, and health-related needs of the greater community in which they serve.
- Partnering with FBOs to develop and implement interventions can lead to broad dissemination of public health initiatives related to increasing PA behavior.
- FBOs often have facilities, communications infrastructure, and volunteers that are integral to the successful delivery and sustainability of PA interventions.
- It is important to involve key stakeholders from FBOs, especially clergy, during all stages of intervention planning and development to ensure the intervention aligns with the mission and values of the FBO.

Resources

- The Association for Religious Data Archives provides access to multiple sources of data on religion:
  www.thearda.com
- The Barna Group is a leading research firm on matters of faith and culture in the United States:
  www.barna.com
- The *Let's Move Faith and Communities* tool kit:
  www.hhs.gov/sites/default/files/lets_move_toolkit.pdf

- Community Preventive Services Task Force recommendations for PA promotion:
  www.thecommunityguide.org/content/task-force-findings-physical-activity
- The National Physical Activity Plan Alliance faith-based sector:
  www.physicalactivityplan.org/theplan/faithbased.html

▓ References

1. Scott JD. *The Scope and Scale of Faith-Based Social Services: A Review of the Research Literature Focusing on the Activities of Faith-Based Organizations in the Delivery of Social Services. Roundtable on Religion and Social Welfare Policy.* 2nd ed. New York, NY: Rockefeller Institute of Government; 2003.
2. Sider RJ, Unruh HR. Typology of religious characteristics of social service and educational organizations and programs. *Nonprofit Volunt Sect Q.* 2004;33(1):109–134. doi:10.1177/0899764003257494
3. Frank JD, Frank JB. *Persuasion and Healing: A Comparitive Study of Psychotherapy.* 3rd ed. Baltimore, MD: Johns Hopkins University Press; 1991.
4. Pollak K. *The Healers: The Doctor, Then and Now.* Camden, NJ: Thomas Nelson and Sons, Ltd; 1963.
5. Amundsen DW, Amundsen DW, eds. The medeival Catholic tradition. In: *Care and Curing: Health and Medicine in the Western Religious Traditions.* Baltimore, MD: Johns Hopkins University Press; 1998.
6. Gamwell L, Tomes N. *Madness in America: Cultural and Medical Perceptions of Mental Illness Before 1914.* New York, NY: State University of New York at Binghamton and Cornell University Press; 1995.
7. Walsh JJ. *Religion and Health.* Boston, MA: Little, Brown, and Company; 1920.
8. Koenig HG, King M, Larson DB. *The Handbook of Religion and Health.* 2nd ed. New York, NY: Oxford University Press; 2012.
9. Gonnerman ME Jr, Lutz GM, Yehieli M, et al. Religion and health connection: a study of African American, protestant christians. *J Health Care Poor Underserved.* 2008;19(1):193–199. doi:10.1353/hpu.2008.0020
10. Levin JS. Religion and health: is there an association, is it valid, and is it causal? *Soc Sci Med.* 1994;38(11):1475–1482. doi:10.1016/0277-9536(94)90109-0
11. Sloan RP, Bagiella E, Powell T. Religion, spirituality, and medicine. *Lancet.* 1999;353(9153):664–667. doi:10.1016/S0140-6736(98)07376-0
12. Koenig HG, Hooten EG, Lindsay-Calkins E, et al. Spirituality in medical school curricula: findings from a national survey. *Int J Psychiatry Med.* 2010(4):391–398. doi:10.2190/PM.40.4.c
13. Grammich C, Hadaway K, Houseal R, et al. 2010 U.S. Religion Census. Religious Congregations & Membership Study. 2012. Available at: http://www.thearda.com/rcms2010/ Accessed September 5, 2017.
14. Pew Research Center. U.S. Religious Landscape Study. 2014. Available at: http://www.pewforum.org/religious-landscape-study/ Accessed September 1, 2017.
15. Ammerman A, Corbie-Smith G, St George DM, et al. Research expectations among African American church leaders in the PRAISE! project: a randomized trial guided by community-based participatory research. *Am J Public Health.* 2003;93(10):1720–1727. doi:10.2105/AJPH.93.10.1720
16. Campbell MK, Resnicow K, Carr C, et al. Process evaluation of an effective church-based diet intervention: body & soul. *Health Educ Behav.* 2006;34(6):864–880. doi:10.1177/1090198106292020
17. Taylor RJ, Chatters LM, Levin J. Socio-historical role of the church. In: *Religion in the Lives of African Americans: Social, Psychological, and Health Perspectives.* Thousand Oaks, CA: Sage Publications; 2003:21.

18. Pew Research Center. The Shifting Religious Identity of Latinos in the United States. Available at: http://www.pewforum.org/2014/05/07/the-shifting-religious-identity-of-latinos-in-the-united-states. May 7, 2014. Accessed September 5, 2017.

19. Perez A, Fleury J, Shearer N. Salud de Corazon: cultural resources for cardiovascular health among older Hispanic women. *Hisp Health Care Int*. 2012;10(2):93–100. doi:10.1891/1540-4153.10.2.93

20. Rifat M, Rusen I, Mahmud MH, et al. From mosques to classrooms: mobilizing the community to enhance case detection of tuberculosis. *Am J Public Health*. 2008;98(9):1550–1552. doi:10.2105/AJPH.2007.117333

21. Bader A, Musshauser D, Sahin F, et al. The Mosque Campaign: a cardiovascular prevention program for female Turkish immigrants. *Wien Klin Wochenschr*. 2006;118(7):217–223. doi:10.1007/s00508-006-0587-0

22. Padela AI, Killawi A, Heisler M, et al. The role of imams in American Muslim health: perspectives of Muslim community leaders in Southeast Michigan. *J Relig Health*. 2011;50(2):359–373. doi:10.1007/s10943-010-9428-6

23. Grace C, Begum R, Subhani S, et al. Prevention of type 2 diabetes in British Bangladeshis: qualitative study of community, religious, and professional perspectives. *BMJ*. 2008;337:a1931. doi:10.1136/bmj.a1931

24. Moberg D. *The Church as a Social Institution: The Sociology of American Religion*. Englewood Cliffs, NJ: Prentice-Hall, Inc.; 1962.

25. Pattillo-McCoy M. Church culture as a strategy of action in the black community. *Am Sociol Rev*. 1998;63(6):767–784. doi:10.2307/2657500

26. Wuthnow R. *Boundless Faith: Global Outreach of the American Church*. Berkeley, CA: University of California Press; 2009.

27. Olson LM, Reis J, Murphy L, et al. The religious community as a partner in health care. *J Community Health*. 1988;13(4):249–257. doi:10.1007/BF01324237

28. Bass BG. Faith-based programs and their influence on homelessness. *Fam Community Health*. 2009;32(4):314–319. doi:10.1097/FCH.0b013e3181b91f25

29. Sutherland M, Hale CD, Harris GJ. Community health promotion: the church as partner. *J Prim Prev*. 1995;16(2):201–215. doi:10.1007/BF02407340

30. Weaver AJ, Flannelly KJ, Flannelly LT, et al. Collaboration between clergy and mental health professionals: a review of professional health care journals from 1980 through 1999. *Couns Values*. 2003;47(3):162–171. doi:10.1002/j.2161-007X.2003.tb00263.x

31. Elder J, Haughton J, Perez L, et al. Promoting cancer screening among churchgoing Latinas: Fe en Acción/faith in action. *Health Educ Res*. 2017;32(2):163–173. doi:10.1093/her/cyx033

32. Saunders DR, Holt CL, Whitehead TL, et al. Development of the men's prostate awareness church training: church-based workshops for African American men. *Fam Community Health*. 2013;36(3):224–235. doi:10.1097/FCH.0b013e318292eb40

33. Cornelius JB, Appiah JA. A 5-year review of faith-based sexuality education and HIV prevention programs. *Curr Sex Health Rep*. 2016;8(1):27–38. doi:10.1007/s11930-016-0062-5

34. Gutierrez J, Devia C, Weiss L, et al. Health, community, and spirituality: evaluation of a multicultural faith-based diabetes prevention program. *Diabetes Educ*. 2014;40(2):214–222. doi:10.1177/0145721714521872

35. Boltri JM, Davis-Smith YM, Seale JP, et al. Diabetes prevention in a faith-based setting: results of translational research. *J Public Health Manag Pract*. 2008;14(1):29–32. doi:10.1097/01.PHH.0000303410.66485.91

36. Sattin RW, Williams LB, Dias J, et al. Community trial of a faith-based lifestyle intervention to prevent diabetes among African-Americans. *J Community Health*. 2016;41(1):87–96. doi:10.1007/s10900-015-0071-8

37. Yeary KH-cK, Cornell CE, Moore P, et al. Peer reviewed: feasibility of an evidence-based weight loss intervention for a faith-based, rural, African American population. *Prev Chronic Dis*. 2011;8(6):A146.

38. Yanek LR, Becker DM, Moy TF, et al. Project Joy: faith based cardiovascular health promotion for African American women. *Public Health Rep*. 2001;116(suppl 1):68–81. doi:10.1093/phr/116.S1.68

39. Bopp M, Peterson J, Webb B. A comprehensive review of faith-based physical activity interventions. *Am J Lifestyle Med.* 2012;6(6):460–478. doi:10.1177/1559827612439285

40. Whitt-Glover MC, Goldmon MV, Gizlice Z, et al. Learning and Developing Individual Exercise Skills (LADIES) for a better life: a church-based physical activity intervention-baseline participant characteristics. *Ethn Dis.* 2017;27(3):257. doi:10.18865/ed.27.3.257

41. Baltic RD, Weier RC, Katz ML, et al. Study design, intervention, and baseline characteristics of a group randomized trial involving a faith-based healthy eating and physical activity intervention (Walk by Faith) to reduce weight and cancer risk among overweight and obese Appalachian adults. *Contemp Clin Trials.* 2015;44:1–10. doi:10.1016/j.cct.2015.06.017

42. Arredondo EM, Haughton J, Ayala GX, et al. Fe en Acción/faith in action: design and implementation of a church-based randomized trial to promote physical activity and cancer screening among churchgoing Latinas. *Contemp Clin Trials.* 2015;45:404–415. doi:10.1016/j.cct.2015.09.008

43. Personal Responsibility and Work Opportunity Reconciliation Act, 110.2105 (1996).

44. Bush GW. Executive Order 13199: Establishment of White House Office of Faith-Based and Community Initiatives. 2001. Available at: https://georgewbush-whitehouse.archives.gov/news/releases/2001/01/20010129-2.html. Accessed September 6, 2017.

45. Obama B. Executive Order 13498—Amendments to Executive Order 13199 and Establishment of the President's Advisory Council for Faith-Based and Neighborhood Partnerships. 2009. Available at: https://www.gpo.gov/fdsys/pkg/FR-2009-02-09/pdf/E9-2893.pdf. Accessed September 6, 2017.

46. Obama M. About Let's Move. 2010. Available at: https://letsmove.obamawhitehouse.archives.gov/about. Accessed September 6, 2017.

47. White House Task. Force on Childhood Obesity. Solving the problem of childhood obesity within a generation: White House Task Force on Childhood Obesity report to the president. 2010. Available at: https://letsmove.obamawhitehouse.archives.gov/sites/letsmove.gov/files/TaskForce_on_Childhood_Obesity_May2010_FullReport.pdf. Accessed September 7, 2017.

48. U.S. Supreme Court. *Trinity Lutheran Church of Columbia, Inc v Comer*, 2017: 587 US.

49. U.S. Department of Health and Human Services. Healthy People 2020. 2010. Available at: www.healthypeople.gov. Accessed September 1, 2017.

50. Community Preventive Services Task Force. Task force findings for physical activity. 2001. Available at: https://www.thecommunityguide.org/content/task-force-findings-physical-activity. Accessed September 7, 2017.

51. National Physical Activity Plan Alliance. National Physical Activity Plan. 2016. Available at: http://www.physicalactivityplan.org/index.php. Accessed July 21, 2016.

52. Community Preventive. *Services Task Force. The Guide to Community Preventive Services.* New York, NY: Oxford University Press; 2005.

53. Methodist Le Bonheur Healthcare. Congregational Health Network. 2017. Available at: http://www.methodisthealth.org/about-us/faith-and-health/congregational-health-network/. Accessed September 8, 2017.

54. Agency for Healthcare Research and Quality. Church-health system partnership facilitates transitions from hospital to home for urban, low-income African Americans, reducing mortality, utilization, and costs. 2011. Available at: https://innovations.ahrq.gov/profiles/church-health-system-partnership-facilitates-transitions-hospital-home-urban-low-income. Accessed September 14, 2017.

55. Resnicow K, Baranowski T, Ahluwalia JS, et al. Cultural sensitivity in public health: defined and demystified. *Ethn Dis.* 1999;9(1):10–21. doi:10.1177/014572170202800607

56. DeHaven MJ, Hunter IB, Wilder L, et al. Health programs in faith-based organizations: are they effective? *Am J Public Health.* 2004;94(6):1030–1036. doi:10.2105/AJPH.94.6.1030

57. Lancaster K, Carter-Edwards L, Grilo S, et al. Obesity interventions in African American faith-based organizations: a systematic review. *Obes Rev.* 2014;15(suppl 4):159–176. doi:10.1111/obr.12207

58. Wilcox S, Laken M, Parrott AW, et al. The faith, activity, and nutrition (FAN) program: design of a participatory research intervention to increase physical activity and improve

dietary habits in African American churches. *Contemp Clin Trials.* 2010;31(4):323–335. doi:10.1016/j.cct.2010.03.011

59. Wilcox S, Laken M, Bopp M, et al. Increasing physical activity among church members: community-based participatory research. *Am J Prev Med.* 2007;32(2):131–138. doi:10.1016/j.amepre.2006.10.009

60. Campbell MK, Motsinger BM, Ingram A, et al. The North Carolina Black Churches United for Better Health Project: intervention and process evaluation. *Health Educ Behav.* 2000;27(2):241–253. doi:10.1177/109019810002700210

61. Baruth M, Wilcox S, Laken M, et al. Implementation of a faith-based physical activity intervention: insights from church health directors. *J Community Health.* 2008;33(5):304–312. doi:10.1007/s10900-008-9098-4

62. Baruth M, Wilcox S, Saunders RP. The role of pastor support in a faith-based health promotion intervention. *Fam Community Health.* 2013;36(3):204–214. doi:10.1097/FCH.0b013e31828e6733

63. Bopp M, Fallon EA. Individual and institutional influences on faith-based health and wellness programming. *Health Educ Res.* 2011;26(6):1107–1119. doi:10.1093/her/cyr096

64. Fallon EA, Bopp MJ, Webb B. Factors associated with faith-based health counseling in the United States: implications for dissemination of evidence-based behavioral medicine. *Health Soc Care Community.* 2012;21(2):129–139. doi:10.1111/hsc.12001

65. Webb B, Bopp M, Johnson D. Practicing what they preach? Physical activity promotion practices of clergy. Under review.

66. Harmon BE, Blake CE, Armstead CA, et al. Intersection of identities. Food, role, and the African-American pastor. *Appetite.* 2013;67:44–52. doi:10.1016/j.appet.2013.03.007

67. Webb B, Bopp M, Fallon EA. Factors associated with obesity and health behaviors among clergy. *J Health Behav Public Health.* 2013;3(1):20–28. doi:10.1177/2158244017710840

68. Proeschold-Bell RJ, LeGrand S. High rates of obesity and chronic disease among United Methodist clergy. *Obesity.* 2010;18(9):1867–1870. doi:10.1038/oby.2010.102

69. Halaas GW. *Ministerial Health and Wellness.* Chicago, IL: Evangelical Lutheran Church in America; 2002.

70. Webb BL, Bopp MJ. Results of walking in faith: a faith-based physical activity program for clergy. *J Relig Health.* 2016;1–14. doi:10.1007/s10943-016-0255-2

71. Proeschold-Bell RJ, Turner EL, Bennett GG, et al. A 2-year holistic health and stress intervention: results of an RCT in clergy. *Am J Prev Med.* 2017;53(3):290–299. doi:10.1016/j.amepre.2017.04.009

72. Chavez M. *Congregations in America.* Cambridge, MA: Harvard University Press; 2004.

73. Israel BA, Eng E, Schulz AJ, et al. *Methods in Community-Based Participatory Research for Health.* San Francisco, CA: Jossey-Bass; 2005.

74. Wilcox S, Parrot A, Baruth M, et al. The faith, activity, and nutrition program: a randomized controlled trial in African-American churches. *Am J Prev Med.* 2013;44(2):122–131. doi:10.1016/j.amepre.2012.2009.2062

PROMOTING PHYSICAL ACTIVITY IN THE HEALTHCARE SECTOR

MARK STOUTENBERG | ELIZABETH A. RICHARDS

LEARNING OBJECTIVES

By the end of this chapter, the student should be able to

1. Explain four strategies that healthcare can use to promote physical activity (PA).
2. Discuss how the stages of change can be used in a healthcare setting.
3. Apply lessons learned for previous interventions in healthcare settings to develop new interventions.
4. Assess PA as a vital sign.
5. Develop a basic PA prescription

▦ Importance of the Healthcare Sector for Promoting Physical Activity

The Role of the Healthcare Setting in Promoting Physical Activity

Healthcare providers play an important role in positively impacting a large segment of our society through the promotion of physical activity (PA). More than 80% of U.S. adults visit a healthcare provider at least once annually (1). The primary care setting, which accounts for approximately 52.2% of all office visits, is a particularly valuable location for health promotion interventions (2). Primary care providers have taken on the responsibility of providing care not only for acute and chronic illnesses, but also for preventive services and, therefore, are a powerful influence on individual lifestyle behaviors. Further, the bond of the clinician–patient relationship increases the potential of healthcare settings to effectively promote healthy behaviors. The U.S. Department of Health and Human Services acknowledged the potential of the healthcare setting in promoting PA at a population level by adding physician PA counseling as a Healthy People 2020 objective (3). The goal is "to increase the proportion of physician office visits made by patients with a diagnosis of cardiovascular disease, diabetes, or hyperlipidemia that include counseling or education related to physical activity" by at least 10%.

Call to Action for the Promotion of PA in Healthcare Settings

The U.S. National Physical Activity Plan (NPAP) (4), which was first released in May 2010 and later updated in April 2016, describes the promotion of PA through nine different societal sectors, one of which is healthcare (5). Similarly, the International Society for Physical Activity and Health released the Toronto Charter at the 3rd International Congress on Physical Activity and Public Health in 2010 (6). The Toronto Charter is a global call to action that provides a framework for initiating and expanding population-based approaches to increase PA levels. The third section of the Charter outlines several strategies for increasing PA in health settings including: reorienting health services and funding systems toward PA, screening of patient PA levels at every primary care consultation, and providing brief, structured advice and referral to community programs for insufficiently active patients. Further, the Toronto Charter recommends that national organizations should advocate for greater health sector funding for PA-related promotion campaigns and programs (Box 11.1).

BOX 11.1

The Healthcare Sector of the NPAP

The NPAP outlines four strategies in which the healthcare sector can promote PA:

1. Increase the priority of PA assessment, advice, and promotion
2. Encourage healthcare systems and professional societies to recognize physical inactivity as treatable and preventable with profound health and cost implications
3. Develop partnerships between healthcare systems and other societal sectors to promote access to evidence-based, PA-related services that increase health equity
4. Include PA education in the training of all healthcare professionals

NPAP, National Physical Activity Plan; PA, physical activity.

In 2014, the U.S. Preventive Services Task Force (USPSTF) released a statement on behavioral counseling for cardiovascular disease prevention in at-risk adults (7). They suggested that there was adequate evidence that intensive behavioral counseling interventions moderately increased PA levels in overweight or obese adults who are at increased risk for cardiovascular disease. The USPSTF reported that intensive behavioral counseling (over 12–24 months), conducted with patients having a body mass index (BMI) of 30 kg/m² or greater, resulted in small, but important, changes in health behavior outcomes, body weight, and selected clinical outcomes. The USPSTF concluded that the proportion of overweight to obese individuals meeting national PA guidelines increased by 10% (from a baseline level of 15% based on self-report measures) after receiving intensive behavioral counseling.

Over time, these overarching guidelines have been supported by additional calls to action by medical societies (8) and leading health professionals (9, 10) for greater integration of PA in healthcare settings.

Initial Trials Integrating PA Counseling in Healthcare Settings

One of the first trials to examine PA promotion in a health setting was the Physician-Based Assessment and Counseling for Exercise (PACE) trial (11). PACE was conducted in the 1990s in San Diego, California, where 17 physicians from diverse ethnic backgrounds and practice types were recruited to participate—10 in the intervention arm and 7 as controls. Physicians in the PACE intervention arm received training in small groups, a study training manual, and conducted role-playing with mock patients. Eligible patients who had appointments with physicians in the intervention arm completed a PACE questionnaire that assessed their behavioral stage of change in the waiting room before their visit. Patients were classified as being in precontemplation, contemplation, or currently active (see Box 11.2). Physicians then spent 3 to 5 minutes of the office visit discussing stage-relevant information and strategies for becoming more active with the patient. A health educator followed up the counseling session with a "booster" phone call to reinforce information provided during the clinic visit. A significant proportion of patients who visited physicians in the PACE intervention arm moved from contemplation to the active stage, with 52% reporting being regularly active (compared to only 12% of the control patients). Patients receiving the PACE intervention significantly increased their walking time by 40 minutes a week, a 100% increase over baseline activity levels (compared to a 10-minute per week increase in the control patients). The PACE study set a historical precedent by showing that 3 to 5 minutes of counseling, matched to a patient's needs and current motivation level, can lead to important changes in PA levels.

BOX 11.2

Stages of the TTM

Stage 1—Precontemplation. Individuals in this stage are not thinking about becoming more active in the next 6 months. They may not see being inactive as a problem and the benefits of becoming active do not outweigh the consequences.

Stage 2—Contemplation. Individuals in this stage are considering the possibility of becoming more active in the near future, but may still feel ambivalent about taking the next step. The benefits of being active do not yet outweigh the consequences enough for them to take action.

Stage 3—Preparation. Individuals in this stage have made, or are making, attempts to become more active. Although they are taking steps toward being more active (i.e.,

(continued)

(continued)

> purchasing a gym membership), they have not increased their PA levels sufficiently to meet national guidelines.
>
> Stage 4—Action. Individuals in this stage are actively taking steps to increase their PA levels and are making great steps toward meeting national PA guidelines, but have done so for less than 6 months.
>
> Stage 5—Maintenance. Individuals in this stage have now met national PA guidelines for a sustained period of time (i.e., 6 months or longer). They are better equipped to avoid temptations to return to an inactive lifestyle by anticipating temptations and learning to cope with life challenges.
>
> TTM, transtheoretical model.

Following in the footsteps of the PACE trial, the Activity Counseling Trial (ACT) investigated the effectiveness of different PA counseling interventions compared to current practices in the primary care setting (12). In this study, 874 inactive adults, with relatively equal numbers of males and females, received one of three interventions: Advice; Assistance; or Counseling. All patients completed an initial visit with their primary care physician, as well as a follow-up visit at the end of the study to discuss their progress. The *Advice group* received advice from their primary care physicians based on the national guidelines, as well as educational material from health educators. The *Assistance group* received the same advice plus additional behavioral counseling. The *Counseling group* received the same components as the Assistance group, as well as health educator-initiated telephone counseling biweekly for 3 weeks, then monthly for the first year of intervention. At the end of the study, patients, especially the females in the *Assistance* and *Counseling* groups, equally increased their PA levels. For the male patients, more in-depth counseling proved to be no more effective than receiving advice only, suggesting that a more comprehensive approach involving the integration of community resources and exercise professionals may be necessary to engage men in greater levels of PA.

In both the PACE and ACT trials, the study physicians reported that they did not feel an extra burden in addressing their patient's PA habits. Further, they believed that their efforts were beneficial to the patients and their practice. Numerous other studies have shown similar results regarding the effectiveness of physician counseling efforts to increase patient PA levels (13–15) (Box 11.3).

BOX 11.3

Lessons Learned From PA Interventions in Healthcare Settings

1. Promoting PA through the healthcare setting is feasible without unduly burdening healthcare providers and can lead to meaningful increases in patient PA levels.
2. Using specific behavior change strategies with patients is an essential component of any behavior change intervention.
3. It is important to consider how patient responses to the advice and counseling provided to them by their healthcare teams may vary by gender.

(continued)

(continued)

4. The optimal way to intervene and encourage patients to be physically active is unknown, but likely varies across a number of different factors, such as gender, socioeconomic status, education level, and patient neighborhood characteristics.

PA, physical activity.

Challenges in Promoting PA in Healthcare Settings

Despite these calls to action and the initial success of the PACE and ACT trials, rates of PA counseling in the clinic setting remain low. Data from the National Health Interview Survey (NHIS) indicates that only 23% of patients surveyed in 2000 had been advised by their healthcare provider to begin, or continue, a PA program (16). Reported levels of PA counseling increased slightly to 29% in 2005 and further to 34% by 2010. Another source of information on physician counseling rates comes from the National Committee for Quality Assurance (NCQA). In 2004, the NCQA added two questions on PA to the Healthcare Effectiveness Data and Information Set (HEDIS) measure for older adults (17). The HEDIS tool is used by nearly all of U.S. health plans to measure performance on different dimensions of care and service. Despite formal inclusion as a HEDIS measure, national compliance with these PA measures by healthcare teams has hovered between 53% and 56% over the past decade (18).

The most common barrier to PA counseling in the clinic setting is the limited amount of time physicians have with each of their patients. The typical primary care patient visit lasts approximately 17 to 21 minutes, during which an average of six different topics are addressed (19, 20). The most important topics receive approximately 5 minutes of time, during which the physician speaks for only 2 minutes. The most common major topics discussed include mental health (initiated by the physician) and biomedical issues (initiated by the patient) (19). With a greater number of patients presenting with multiple comorbidities, more topics must be addressed in a single visit, diminishing the amount of time spent on any one topic. While 3 to 5 minutes is often recommended as the minimum amount of time for effective behavior change counseling, this would amount to 30% to 35% of the clinic visit dedicated to a single topic; something that may not be feasible in a real-world setting. Therefore, changes in provider reimbursement rates and workflow are likely necessary to ensure greater time and higher quality counseling efforts with each patient (20). Low PA counseling rates are also attributed to a lack of formal education in providing PA counseling, perceived effectiveness of their efforts, patient and professional materials, staff to assist with counseling efforts, and support from their clinic administration (21, 22). PA assessment and counseling is also limited by a lack of pragmatic strategies and fully developed protocols through which PA interventions can be feasibly implemented in the healthcare setting.

When designing interventions for the clinic setting, it is important for public health practitioners to be aware of the context of the clinic setting that influences the responsibilities and actions of healthcare providers. PA is typically not a priority for either the patient or the provider, with more immediate, or acute, health concerns taking precedence. Therefore, the key to integrating PA is to systematically involve all members of the healthcare team before, during, and after the clinician–patient encounter to leverage the effect of this time-limited, but crucially important, interaction. Further, intervention strategies must be brief and built into the standard patient workflow. Throughout the remainder of this chapter, we will present various pragmatic strategies through which PA can be integrated into patient care in a standardized manner across healthcare systems.

Best Practices for Establishing PA Promotion in a Healthcare Setting

Getting Things Started—Assessing Patient PA Levels

Assessing patient PA levels is the cornerstone to subsequent PA counseling, prescription, and referral in the healthcare setting (23). As with any other clinical indicator, the initial diagnosis is crucial. By incorporating PA as an officially recognized "vital sign," healthcare teams emphasize the importance of PA as being equal to that of traditional vital signs, such as blood pressure and heart rate, and highlight the importance of maintaining favorable PA levels as a means to achieve optimal health. When included as a formal vital sign, PA levels can be tracked and monitored over time, identifying physically inactive individuals as an at-risk population.

Several different tools have been tested for use in clinical practice. However, these tools are often evaluated in controlled research settings, use ancillary staff, and require additional time and resources that are not feasible for routine clinical practice (24). To increase their clinical feasibility and acceptability, PA assessment tools must be brief, easy to use, and yield clinically meaningful and actionable information. Further, given the limited time that physicians are able to spend with patients, the entire clinic staff must be trained and capable of using the selected PA tool. The Physical Activity Vital Sign (PAVS) is a tool that is brief, takes no longer than 30 seconds to complete, can be administered by any member of the healthcare team, and is effective in identifying whether patients are meeting national PA guidelines (see Box 11.4).

BOX 11.4

The Physical Activity Vital Sign

1. On average, how many days per week do you engage in moderate to strenuous PA (like a brisk walk)?	_____ days
2. On average, how many minutes do you engage in PA at this level?	_____ minutes
Total minutes per week of PA (multiply #1 by #2)	_____ **minutes per week**

PA, physical activity; PAVS, Physical Activity Vital Sign.

The PAVS has been integrated into multiple large healthcare systems across the country (25, 26), contributing, in part, to a recommendation by the National Academy of Medicine that electronic medical records (EMRs) be used to capture (assess and record) patient PA levels (27). In Kaiser Permanente Southern California, the PAVS was shown to have good face and discriminant validity in properly identifying physically inactive individuals across gender, age groups, and disease conditions (26). Further, significant associations were reported between self-reported PA levels and cardiometabolic risk factors, such as blood pressure and fasting blood glucose (28). Other studies demonstrated strong associations between results from the PAVS and patient BMI, as well as moderately strong associations with patient disease burden (29). The use of the PAVS also resulted in greater exercise-related progress note documentation and exercise referrals compared to patient visits when the PAVS was not administered (30). Further, patients were more likely to report receiving exercise counseling during their clinic visit if their PA levels were assessed.

Typically, the PAVS asks patients only about their aerobic activity levels. However, it may also be useful to ask patients about their muscle-strengthening habits. A single question, such as "In a typical week, how many days do you engage in muscle strengthening activities?" can further assist practitioners in determining whether their patients are meeting the resistance training component of the national PA guidelines (i.e., incorporating strength training at least 2 days per week) and guide them in customizing their PA recommendations.

More recently, the American Heart Association has advocated for the assessment of cardiorespiratory fitness in the clinic setting given its strong association with all-cause and cardiovascular mortality (31). A barrier to the widespread assessment of cardiorespiratory fitness is that it is best done through cardiopulmonary testing and the measurement of ventilator gases. While this testing is acceptable and often necessary to ensure the safety of individuals with chronic diseases, it is not a highly pragmatic option for the primary care setting due to its associated costs, specialized equipment, and need for trained personnel. Instead, other methods (submaximal and field testing) have been proposed as alternatives for estimating cardiorespiratory fitness. One pragmatic option for the clinic setting may be the estimation of cardiorespiratory fitness using nonexercise equations (32–35) that can be calculated as a part of annual health examinations (31). However, these equations currently tend to under- and overestimate fitness levels at the upper and lower ends of the distribution, respectively. More recent work is examining the use of data from wearable sensors to better estimate cardiorespiratory fitness (36).

Providing Patients With a Basic PA Prescription

After patients have their current PA levels assessed, the next step is to provide them with a PA prescription. Based on the assessed PA levels, it is recommended that prescriptions are given to all patients not meeting current recommendations (i.e., 150 minutes per week of moderate-intensity aerobic activity + 2 days per week of strength training). The PA prescription can be modified based on the patient's current activity level and motivational readiness. When writing PA prescriptions, providers should consider a gradual, stepwise approach. Instead of recommending that patients go from low levels of activity directly to 150 minutes a week, a more individualized approach involves prescribing slow, incremental increases over successive clinic visits to ensure a safer, more feasible process to becoming more active.

The Green Prescription in New Zealand is an example of one of the longest and best-known PA prescription programs. Started in 1998 by Sport and Recreation New Zealand, the Green Prescription program was officially adopted by the Ministry of Health in 2009 (37). The Green Prescription involves health professionals (i.e., a general practitioner or nurse) giving medically stable patients an exercise prescription that is either written or issued electronically. If the patient desires more support and guidance, the prescription is forwarded to the nearest Green Prescription PA provider. Early findings showed that patients receiving a Green Prescription increased their recreational activity compared to those who received only verbal advice (38). Subsequent work showed that patients receiving a Green Prescription, as compared to those receiving usual care, were more likely to meet national PA guidelines, increased their weekly activity by 34 minutes, and achieved a higher weekly energy expenditure (39). More recently, research has shown that the benefits of receiving a Green Prescription extend as far as 2 to 3 years after original receipt (40) (Box 11.5).

BOX 11.5

PAP in Sweden

In Sweden, the physical activity on prescription (PAP) program encourages healthcare providers to write individual PA prescriptions for their patients to prevent and treat illness (41). To aid practitioners in implementing the program in their local health settings, a PAP textbook was created in 2012 and recently updated in 2017 (42). The textbook outlines suggested routines for prescribing PA activity that resemble prescriptions for medicine as a way to enhance their significance.

An evaluation of the PAP program in the Östergötland region of Sweden was conducted in 2004-04 (43). The evaluation involved 38 of the 42 primary health centers in the region and a variety of healthcare professionals (i.e., physicians, nurses, physiotherapists, occupational therapists). Patients were eligible to receive the PA prescriptions if they were either sedentary or had a medical diagnosis for which PA would be beneficial (e.g., high blood pressure, diabetes). Patients were provided with a written PA prescription and a copy was kept in their medical record. The single-page prescription included their current activity levels, information regarding the prescription, and recommended activities. If the prescribed activity was facility based, a copy of the prescription was sent to a coordinator at one of the PA organizations in the network. More than 80% of the primary health centers established community-based networks to assist patients in gaining access to local PA resources. The PA coordinators contacted the patients by phone or letter after 5 weeks to check whether they had attended the suggested activities.

Over the 2-year study, 6,300 patients in Östergötland received a PA prescription (1.5% of all residents). At entry into the program, one-third of all patients were categorized as inactive, while only 22% met current PA recommendations. At the 3- and 12-month follow-ups, the proportion of inactive patients had declined to 17% and 20%, respectively. The number of regularly active patients increased to 33% and 30%, respectively. In total, more than half of the patients (52%) receiving PA prescriptions reported increasing their PA levels. The results of this study show that prescribing PA is effective in increasing both short- (3 months) and long-term (12 months) activity levels. More than half of the participating patients in Östergötland increased their PA, with the largest increases occurring in patients who were least active at baseline and needed assistance the most. This study involved typical patients, recruited by existing staff during regular appointments at the primary health centers. Further, the study involved no extra medical or research personnel other than the PA coordinator, who followed up with patients and encouraged them to participate in the PA programs.

PA, physical activity; PAP, physical activity on prescription.

Practical Strategies for Giving PA Prescriptions

The PA prescription sends a reinforcing message to patients about the importance of PA as a part of their overall wellness plan. All eligible patients (i.e., those not meeting the PA guidelines) should receive a PA prescription. Healthcare providers can give their patients a PA prescription using a number of different strategies. First, basic PA guidance can be given to patients in the form of a simple, written prescription—a format that patients are accustomed to and comfortable with. Several exercise "prescription pads" have been developed and are publicly available (44, 45). With the widespread use of EMRs in healthcare settings, patients may also wish to receive their PA prescription in an electronic format that is conveniently emailed to them. A final method to provide patients with semicustomized PA guidance is through the distribution of the "Prescription for Health" series developed by Exercise is Medicine (EIM) (46). These "prescriptions" are designed to provide patients with customized guidance on being physically active, as well as contraindications and special considerations, based on their current health condition. Regardless of the delivery method, the provision of a PA prescription should be noted in the patient's EMR (i.e., notes section) to allow healthcare providers to follow up on the original prescription at subsequent patient visits.

Scope of Practice Considerations

A final consideration in providing PA prescriptions involves the scope of practice of healthcare providers. The term "scope of practice" describes the procedures, actions, and processes that a provider is permitted to undertake based on his/her level of education, training, and competency in performing services in the clinic setting. Defining a scope of practice is critical in achieving safe, quality care for patients. When it comes to PA, there are no set guidelines defining the scope of practice for healthcare providers. Some associations, such as the American Society of Exercise Physiologists, have developed standards of practice for exercise physiologists that include academic training and proficiency of a number of job-based skills (47). Similarly, the American College of Sports Medicine developed the EIM® Credential to ensure that exercise professionals have the proper skills and knowledge to safely develop and implement PA programs with patients referred from healthcare systems (48).

Many physicians and other healthcare providers receive little to no formal education in PA during their professional training (49), often leaving them unprepared to properly prescribe PA. There should not be an expectation that providers can, or should, give detailed, comprehensive PA prescriptions. Instead, providers can be reasonably expected to assess the risks and benefits to their patients when exercising, clearly outline contraindications based on their current health status, identify issues that must be addressed when devising personalized activity plans, and provide simple messages that reinforce the importance of PA as a necessary and valued part of their overall wellness. Healthcare providers should then feel comfortable referring their patients to qualified exercise professionals who have years of specialized training in developing PA programs for individuals with a variety of different health conditions.

PA Counseling in the Clinic Setting

ACT and PACE trials, as well as several other trials that followed in their footsteps, healthcare providers have been called upon to provide specialized PA counseling to their patients (10, 21, 50). Given the time constraints of office visits, it is important that counseling strategies be brief, yet effective. Minimal intervention strategies, such as the 5As (ask, advise, assess, assist, arrange), can be used to facilitate PA behavior change (51) (see Table 11.1). The 5As is a proven framework for providers to ask about current PA behavior, advise about a change in behavior, assess readiness for behavior change, assist with PA goal setting, and arrange for follow-up (15, 52).

Another proven PA counseling strategy that healthcare providers are often encouraged to use is motivational interviewing (53, 54). Motivational interviewing is a method for approaching patients who are ambivalent about making a health behavior change and is considered to be more effective than traditional, advice-giving, counseling strategies (55, 56). The goal of motivational interviewing is to encourage patients to express their own reasons for behavior change by fostering internal motivation. Motivational interviewing typically encompasses four key phases:

- **Engaging:** The healthcare provider and the patient establish a strong working relationship. Early in this phase, the provider should make it clear that his or her intention is to form a partnership with the client.
- **Focusing:** The healthcare provider helps the patient identify a specific area which he or she is unsure about or struggling with to make a behavior change.
- **Evoking:** The healthcare provider draws out the patient's thoughts, ideas, and personal motivation regarding behavior change.
- **Planning:** This is the "how" phase where the provider continues to foster a commitment to change and assists in forming a specific action plan for behavior change.

TABLE 11.1. The 5As to PA counseling

5AS CONCEPT	DESCRIPTION	EXAMPLE
Ask	Ask about or assess current PA behavior (type, frequency, intensity, duration)	"Tell me about your current level of physical activity or exercise."
Advise	Provide clear, structured, tailored counseling about changing PA behavior	"You need to get 30 minutes of physical activity at least 5 days a week."
Assess	Assess patient readiness to change PA behavior	"Do you see yourself getting more exercise in the next few weeks?"
Assist	Assist with behavior change by providing a PA prescription, support materials, and/or self-monitoring tools.	"What might interfere with your plans to increase your physical activity?"
Arrange	Arrange for referral or follow-up either in-person, via telephone, or by email.	"I will arrange for a referral to (a community resource), this program is excellent at helping others increase physical activity."

NOTE: PA, physical activity.

During motivational interviewing, several core components are utilized (see Table 11.2). When healthcare providers utilize communication styles, such as motivational interviewing, which actively engage patients in decision making, the result is an increase in adherence to treatment plans and enhanced patient satisfaction (57). A recent review of 10 interventions using motivational interviewing in patients with chronic conditions demonstrated small effect sizes in increasing PA relative to comparison groups (53).

Linking Patients to PA Resources

Before leaving the clinic setting, eligible patients should be provided with a referral to a network of available PA resources, offered both through the health system and in the local community. Given the barriers to providing PA counseling in the clinic setting,

TABLE 11.2. Core components of motivational interviewing

SKILL	DEFINITION	EXAMPLE
Respect patient autonomy	Recognize that the patient is in charge of his/her own behavior change.	*"Is it OK if we talk about your current physical activity?"*
Collaboration	The healthcare provider creates an environment free of coercion that is built on principles of partnership.	*"What reasons do you have to increase your physical activity?"*
Express empathy	Ability to relate to the patient's perceptions and experiences	*"I can understand why it seems difficult to be physically active after work."*
Use of open-ended questions	Questions which require more thought and response than a simple yes or no. Designed to encourage a full and meaningful answer using the patient's own feelings and knowledge.	*"What makes you think it might be time for a change in your level of physical activity?"* *"How could an increase in your physical activity level benefit you?"*
Support patient self-efficacy	Supporting the patient to increase his or her confidence in the ability to increase his or her PA.	Ask patients about the changes they have made: *"It seems you've been working hard to increase your physical activity."* Follow-up with questions about how he/she feels about this change: *"How do you feel about the changes you made?"*
Use of reflective listening	A two-step communication strategy where the provider attempts to understand the patient's statements and then confirms with the patient that the provider has correctly understood.	*"It sounds like . . . ."* *"It seems as if . . . ."* *"What I hear you saying is . . . ."*

NOTE: PA, physical activity.

connecting patients to appropriate PA resources takes on added importance. Linking patients to these resources "extends" the typical boundaries of the healthcare team beyond the clinic setting to include outside PA programs and professionals. However, developing these PA "networks" can be difficult and time consuming, especially when connecting patients to community-based resources. Following, we discuss a number of strategies for developing and implementing referral systems to connect patients to existing PA resources.

Referring Patients to PA Resources Within a Health System

Many health systems may prefer to keep their patients "in-house" and encourage participation in programs under their control using their own trained personnel. This gives the health system a greater sense of quality control and provides a reduced sense of liability risk when referring patients to PA resources. Within each health system, there are generally a number of resources available to patients to guide and support them in becoming more physically active. Key to developing an "internal" referral network is maintaining an updated registry of existing resources that can be easily accessed by healthcare teams and provided to their patients (see Table 11.3).

Referring Patients to PA Resources Outside of the Health Setting

While health systems may initially attempt to utilize existing, internal PA resources, their capacity to provide high-quality options for a large number of patients may be limited considering the high prevalence of patients that are overweight/obese, have chronic diseases, and require PA guidance and support. Therefore, the referral process will likely need to link patients to external community resources. When developing a network of community-based PA resources, healthcare leaders should consider all available *places* (e.g., YMCAs), evidence-based *programs*, and credentialed exercise *professionals* for inclusion. In some instances, a quality control framework may be required to ensure that the programs, places, and professionals in a network meet preestablished standards in order to be eligible to receive patients from a healthcare system (Table 11.3).

Examples of Existing Exercise Referral Schemes

One of the largest exercise referral schemes (ERSs) was first established by the National Institute for Health and Care Excellence (NICE) in the United Kingdom in the 1990s (58). The ERS involved an initial physical assessment to screen for physical inactive individuals, followed by the healthcare professional referring his or her patients to a PA professional or program. As part of the NICE recommendations, ERSs are most effective with patients who are sedentary or inactive *and* have existing health conditions, putting them at an increased long-term health risk. Participating exercise professionals and programs are then encouraged to conduct personal assessments to determine the specific activity needs of the patient. Since their inception, ERSs have proliferated throughout the United Kingdom with more than 600 individual ERS in existence in 2011 (59). Studies show that the use of ERSs can increase the PA levels of patients, result in lower levels of depression and anxiety, and are moderately cost-effective relative to current payer thresholds (59, 60). A more recent review in 2015, commissioned by the National Institute for Health Research Health Technology Assessment program, supported these findings and suggested that ERSs lead to improvements in self-reported levels of PA when

TABLE 11.3. Potential referral sources for PA guidance and support

PA RESOURCES IN THE HEALTHCARE SETTING	PA RESOURCES IN THE COMMUNITY SETTING
▪ Cardiac rehabilitation ▪ Disease prevention and management programs ▪ Employee wellness programs ▪ Hospital-based walking programs ▪ Hospital-based wellness center or exercise facilities ▪ Physical therapy	▪ Boys & Girls Clubs of America ▪ City bike rental programs ▪ Community centers ▪ Joint-use facilities (i.e., school gyms open after school hours) ▪ Local gyms ▪ Outdoor exercise gyms ▪ Park and recreation facilities ▪ Pools ▪ Silver Sneaker programs ▪ University wellness centers ▪ YMCAs

NOTE: PA, physical acitivity.

compared to patients receiving advice only, particularly in older patients and patients with a greater number of cardiovascular disease risk factors (61).

Another example of a large-scale exercise referral program took place in Cuernavaca, Mexico, involving 108 physicians across four different primary healthcare centers (62). Inactive adults, 35 to 70 years of age and with hypertension, received either brief PA counseling by a primary care nurse in the clinic setting or were referred to group-based, PA interventions at the local Social Security center where they participated in group-based PA interventions guided by trained and certified exercise professionals. At the end of the trial, both groups had successfully increased the proportion of individuals meeting national PA guidelines. However, patients receiving the PA referrals were more successful in limiting their sedentary behavior compared to the patients receiving the brief PA counseling. These results demonstrate that providing patients with a PA referral to local community-based resources is equally, or more, effective in increasing activity levels as compared to the more resource-intensive provision of behavior counseling.

Self-Directed or Less Resource-Intensive Activities

In addition to referring patients to internal programs within a health system or to a network of community-based resources, it may also be useful to consider using self-directed, and other less resource-intensive, PA programs. For many patients, these options are more convenient, feasible, and acceptable than gym-based options. Other patients may not have the resources to hire exercise professionals to design and supervise their workouts. Self-directed programs may include individual or group walking programs, following (evidence-based) programs delivered via the Internet, or apps that guide patients through exercise routines and facilitate monitoring of their daily activity levels. One potential strategy is to initially refer patients, who are reluctant to join formal activity programs, to self-directed programs. If at the next follow-up visit their PA levels have not improved, then referral to supervised programs may be indicated.

Most urban centers have a number of less resource-intensive PA opportunities in the form of outdoor exercise equipment, city parks, and active transportation options. As an example, the Boston Medical Center formed a partnership with Boston Bikes. Their "prescribe-a-bike" program allowed physicians to give low-income residents a prescription for purchasing an annual pass for the city bikes for $5, instead of the regular price of $85. These prescriptions assisted patients in moving throughout the city while simultaneously improving their health (63). Another example of using existing PA resources is the National Park Prescription program (64). The National Park Prescription program involves a collaboration between health clinics, park agencies, and public health departments as part of an effort to use nature and public lands to improve individual and community health. To encourage outdoor activity, patients are given a prescription by their healthcare provider to specific programs at their local park that are led by trained park staff.

Utilizing PA Networks

Poor referral practices limit the overall effectiveness of any PA/ERS. The referral process should include an agreed upon set of criteria and procedures that are simple to implement and do not require providers to take on additional responsibilities for which they are ill-equipped. In some situations, the delivery and explanation of the PA referral process to patients may involve other members of the healthcare team, such as care coordinators or nurse managers. To ensure that the healthcare team is on the same page and engaged in the referral of patients, all team members should have the opportunity to provide input on the referral process and receive standardized training prior to its implementation.

When a network of internal and external PA resources is developed and activated, patients need to be referred to the appropriate PA resources according to their current health status. A "stepped approach" may involve the initial delivery of brief PA counseling, plus referral to self-directed programs, to assist patients in becoming more active. If ineffective, then healthier, stable patients can be referred to a wider array of group-based, community programs. Patients with a greater number of cardiovascular disease risk factors or other medical conditions that might inhibit them from being active (i.e., increasing frailty) will require referral to programs and professionals with greater levels of training and specialization (i.e., cardiac rehabilitation specialists or clinical exercise professionals). Having a range of activities and programs can better meet the diverse needs of a large patient population. Group-based programs are typically more cost-effective, providing greater access to a wider range of patients, particularly those in lower resources communities who may not be able to afford more costly programs or individualized guidance.

A final consideration when implementing a PA referral network is the transfer of relevant information between healthcare teams and the exercise professionals conducting the PA interventions. Healthcare providers should have a means to deliver general prescriptions, as well as advice concerning the health conditions of their patients, to exercise professionals. Ideally, the communication pathway will allow exercise professionals to provide information back to the healthcare team on the patient's progress and note any problems encountered throughout the program in a simple and easily accessible format (Box 11.6).

BOX 11.6

Comprehensive PA Integration in a Healthcare Setting—Adoption of PA by The Greenville Health System

The Greenville Health System, an academic healthcare delivery system that provides care for more than 3.6 million outpatient visits a year, is one of the first major U.S. health systems to commit to implementing an integrated and comprehensive model for promoting PA as a standard of care with all of their patients. This widespread integration first began with the addition of PA training embedded in all 4 years of the undergraduate medical education program at the University of South Carolina Greenville School of Medicine (65). PA was the first health behavior targeted for integration within the undergraduate medical curriculum with the goal of ensuring that students understand the physiological mechanisms behind exercise and disease prevention, improve their skills in guiding patient behavior change, and learn how to become "partners in care" with community PA resources. Tool kits were made and disseminated to all practicing physicians in the Greenville Health System, as part of an effort to train them to council patients on PA and effectively refer them to certified exercise professionals. Next, the Greenville Health System adopted the EIM Solution. The PAVS was integrated into their EMR to allow healthcare teams to systematically screen patient PA levels. Inactive patients receive an "order set" consisting of predeveloped exercise prescriptions for their specific medical condition. The patients are referred to one of the YMCAs in the Greenville area to participate in group-based PA interventions, led by exercise professionals with the EIM Credential, who have specialized training on working with health systems and patients with chronic diseases. Scholarships are provided by the Greenville Health System to patients who are unable to afford the cost of the YMCA group-based activity programs.

EIM, Exercise is Medicine; EMR, electronic medical record; PA, physical activity; PAVS, Physical Activity Vital Sign.

■ Strategies for Utilizing the Entire Healthcare Team

To effectively promote PA in clinic settings, health systems need to leverage what their primary care clinicians do well, combined with the strengths of practice staff, healthcare systems, and community agencies (66). There is no question that physicians play an important component in PA promotion across the life span. However, physicians often have inadequate time during patient visits to sufficiently address prevention and the optimization of healthy lifestyles. Therefore, it is necessary to utilize the entire healthcare team in the promotion of PA in these settings. As an example, the 5As do not all need to be performed by clinicians as the assessment of PA levels and readiness to change can be done by patients independently or medical staff using prespecified tools (67). The advising and agreeing steps build on the patient, family, and community relationships of primary care; the assisting and arranging steps could be coordinated with primary care staff, or community or healthcare system partners, depending on individual or local circumstances.

PA Promotion Efforts by Nurses, Nurse Practitioners, and Physician Assistants

The 3.1 million RNs in the United States make up the country's largest healthcare profession (68). Nurses are known as one of the most trusted health professions and serve as an important source of health-related advice, both inside and outside of the workplace. Because of their frequent contact with patients and proven ability to develop trusting, therapeutic relationships, nurses need to be considered as key players in PA promotion (69). The role of RNs may vary from basic assessment of PA to provision of PA counseling to leading exercise training and/or monitoring PA programs. PA assessment should be done at every routine patient encounter. Studies have shown that nurses can be specifically trained to deliver PA interventions in a variety of settings (e.g., in-home, community) (70–73). Not only have these interventions been successful in increasing PA, but these interventions have also shown to be cost-effective.

Similar to RNs, the advanced practice role of nurse practitioners and physician assistants focuses on preventive care and health promotion; as such, these healthcare providers also play a key role in promotion of PA among their patient populations. As fewer physicians are entering the primary care setting, nurse practitioners and physician assistants are filling the gap in healthcare provision. In fact, nurse practitioners are the quickest growing group of primary care providers, providing approximately 600 million patient visits per year (74). Furthermore, care provided by nurses and nurse practitioners has been shown to often be more cost-effective than physicians (75). Therefore, utilizing these healthcare providers in PA promotion could be a cost-effective way to increase population levels of PA. However, as many as 50% of advanced practice providers reported not receiving training in PA counseling (76). As such, the NPAP includes tactics to enhance PA education in the training of all healthcare professionals.

Opportunities and Roles for Medical Assistants and Other Clinic Staff

Medical assistants are allied health professionals present in numerous healthcare settings. Medical assistants typically have 1 year of training postsecondary school and are able to perform a variety of clinical duties in outpatient settings. Clinic-based health promotion programs have begun to examine the role of medical assistants in health coaching to improve health behaviors, including PA (77, 78). Ferrer and colleagues (78) examined a medical assistant-driven program of screening and referral for four health behaviors, including PA, compared to usual care. Medical assistants administered the International Physical Activity Questionnaire (IPAQ), informed patients of their health behavior risks, and referred patients to existing behavioral interventions. To address physical inactivity, patients could choose between a community-based walking program or a supervised 8-week low-impact aerobics program. At 1-year follow-up, patients who chose to address PA were twice as likely to attend a referral program compared to the control group.

Healthcare assistants, also known as nursing assistants, work under the guidance of nurses. Pears and colleagues (79) demonstrated that healthcare assistants can be instrumental in delivering brief PA interventions in the primary care setting. A feasibility study examined four brief PA interventions focused on motivation, action planning, pedometer use, or PA diaries. On average, each strategy took 5 minutes or less to implement during the patient visit and each strategy was rated as effective, acceptable, and feasible by both the patients and the healthcare assistants.

Home care aides are nonmedical paid caregivers who provide in-home services such as assistance with activities of daily living (ADLs) (i.e., bathing, dressing, eating). Home care aides have been utilized to implement home-based, low-intensity PA interventions (80, 81). In the Healthy Moves for Aging Well program, home care aides and other volunteer coaches delivered a tailored PA program to frail, high-risk sedentary seniors living at home with the goal of enhancing PA levels (80). Program participants maintained increases in PA 6 months after the end of the program (82) and reported a decrease in falls, depression, and pain (80).

Although several barriers to implementing PA promotion in the healthcare setting exist, many of these barriers can be overcome by fully utilizing the entire healthcare team in PA promotion. This includes office staff, who should also receive education and resources to facilitate PA promotion with clinic patients. The utilizations of existing exercise resources, such as the *Healthcare Providers Action Guide* developed by EIM®, can further assist all healthcare providers in integrating PA into the clinic setting. Furthermore, sustained, long-term change in implementing PA counseling in the clinic setting requires a commitment, not only from the entire healthcare team, but also from senior leaders of the health system. Healthcare leaders have the ability to increase capacity, introduce quality improvement initiatives, and incentivize their healthcare teams (i.e., through value recognition programs). This also involves understanding the long-term clinic practices that have been in place for years and developing innovative strategies for change supported by efficient decision support processes and the appropriate information technology.

Integrating PA for Disease Prevention and Treatment

The promotion of PA in health settings can be effective in addressing all three levels of public health prevention for a multitude of chronic diseases and health conditions. Here we will provide examples of these prevention strategies as they relate to PA promotion and health settings (Table 11.4).

Primary Prevention

It is well known that a physically active lifestyle is essential for the prevention of many chronic diseases and conditions. Further, PA activity reduces fall risk in older adults (83). Given that falls are the leading cause of injury-related deaths in older adults (84), prevention of falls and related injuries reduces disability, improves quality of life, and reduces healthcare costs. Therefore, the primary prevention of falls is a priority for the health and well-being of older adults. The USPSTF recommends PA as a strategy to prevent falls in community-dwelling older adults and recognizes the healthcare system as a key place to intervene during routine care provision (85). The National Institute on Aging's Frailty and Injuries: Cooperative Studies of Intervention Techniques (FICSIT) initiative represents a set of eight different clinical trials concerning physical frailty and injuries in later life (Box 11.7).

TABLE 11.4. Levels of prevention definitions and PA examples

LEVEL OF PREVENTION	GOAL	PA-SPECIFIC EXAMPLE
Primary	Prevent disease or health outcome before it occurs by addressing risk factors	▪ Provider encouragement for continuing an active lifestyle ▪ Provider assessment of current PA and, if not meeting recommended levels, provide PA counseling, prescription, and referral
Secondary	Early identification of disease or health outcome and prompt treatment in order to limit impact	▪ Chronic disease management plans include a focus on PA ▪ Prevention of treatment-related symptoms by increasing PA levels
Tertiary	Improve quality of life and reduce the long-term impact of a disease or health outcome	▪ Cardiac rehabilitation ▪ Home health programs that include low-intensity PA

NOTE: PA, physical activity.

BOX 11.7

The Seattle FICSIT/MoveIT study

The Seattle FICSIT/MoveIT study examined the effects of different intensities of endurance and strength training on outcomes of gait, balance, and fall risk. Patients, between 68 and 85 years of age, were recruited from primary care providers practicing in a large HMO system. The "FICSIT" part of the study compared strength and endurance training for 6 months across three groups: strength training only, endurance training only, or combined strength and endurance training. The "MoveIt" part of the study compared three different forms of endurance training: stationary cycling, walking, and aerobic exercise. The exercise groups were designed to simulate typical community programs in terms of frequency and duration of exercise. All groups exercised 3 days per week for approximately 1 hour. It was hypothesized that strength training would be superior to endurance training in improving gait and balance in adults with leg weakness. A second hypothesis was that more movement during exercise (i.e., aerobic

(continued)

(*continued*)

exercise) would promote greater improvement in gait and balance compared to cycling or walking exercise.

In the FICSIT arm, investigators found that exercise reduced the risk of falling by 47% (relative hazard = 0.53, 95% CI = 0.30–0.91). Between 7 and 18 months after randomization, control patients had more outpatient clinic visits ($p < .06$) and were more likely to sustain hospital costs over $5,000 ($p < .05$) (86). After 3 months in the MoveIT arm of the study, a dose–response relationship was found between balance and exercise: no exercise (control group): –6% improvement; low movement (cycle exercise): 3% improvement; medium movement (walking exercise): 7% improvement; and high movement (aerobic movement): 18% improvement (87).

FICSIT, Frailty and Injuries: Cooperative Studies of Intervention Techniques; HMO, health maintenance organization.

Secondary Prevention

There is strong evidence that meeting PA guidelines is related to a decreased risk of breast, endometrial, and colon cancer development (88). Furthermore, increasing and maintaining PA after a cancer diagnosis plays an important role in secondary prevention. For example, being physically active postdiagnosis (both during and after treatment) has been shown to decrease cancer-specific mortality and decrease the side effects of cancer therapy such as fatigue, nausea, and lymphedema (89). As such, exercise programs are an integral part of cancer care (Box 11.8).

BOX 11.8

The Physical Activity during Cancer Treatment (PACT) study

The PACT study examined the effects of exercise training during breast and colon cancer treatment in reducing complaints of fatigue, health service utilization, and sick leave. This 18-week exercise program was delivered in seven outpatient hospital clinics in the Netherlands and included twice weekly, supervised 1-hour exercise classes consisting of a combination of aerobic and muscle-strengthening training. In addition, patients were asked to be physically active for at least 30 minutes per day on three other days in the week. The program was individualized to the patient's personal preferences and current fitness level. The PACT trial was effective in reducing fatigue in both breast and colon cancer patients up to 9 months postintervention (90). Furthermore, cost analysis indicated that for patients with colon cancer, starting the 18-week exercise program as soon as possible after diagnosis was less costly and more effective. The intervention group had less healthcare usage and reported less hours of absence from work compared to usual care (91).

PACT, Physical Activity during Cancer Treatment.

Tertiary Prevention

Not only does a physically active lifestyle help prevent adverse health outcomes, such as diabetes or heart failure, it can also increase physical function, quality of life, and decrease mortality risk after a major health event occurs (i.e., heart attack, stroke, open heart

TABLE 11.5. The phases of cardiac rehabilitation

PHASE	SETTING	DURATION	DESCRIPTION
1: The acute phase	Inpatient	~3–5 d	Graded exercises (lasting 3–5 min or as tolerated), include early mobilization postsurgery.
2: The subacute phase	Outpatient rehab	~4–12 wk	Supervised exercise program, typically three times a week. Patient also receives prescription for at-home exercises
3: Intensive outpatient therapy	Outpatient rehab	6 mo	Patient begins to assume responsibility for self-monitoring exercise. Sessions are two to three times a week.
4: Maintenance	Home/ community	Indefinite	Patients have established exercise route that can be done independently at home or at an exercise facility.

surgery). Cardiac rehabilitation, or cardiac rehab, is a tailored, structured, medically supervised program for patient's postcardiac event. Cardiac rehab is a team approach and includes doctors, nurses, exercise specialists, physical therapists, dietitians, and other members of the healthcare team. Among the many patient goals in cardiac rehab, a major one is to teach the patient how to exercise safely and assist the patient in increasing his or her PA levels. (Table 11.5).

■ Adaptations for Low-Income Communities

Several subpopulations are less active than the population overall and warrant more focused promotion efforts. For example, more non-Hispanic white adults (23%) meet PA guidelines than non-Hispanic black (18%) and Hispanic (16%) adults (92). Furthermore, adults with less education and whose income is at or near the poverty level are also less likely to meet PA guidelines. When you couple these disparities in PA behavior with the fact that these vulnerable populations are also at greater risk of chronic conditions, such as obesity, diabetes, and cardiovascular disease, the need for PA promotion becomes even more urgent. Not only should PA be integrated in our larger health systems, but it is vital that efforts also focus on promoting PA at the community health clinics that often serve these vulnerable populations.

Federally Qualified Health Centers and Community Health Centers

Federally Qualified Health Centers (FQHCs), funded under the Public Health Service Act in 1944, provide comprehensive healthcare services in underserved areas across the country. In 2015, FQHCs provided approximately 97 million patient visits across nearly 10,000 service sites (93). FQHCs are a critical component of the U.S. healthcare system, providing primary and preventive care to various vulnerable populations. Currently, Medicaid and Medicare beneficiaries receive coverage for Annual Wellness Visits (AWV), which focus on preventive health and preventive activities, such as PA counseling. In addition, many FQHCs are involved in novel, grassroots PA promotion efforts. Following, we present two exemplars through which PA can be successfully integrated into FQHCs. Table 11.6 provides a list of potential PA resources for low-income communities.

The Community Free Clinic and the Cabarrus Health Alliance

Community Free Clinics provide comprehensive medical services at no cost to low income, uninsured residents (94). The Community Free Clinic in Cabarrus County, North Carolina, was founded in 1994 and is operated by part- and full-time staff that includes physicians, nurses, pharmacists, lab technicians, and a large volunteer team. Among those served by the Free Clinic are adults who have high blood pressure, diabetes, heart disease, and other chronic health conditions (95). In an effort to better serve their patients and the local community, the Community Free Clinic partnered with the Cabarrus Health Alliance (CHA) to integrate PA into their patient care. Clinic leadership and medical staff received training on assessing patient PA levels, providing PA counseling, and connecting patients to a database of county resources that the CHA had catalogued. Further, the CHA helped customize an "exercise prescription pad" for

TABLE 11.6. Resources for low-income communities

Walk With a Doc (96)	Started in 2005 by Dr. David Sabgir, the Walk With a Doc program is a grassroots effort to encourage healthcare providers to be active alongside their patients. A typical Walk With a Doc session starts with a brief presentation on a health topic by a healthcare provider who then leads participants on a walk at their own pace.
Park Prescription (64)	The National ParkRx Initiative consists of agencies dedicated to using nature and public lands to improve individual and community health. Park prescription is a movement to strengthen the connection between healthcare and parks with the goal of improvement of physical and mental health in individuals and communities. Park prescriptions offer an alternative to treating or preventing health problems through traditional medicine by connecting patients with parks and nature to increase levels of PA and reduce levels of stress.
Medicaid Wellness Visit (97)	Many Medicaid beneficiaries have access to one preventive health visit each calendar year. The AWV focuses on preventive health and the development of a written personalized prevention plan. During the AWV, clinicians can use standardized questionnaires recognized by national professional medical organizations to assess topics such as performance of ADLs and fall risk. Clinicians can also obtain the following measurements: height, weight, BMI (or waist circumference, if appropriate), and blood pressure. This visit can also include referrals to educational and counseling services or community-based lifestyle interventions to reduce health risks and promote self-management including: nutrition, PA, and weight loss. *Exact health coverage varies by state.*
Medicare Yearly Wellness Visit (98)	This visit is covered by Medicare once every 12 months and includes the completion of a health risk assessment addressing health behaviors such as PA and also includes a tailored discussion of preventive care.

NOTE: ADL, activities of daily living; AWV, Annual Wellness Visit; BMI, body mass index; PA, physical activity.

Date: ___ / ___ / ___   The Community Free Clinic ♡

Patient's name: _____   DOB: ___ / ___ / ___

Walk or exercise _____ minutes _____ days per week

for a total of _____ minutes per week.

Remember, you don't have to do all of your activity at once. Try three, 10 minute sessions throughout the day for a total of 30 minutes.

Ask about The Community Free Clinic's Free Exercise Class

Provider Signature: _____   Exe℞cise is Medicine®
                                                                    Your Prescription for Health

For office use only:

How many days/week of moderate to strenuous exercise?   *Find more exercise resources by clicking*
0   1   2   3   4   5   6   7

How many minutes per day?   *on the* 👟 *icon at*
0   10   20   30   40   50   60   90   120 or 150 or greater

Referral   **www.cabarrushealth.org/EIM**
CFC   Other _____

use by clinic practitioners. These efforts were launched in the second half of 2014 and many aspects of this program are still used today at the Community Free Clinic.

An evaluation of medical records between August 2015 and July 2016 revealed that the Community Free Clinic served 523 unique patients over a total of 2,790 visits to their Chronic Care Clinic. During this time, 44% of the patients discussed PA with their healthcare provider and received a written exercise prescription. Across all patients, a net weight loss of 0.25 pounds was observed, a remarkable feat considering that most adults typically gain weight over time and that the greatest levels of overweight and obesity are often observed in underserved populations. These initial efforts made by the Community Free Clinic, with assistance from the CHA, show just how critical the promotion of PA and a healthy lifestyle can be in positively impacting the health of uninsured and underserved populations.

The Piedmont Siler City Community Health Center

In Chatham County, North Carolina, the Chatham County Health Department partnered with the Piedmont Siler City Clinic (an FQHC) to integrate the EIM Solution into their clinic flow. The integration of the EIM Solution into the Piedmont Siler City Community Health Center consisted of five basic components: assessing patient PA levels, prescribing PA, referring patients to the EIM Referral Network, incorporating notes from the patient encounter into the EMR, and texting cues to action to the patients after their initial visit.

Patients at the Piedmont Siler City Community Health Center were eligible to receive PA counseling if they were 18 years or older, not pregnant or planning to become pregnant, and their physician felt it was safe for them to exercise. Patient PA levels were assessed using the PAVS. If a patient completed less than 150 minutes per week of moderate-intensity PA, it was marked on his or her "Pre-Visit Planning Form" (a standard form used for all patient visits), and the patient was offered the opportunity to participate in the EIM program. This indication alerted providers to review the patient's current PA levels and provide him or her with a written prescription based on the patient's readiness to change and PA preferences. Patients were then referred to the clinic care manager, who provided counseling to the patients, as well as access to a listing of all community-based PA resources that had agreed to participate in an EIM Referral Network. The patient was given a hard copy of the prescription and the referral with instructions to "fill" the prescription at one of the specified EIM Referral Network sites.

All PA prescriptions and EIM referrals were faxed to the Chatham County Health Department for follow-up. At 6, 18, and 24 weeks, patients were contacted by phone to provide feedback on their PA habits and use of the PA prescription. At subsequent office visits, patient PA levels were reassessed along with the other vital signs. Providers continued to discuss PA with their patients, adjusting the patient's PA prescription to meet their needs in helping them achieve and maintain 150 minutes of moderate to vigorous aerobic activity a week. The information recorded in the EMR system was pulled during chart reviews by Piedmont staff and provided to the Chatham County Health Department on an ongoing basis for evaluation purposes.

▓ Utilizing Technology to Promote PA in Healthcare Settings

EMR or electronic health records (EHRs) are digital versions of patients' medical history. Approximately 90% of office-based healthcare providers utilize EMRs (99), making this technology not only important in patient care, but its use also provides new opportunities for health promotion efforts. EMRs allow healthcare providers to track and manage patient data electronically. As mentioned earlier in this chapter, EMRs allow for the seamless integration of self-reported PA levels as a vital sign. Health systems are also developing the capability to collect real-time, patient-generated health data that can be directly imported into the EMR. Data from mobile health (mHealth) technologies has the potential to provide objective tracking of patient PA data, with the goal of eventually replacing self-reported data and its inherent flaws. However, the rapidly growing market of monitoring devices and remote sensing technologies has led to a lack of uniformity in PA data acquisition (i.e., different devices), representation (i.e., displayed in different manners, such as minutes per week vs. steps per day), and uniformity, posing a challenge for health systems to pragmatically upload and interpret this data (100). For health systems to use objective PA data obtained from consumer devices, this information must be transformed into clinically pertinent information that is easily usable and uploaded into patient EMRs for review by the healthcare team. Until these advancements are made, wide-scale deployment of mHealth technologies for assessing patient PA levels will be limited. More pragmatic tools, such as the PAVS, should continue—for the time being—to serve as the foundation for PA assessment in health systems.

Once organized within the EMR, PA data can be utilized by health systems to identify inactive individuals, trigger alerts, and support clinical counseling conducted by the healthcare team. Automated programs can provide patients with educational materials, such as the delivery of written or electronic PA prescriptions. Chronic disease prevention programs have already tapped into mHealth technology to send patients monthly reports, text reminders, and to facilitate interactions with a digital care team made up of health coaches (101). Research suggests that patients with chronic diseases are 50% more likely to fill a prescription for a health app than for a prescribed medication (102). Health systems may also design electronic systems (i.e., Internet-based programs or apps) that provide patients with real-time options to "fill" their exercise prescription.

With the capability to accurately monitor PA levels and provide real-time adaptive and personalized feedback, mHealth offers novel intervention strategies for patients and healthcare providers to impact long-term behavior change. Daily monitoring of PA levels (i.e., daily step counts) can engage patients in their own self-care, provide mechanisms for early intervention, and can be used to directly educate patients (102). Tailoring mHealth PA interventions, using real-time feedback, can provide context-specific, just-in-time support for behavior change delivered directly from the clinic setting (103). An mHealth intervention involving outpatients from a cardiovascular disease clinic examined the delivery of real-time PA level data (i.e., current step count and activity levels) from their wearable device, along with automated text messaging. Patients that received real-time information, compared to those receiving only automated messages, increased their PA levels by more than 2,500 steps per day (104). Increased use of mHealth technologies also facilitates more active communication between patients, their families, friends, and peers through social media and other networking sites (101), all of which can be targeted by interventions to increase PA levels. Overall, the opportunities for broad PA initiatives utilizing a growing array of patient-friendly "consumer" technologies have the capacity to transform healthcare and more effectively manage the growing sedentary behavior epidemic.

▨ Opportunities for the Future—Integration of Lifestyle Medicine

PA promotion in the clinic setting rarely takes place in isolation. There is increasing awareness of the equally important roles that other lifestyle habits, such as diet, sleep, and stress, play in our health and well-being. As such, many health systems are looking to take a more holistic, comprehensive approach in the preventive care of their patients. The growth of "lifestyle medicine" has been fueled by different think tanks and working groups that are pushing to increase the awareness of lifestyle medicine into medical schools and clinic practices (105). Following, we outline a case study that focuses on the role of PA as a part of the prevention strategy for type 2 diabetes (Box 11.9).

BOX 11.9

The National DPP

The National DPP was established by the Diabetes Prevention Act of 2009 and is supported by the CDC (106). The National DPP is a partnership of public and private organizations who share the common goal of reducing the national prevalence of type 2 diabetes. The National DPP provides evidence-based, affordable, and high-quality lifestyle change programs to reduce type 2 diabetes risk. A key component of the National DPP is the provision of a yearlong lifestyle modification program that focuses on nutrition, stress reduction, and increasing PA. The intervention is delivered by trained lifestyle coaches who help build participants' skills and

---

(continued)

(*continued*)

confidence to make lasting lifestyle changes. The lifestyle modification program consists of 16 sessions offered over 6 months (followed by monthly booster sessions thereafter) that provide participants with information and homework assignments, and offer feedback to optimize behavioral change. The PA-specific components of the lifestyle modification program include

- Introduction to PA
- Overcoming barriers to PA
- Environmental cues to eating and PA
- Dealing with slips in lifestyle change
- Mixing up your PA: aerobic fitness
- Tips for staying motivated
- How to make active choices
- PA barriers
- Preventing relapse

CDC, Centers for Disease Control and Prevention; National DPP, National Diabetes Prevention Program; PA, physical activity.

Summary

While integrating PA into health settings is certainly not a simple task, the overall population reach and long-term implications of these efforts have the potential to significantly impact a large and diverse population of individuals across the entire life span, nearly every health condition, and all socioeconomic groups. Given the wide body of evidence for primary, secondary, and tertiary disease prevention, providing PA guidance in health settings needs to become a standard part of the medical duty of care. With several major U.S. health guidelines including PA recommendations for the maintenance of good health, <u>not</u> providing this guidance to patients might be considered medical neglect, similar to failing to treat hypertensive patients or individuals with diabetes. In order to make PA promotion in healthcare a reality, a standard set of guidelines for providing PA counseling as a part of clinic care needs to be established so that change becomes a part of the institutional culture. This includes establishing a quality assurance framework that promotes best practices, guides planning and implementation, facilitates coordination of efforts at all levels of the health system, and encourages providers to meet specific benchmarks.

These changes will not happen all at once or in isolation. With medical practices hardwired after years of practice, transformational change requires a series of incremental, systemic changes performed gradually over time. Initial changes should be those that are most easily adoptable and require limited investment from the healthcare system. This may include providing brief PA trainings to the healthcare team during lunch-and-learn sessions or as a part of staff meetings to begin earning buy-in from key members of the healthcare team. Subsequent steps may include integrating tools for PA assessment into the clinic workflow and encouraging providers to emphasize the importance of PA to their inactive patients. More downstream strategies can then include writing PA prescriptions, providing formal behavior change counseling, and ensuring that all eligible patients receive a PA referral. At the end of the day, the goal is to ensure that healthcare providers and their teams engage in the "right thing to do, the easy thing to do" when working with their patients.

▣ Things to Consider

- ▪ Promoting PA in healthcare settings starts with the systematic assessment and recording of patient PA levels.
- ▪ To optimize PA promotion in healthcare settings, the entire healthcare team, from the administrative assistants to the executive leadership, must be involved.
- ▪ It is necessary for health settings to use all available PA resources at their disposal, located both internally and externally to their clinics.
- ▪ Connecting patients to supportive resources for PA is essential for their long-term engagement and positive health improvements.

▣ Resources

Resources available from Exercise is Medicine® at: http://www.exerciseismedicine.org/support_page.php/resources

- i. Assessing physical activity levels—The Physical Activity Vital Sign (PAVS)
    1. http://www.exerciseismedicine.org/assets/page_documents/The%20 Physical%20Activity%20Vital%20Sign%20without%20Strength_2015_07_09_PDF .pdf
- ii. Exercise Prescription Pads
    1. http://exerciseismedicine.org/assets/page_documents/EIM%20Prescription %20pad%201-up.pdf
    2. http://www.exerciseismedicine.org/canada/assets/page_documents/ EIMC_Pad_ENnewlogo_v3.0_1_copy.pdf
- iii. Exercise guidance for individuals with various health conditions—the EIM Prescription for Health series
    1. http://www.exerciseismedicine.org/support_page.php/your-rx-for-health-series
- iv. The Exercise is Medicine Healthcare Providers Action Guide
    1. http://exerciseismedicine.org/assets/page_documents/HCP_Action_Guide%285% 29.pdf

The National Physical Activity Plan—The Healthcare Setting

- i. http://www.physicalactivityplan.org/theplan/healthcare.html

Prescribing exercise for individuals with disabilities

- i. Foundation of Physical Medicine & Rehabilitation (FPM&R). Americans with fund: Rx for exercise. http://foundationforpmr.org/rx-for-exercise
- ii. National Center on Health, Physical Activity and Disability (NCHPAD). http://www.nchpad.org.

A tool kit for the design, implementation, and evaluation of exercise referral schemes. The British Heart Foundation National Centre for Physical Activity and Health. Loughborough University. 2011. http://www.ssehsactive.org.uk/exercisereferral/index.html.

Resources for motivational interviewing in the clinic setting

i. Rosengren DB. *Building Motivational Interviewing Skills: A Practitioner Workbook (Applications of Motivational Interviewing). 1st ed. New York, NY: The Guilford Press; 2009.*

ii. Levounis P, Arnaout B, Marienfeld C. *Motivational Interviewing for Clinical Practice.* 1st ed. Arlington, VA: American Psychiatric Association Publishing; 2017.

References

1. Blackwell DL, Villarroel MA. Tables of summary health statistics for U.S. adults: 2015. *National Health Interview Survey. National Center for Health Statistics.* 2016. http://www.cdc.gov/nchs/nhis/SHS/tables.htm. Accessed January 22, 2018.
2. Rui P, Hing E, Okeyode T. *National Ambulatory Medical Care Survey: 2014 State and National Summary Tables.* Available at: http://www.cdc.gov/nchs/ahcd/ahcd_products.htm. Accessed January 22, 2018.
3. Department of Health & Human Services. Healthy People website. Available at: https://www.healthypeople.gov. Accessed January 22, 2018.
4. The U.S. National Physical Activity Plan. Available at: http://www.physicalactivityplan.org. Accessed January 22, 2018.
5. Patrick K, Pratt M, Sallis RE. The healthcare sector's role in the U.S. national physical activity plan. *J Phys Act Health.* 2009;6(suppl 2):S211–S219. doi:10.1123/jpah.6.s2.s211
6. Bull FC, Gauvin L, Bauman A, et al. The Toronto charter for physical activity: a global call for action. *J Phys Act Health.* 2010;7(4):421–422. doi:10.1123/jpah.7.4.421
7. LeFevre ML. U.S. Preventive Services Task Force. Behavioral counseling to promote a healthful diet and physical activity for cardiovascular disease prevention in adults with cardiovascular risk factors: U.S. Preventive Services Task Force recommendation statement. *Ann Intern Med.* 2014;161(8):587–593. doi:10.7326/M14-1796
8. Jacobson DM, Strohecker L, Compton MT, et al. Physical activity counseling in the adult primary care setting: position statement of the American College of Preventive Medicine. *Am J Prev Med.* August 2005;29(2):158–162. doi:10.1016/j.amepre.2005.04.009
9. Sallis RE, Matuszak JM, Baggish AL, et al. Call to action on making physical activity assessment and prescription a medical standard of care. *Current Sports Med Reports.* 2016;15(3):207–214. doi:10.1249/JSR.0000000000000249
10. Vuori IM, Lavie CJ, Blair SN. Physical activity promotion in the health care system. *Mayo Clin Proc.* 2013;88(12):1446–1661. doi:10.1016/j.mayocp.2013.08.020
11. Calfas KJ, Long BJ, Sallis JF, et al. A controlled trial of physician counselling to promote the adoption of physical activity. *Prev Med.* 1996;25:225–233. doi:10.1006/pmed.1996.0050
12. Simons-Morton DG, Blair SN, King AC, et al. Effects of physical activity counseling in primary care: the activity counseling trial: a randomized controlled trial. *JAMA.* 2001;286(6):677–687. doi:10.1001/jama.286.6.677
13. Goldstein MG, Pinto BM, Marcus BH, et al. Physician-based physical activity counseling for middle-aged and older adults: a randomized trial. *Ann Behav Med.* 1999;21(1):40–47. doi:10.1007/BF02895032
14. Eakin EG, Glasgow RE, Riley KM. Review of primary care-based physical activity intervention studies: effectiveness and implications for practice and future research. *J Fam Pract.* 2000;49(2):158–168.
15. Pinto BM, Goldstein MG, Ashba J, et al. Randomized controlled trial of physical activity counseling for older primary care patients. *Am J Prev Med.* 2005;29(4):247–255. doi:10.1016/j.amepre.2005.06.016

16. Barnes PM, Schoenborn CA. Trends in adults receiving a recommendation for exercise or other physical activity from a physician or other health professional. *NCHS Data Brief.* 2012;86:1–8.

17. NCQA adds four new measures to HEDIS 2005. *Qual Lett Healthc Lead.* 2004;16(8):12–13.

18. National Committee for Quality. Assurance. Physical activity in older adults. Available at: http://www.ncqa.org/report-cards/health-plans/state-of-health-care-quality/2017-table-of-contents/physical-activity-in-older-adults. Accessed August 20, 2017.

19. Tai-Seale M, McGuire TG, Zhang W. Time allocation in primary care office visits. *Health Serv Res.* 2007;42(5):1871–1894. doi:10.1111/j.1475-6773.2006.00689.x

20. Chen LM, Farwell WR, Jha AK. Primary care visit duration and quality: does good care take longer? *Arch Intern Med.* 2009;169(20):1866–1872. doi:10.1001/archinternmed.2009.341

21. McPhail S, Schippers M. An evolving perspective on physical activity counselling by medical professionals. *BMC Fam Pract.* 2012;13:31. doi:10.1186/1471-2296-13-31

22. Huijg JM, Gebhardt WA, Verheijden MW, et al. Factors influencing primary health care professionals' physical activity promotion behaviors: a systematic review. *Int J Behav Med.* 2015;22(1):32–50. doi:10.1007/s12529-014-9398-2

23. Stoutenberg M, Shaya GE, Feldman DI, et al. Practical strategies for assessing patient physical activity levels in primary care. *Mayo Clin Proc Inn Qual Out.* 2017;1(1):8–15. doi:10.1016/j.mayocpiqo.2017.04.006

24. Strath SJ, Kaminsky LA, Ainsworth BE, et al. American Heart Association Physical Activity Committee of the Council on Lifestyle and Cardiometabolic Health and Cardiovascular, Exercise, Cardiac Rehabilitation and Prevention Committee of the Council on Clinical Cardiology, and Council. Guide to the assessment of physical activity: clinical and research applications: a scientific statement from the American Heart Association. *Circulation.* 2013;128(20):2259–2279. doi:10.1161/01.cir.0000435708.67487.da

25. Greenwood JL, Joy EA, Stanford JB. The Physical Activity Vital Sign: a primary care tool to guide counseling for obesity. *J Phys Act Health.* 2010;7(5):571–576. doi:10.1123/jpah.7.5.571

26. Coleman KJ, Ngor E, Reynolds K, et al. Initial validation of an exercise "vital sign" in electronic medical records. *Med Sci Sports Exerc.* 2012;44(11):2071–2076. doi:10.1249/MSS.0b013e3182630ec1

27. Institute of Medicine. *Capturing Social and Behavioral Domains and Measures in Electronic Health Records: Phase 2.* Washington, DC: The National Academies Press; 2014.

28. Young DR, Coleman KJ, Ngor E, et al. Associations between physical activity and cardiometabolic risk factors assessed in a Southern California health care system, 2010-2012. *Prev Chronic Dis.* 2014;11:E219. doi:10.5888/pcd11.140196

29. Ball TJ, Joy EA, Gren LH, et al. Predictive validity of an adult physical activity "vital sign" recorded in electronic health records. *J Phys Act Health.* 2016;13(4):403–408. doi:10.1123/jpah.2015-0210

30. Grant RW, Schmittdiel JA, Neugebauer RS, et al. Exercise as a vital sign: a quasi-experimental analysis of a health system intervention to collect patient-reported exercise levels. *J Gen Intern Med.* 2014;29(2):341–348. doi:10.1007/s11606-013-2693-9

31. Ross R, Blair SN, Arena R, et al. Importance of assessing cardiorespiratory fitness in clinical practice: a case for fitness as a clinical vital sign: a scientific statement from the American Heart Association. *Circulation.* 2016;134(24):e653–e699. doi:10.1161/CIR.0000000000000461

32. Jackson AS, Blair SN, Mahar MT, et al. Prediction of functional aerobic capacity without exercise testing. *Med Sci Sports Exerc.* 1990;22:863–870. doi:10.1249/00005768-199012000-00021

33. Mailey EL, White SM, Wójcicki TR, et al. Construct validation of a non-exercise measure of cardiorespiratory fitness in older adults. *BMC Public Health.* 2010;10:59. doi:10.1186/1471-2458-10-59

34. Jackson AS, Sui X, O'Connor DP, et al. Longitudinal cardiorespiratory fitness algorithms for clinical settings. *Am J Prev Med.* 2012;43:512–519. doi:10.1016/j.amepre.2012.06.032

35. Stamatakis E, Hamer M, O'Donovan G, et al. A non-exercise testing method for estimating cardiorespiratory fitness: associations with all-cause and cardiovascular mortality in a

pooled analysis of eight population-based cohorts. *Eur Heart J.* 2013;34:750–758. doi:10. 1093/eurheartj/ehs097

36. Altini M, Casale P, Penders J, et al. Cardiorespiratory fitness estimation using wearable sensors: laboratory and free-living analysis of context-specific submaximal heart rates. *J Appl Physiol.* 2016;120(9):1082–1096. doi:10.1152/japplphysiol.00519.2015

37. New Zealand Ministry of Health. Green Prescriptions. Available at: http://www.health.govt .nz/our-work/preventative-health-wellness/physical-activity/green-prescriptions. Accessed January 22, 2018.

38. Swinburn BA, Walter LG, Arroll B, et al. The Green Prescription study: a randomized controlled trial of written exercise advice provided by general practitioners. *Am J Public Health.* 1998;88(2):288–291. doi:10.2105/AJPH.88.2.288

39. Elley CR, Kerse N, Arroll B, et al. Effectiveness of counselling patients on physical activity in general practice: cluster randomised controlled trial. *BMJ.* 2003;326(7393):793. doi:10. 1136/bmj.326.7393.793

40. Hamlin MJ, Yule E, Elliot CA, et al. Long-term effectiveness of the New Zealand Green Prescription primary health care exercise initiative. *Public Health.* 2016;140:102–108. doi:10. 1016/j.puhe.2016.07.014

41. Swedish National Institute of Public Health. *Final Report of the Government Commissions of the National Evaluation of Physical Activity on Prescription (PAP).* Stockholm, Sweden; 2010.

42. Folkhälsoinstitut S. *Physical Activity on Prescription (PAP)—Individual Written Instructions for Physical Activity.* Stockholm, Sweden: Public Health Agency of Sweden; 2012.

43. Leijon ME, Bendtsen P, Nilsen P, et al. Does a physical activity referral scheme improve the physical activity among routine primary health care patients? *Scand J Med Sci Sports.* 2009;19(5):627–636. doi:10.1111/j.1600-0838.2008.00820.x

44. American College of Sports Medicine. Exercise is Medicine® Prescription Pads. Available at: http://exerciseismedicine.org/assets/page_documents/EIM%20Prescription% 20pad%201-up.pdf. Accessed January 22, 2018.

45. Canadian Society of Exercise Professionals. Exercise is Medicine® Canada Exercise Prescription & Referral Pad. Available at: http://www.exerciseismedicine.org/canada/assets/ page_documents/EIMC_Pad_ENnewlogo_v3.0_1_copy.pdf. Accessed January 22, 2018.

46. American College of Sports Medicine. Exercise is Medicine® Your Prescription for Health Series. Available at: http://www.exerciseismedicine.org/support_page.php/your-rx-for-health-series. Accessed January 22, 2018.

47. American Society of Exercise Physiologists. Standards of practice. Available at: https://www. asep.org/index.php/organization/practice. Accessed January 22, 2018.

48. American College of Sports Medicine. *The Exercise is Medicine® Credential.* Available at: https://www.acsm.org/get-stay-certified/get-certified/specialization/eim-credential. Accessed January 22, 2018.

49. Stoutenberg M, Stasi S, Stamatakis E, et al. Physical activity training in U.S. medical schools: preparing future physicians to engage in primary prevention. *Phys Sportsmed.* November 2015;43(4):388–394. doi:10.1080/00913847.2015.1084868

50. Berra K, Rippe J, Manson JE. Making physical activity counseling a priority in clinical practice: the time for action is now. *JAMA.* 2015;314(24):2617–2618. doi:10.1001/jama. 2015.16244

51. Carroll JK, Fiscella K, Epstein RM, et al. A 5A's communication intervention to promote physical activity in underserved populations. *BMC Health Serv Res.* 2012;12:374. doi:10. 1186/1472-6963-12-374

52. Carroll JK, Antognoli E, Flocke SA. Evaluation of physical activity counseling in primary care using direct observation of the 5As. *Ann Fam Med.* 2011;9(5):416–422. doi:10.1370/ afm.1299

53. O'Halloran PD, Blackstock F, Shields N, et al. Motivational interviewing to increase physical activity in people with chronic health conditions: a systematic review and meta-analysis. *Clin Rehabil.* 2014;28(12):1159–1171. doi:10.1177/0269215514536210

54. VanBuskirk KA, Wetherell JL. Motivational interviewing with primary care populations: a systematic review and meta-analysis. *J Behav Med.* August 2014;37(4):768–780. doi:10.1007/s10865-013-9527-4

55. Rubak S, Sandbæk A, Lauritzen T, et al. Motivational interviewing: a systematic review and meta-analysis. *Brit J Gen Pract.* 2005;55(513):305–312.

56. Miller WR, Rollnick S. *Motivational Interviewing: Helping People Change.* New York, NY: Guilford Press; 2012.

57. Charlton CR, Dearing KS, Berry JA, et al. Nurse practitioners' communication styles and their impact on patient outcomes: an integrated literature review. *J Am Acad Nurse Pract.* 2008;20:382–388. doi:10.1111/j.1745-7599.2008.00336.x

58. National Institute for Health and Care Excellence (NICE). Implementation of Physical Activity Referral Schemes in the United Kingdom. September 2014. *NICE Public Health Guidance 54.* Available at: https://www.nice.org.uk/guidance/ph54/chapter/1-recommendations. Accessed January 22, 2018.

59. Pavey TG, Taylor AH, Fox KR, et al. Effect of exercise referral schemes in primary care on physical activity and improving health outcomes: systematic review and meta-analysis. *BMJ.* 2011;343:d6462. doi:10.1136/bmj.d6462

60. Murphy SM, Edwards RT, Williams N, et al. An evaluation of the effectiveness and cost effectiveness of the National Exercise Referral Scheme in Wales, UK: a randomized controlled trial of a public health policy initiative. *J Epidemiol Community Health.* 2012;66(8):745–753. doi:10.1136/jech-2011-200689

61. Campbell F, Holmes M, Everson-Hock E, et al. A systematic review and economic evaluation of exercise referral schemes in primary care: a short report. *Health Technol Assess.* 2015;19(60):1–110. doi:10.3310/hta19600

62. Gallegos-Carrillo K, García-Peña C, Salmerón J, et al. Brief counseling and exercise referral scheme: a pragmatic trial in Mexico. *Am J Prev Med.* 2017;52(2):249–259. doi:10.1016/j.amepre.2016.10.021

63. Singh V. Boston doctors write "prescriptions" for bike-share program. *CBS News.* April 12, 2014. Available at: https://www.cbsnews.com/news/boston-doctors-write-prescriptions-for-bike-share-program. Accessed January 22, 2018.

64. The National Park Rx Initiative. Available at: www.parkrx.org. Accessed January 22, 2018.

65. Trilk JL, Phillips EM. Incorporating 'Exercise is Medicine' into the University of South Carolina School of Medicine Greenville and Greenville Health System. *Br J Sports Med.* 2014;48:165–167. doi:10.1136/bjsports-2013-093157

66. Stange KC, Woolf SH, Gjeltema K. One minute for prevention: the power of leveraging to fulfill the promise of health behavior counseling. *Am J Prev Med.* 2002;22(4):320–323. doi:10.1016/S0749-3797(02)00413-0

67. Whitlock EP, Orleans T, Pender N, et al. Evaluating primary care behavioral counseling interventions: an evidenced-based approach. *Am J Prev Med.* 2002;22(4):267–284. doi:10.1016/S0749-3797(02)00415-4

68. Health Resources and Services Administration. *The Registered Nurse Population: Findings From the 2008 National Sample Survey of Registered Nurses.* Washington, DC: U.S. Department of Health and Human Services; 2010.

69. Richards E. The evolution of physical activity promotion: implications for nurses. *Am J Nurs.* 2015;115(8):50–54. doi:10.1097/01.NAJ.0000470400.28683.97

70. Ebrahim S, Thompson PW, Baskaran V, et al. Randomized placebo-controlled trial of brisk walking in the prevention of postmenopausal osteoporosis. *Age Ageing.* 1997;26(4):253–260. doi:10.1093/ageing/26.4.253

71. Robertson MC, Gardner MM, Devlin N, et al. Effectiveness and economic evaluation of a nurse delivered home exercise programme to prevent falls. 2: controlled trial in multiple centres. *BMJ.* 2001;32(7288):701–704. doi:10.1136/bmj.322.7288.701

72. Richards E, Cai Y. Integrative review of nurse-delivered physical activity interventions in primary care. *West J Nurs Res.* 2016;38:484–507. doi:10.1177/0193945915581861

73. Richards E, Cai Y. Integrative review of nurse-delivered community-based physical activity promotion. *Appl Nurs Res.* 2016;31:132–138. doi:10.1016/j.apnr.2016.02.004

74. Naylor MD, Kurtzman ET. The role of nurse practitioners in reinventing primary care. *Health Aff (Millwood)*. 2010;29(5):893–899. doi:10.1377/hlthaff.2010.0440

75. Chenoweth D, Martin N, Pankowski J, et al. Nurse practitioner services: three-year impact on health care costs. *J Occup Environ Med*. 2008;50(11):1293–1298. doi:10.1097/JOM.0b013e318184563a

76. Grimstvedt ME, Der Ananian C, Keller C, et al. Nurse practitioner and physician assistant physical activity counseling knowledge, confidence and practices. *Prev Med*. 2012;54:306–308. doi:10.1016/j.ypmed.2012.02.003

77. Djuric Z, Segar M, Orizondo C, et al. Delivery of health coaching by medical assistants in primary care. *J Am Board Fam Med*. 2017;30(3):362–370. doi:10.3122/jabfm.2017.03.160321

78. Ferrer RL, Mody-Bailey P, Jaen CR, et al. A medical assistant-based program to promote healthy behaviors in primary care. *Ann Fam Med*. 2009;7(6):504–512. doi:10.1370/afm.1059

79. Pears S, Morton K, Bikjer M, et al. Development and feasibility study of very brief interventions for physical activity in primary care. *BMC Public Health*. 2015;15:333. doi:10.1186/s12889-015-1703-8

80. Yan T, Wilber KH, Wieckowski J, et al. Results from the healthy moves for aging well program: changes of the health outcomes. *Home Health Care Serv Q*. 2009;28(2-3):100–111. doi:10.1080/01621420903176136

81. Muramatsu N, Yin L, Lin TT. Building health promotion into the job of home care aides: transformation of the workplace health environment. *Int J Environ Res Public Health*. 2017;14(4):doi:10.3390/ijerph14040384

82. Wieckowski J, Simmons J. Translating evidence-based physical activity interventions for frail elders. *Home Health Care Serv Q*. 2006;25(1-2):75–94. doi:10.1300/J027v25n01_05

83. Physical Activity Guidelines Advisory Committee. *Physical Activity Guidelines Advisory Committee Report, 2008*. Washington, DC: U.S. Department of Health and Human Services; 2008.

84. Centers for Disease Control and Prevention. *Stopping Elderly Accidents, Death & Injuries (STEADI)*. 2017. Available at: https://www.cdc.gov/steadi/materials.html. Accessed January 25, 2018.

85. U.S Preventive Services Task Force. *Final Recommendation Statement: Falls Prevention in Older Adults: Counseling and Preventive Medication*. 2016. Available at: https://www.uspreventiveservicestaskforce.org/Page/Document/RecommendationStatementFinal/falls-prevention-in-older-adults-counseling-and-preventive-medication. Accessed January 25, 2018.

86. Buchner DM, Hornbrook MC, Kutner NG, et al. Development of the common data base for the FICSIT trials. *J Am Geriatr Soc*. 1993;41(3):297–308. doi:10.1111/j.1532-5415.1993.tb06708.x

87. Buchner DM, Cress ME, de Lateur BJ, et al. A comparison of the effects of three types of endurance training on balance and other fall risk factors in older adults. *Aging Clin Exp Res*. 1997;9:112–119. doi:10.1007/BF03340136

88. National Cancer Institute. *Physical activity and cancer*. Available at: https://www.cancer.gov/about-cancer/causes-prevention/risk/obesity/physical-activity-fact-sheet. Accessed January 22, 2018.

89. Kushi LH, Doyle C, McCullough M, et al. American Cancer Society guidelines on nutrition and physical activity for cancer prevention. *CA Cancer J Clin*. 2012;62:30–67. doi:10.3322/caac.20140

90. Travier N, Velthuis M, Steins Bisschop C, et al. Effects of an 18-week exercise programme started early during breast cancer treatment: a randomised controlled trial. *BMC Medicine*. 2015;13(1):1–12. doi:10.1186/s12916-015-0362-z

91. May AM, Bosch MJ, Velthuis MJ, et al. Cost-effectiveness analysis of an 18-week exercise programme for patients with breast and colon cancer undergoing adjuvant chemotherapy: the randomized PACT study. *BMJ Open*. 2017;7(3):doi:10.1136/bmjopen-2016-012187

92. Centers for Disease Control and Prevention. *Facts about physical activity*. Available at: https://www.cdc.gov/physicalactivity/data/facts.htm. Accessed January 25, 2018.

93. Kaiser Family Foundation. *Community health center delivery sites and patient visits— 2015.* Available at: http://www.kff.org/other/state-indicator/community-health-center-sites-and-visits/?currentTimeframe=0&sortModel=%7B%22colId%22:%22Location%22,%22sort%22:%22asc%22%7D. Accessed January 22, 2018.
94. The National Association of Free & Charitable Clinics. Available at: http://www.nafcclinics.org Accessed January 22, 2018.
95. The Community Free Clinic. Available at: https://communityfreeclinic.org. Accessed January 22, 2018.
96. Walk With a Doc. Available at: www.walkwithadoc.org. Accessed January 22, 2018.
97. Medicaid.gov. *Prevention.* Available at: www.medicaid.gov/medicaid/benefits/prevention/index.html. Accessed January 22, 2018.
98. Medicare.gov. *Your Medicare coverage.* Available at: www.medicare.gov/coverage/preventive-visit-and-yearly-wellness-exams.html. Accessed January 22, 2018.
99. Jamoom E, Yang N. Table of electronic health record adoption and use among office-based physicians in the U.S., by state: 2015. *National Electronic Health Records Survey.* 2016. Available at: https://www.cdc.gov/nchs/data/ahcd/nehrs/2015_nehrs_web_table.pdf.
100. Lobelo F, Kelli HM, Tejedor SC, et al. The wild wild west: a framework to integrate mHealth software applications and wearables to support physical activity assessment, counseling and interventions for cardiovascular disease risk reduction. *Prog Cardiovasc Dis.* 2016;58(6):584–594. doi:10.1016/j.pcad.2016.02.007
101. Milani RV, Franklin NC. The role of technology in healthy living medicine. *Prog Cardiovasc Dis.* 2017;59(5):487–491. doi:10.1016/j.pcad.2017.02.001
102. Milani RV, Bober RM, Lavie CJ. The role of technology in chronic disease care. *Prog Cardiovasc Dis.* 2016;58(6):579–583. doi:10.1016/j.pcad.2016.01.001
103. O'Reilly GA, Spruijt-Metz D. Current mHealth technologies for physical activity assessment and promotion. *Am J Prev Med.* 2013;45(4):501–507. doi:10.1016/j.amepre.2013.05.012
104. Martin SS, Feldman DI, Blumenthal RS, et al. mActive: a randomized clinical trial of an automated mHealth intervention for physical activity promotion. *J Am Heart Assoc.* 2015;4(11):doi:10.1161/JAHA.115.002239
105. Institute of Lifestyle Medicine. Available at: http://www.instituteoflifestylemedicine.org. Accessed January 22, 2018.
106. Centers for Disease Control and Prevention. *National Diabetes prevention program.* Available at: https://www.cdc.gov/diabetes/prevention/index.html. Accessed January 22, 2018.

PHYSICAL ACTIVITY PROMOTION IN SCHOOLS

RUSSELL L. CARSON | JAIMIE MCMULLEN | BRIAN D. DAUENHAUER |
DANIELLE R. BRITTAIN

LEARNING OBJECTIVES

By the end of this chapter, the student should be able to

1. Describe what a comprehensive school physical activity program includes.
2. Discuss PA interventions in schools that work.
3. Compare school-based policies for PA promotion.
4. Appraise areas where culture needs to be considered in developing school-based interventions.
5. Develop a multicomponent school-based PA intervention.

▨ Introduction

I do believe it is both fair and indeed essential that our schools lead the way and do everything they reasonably can do to help increase physical activity among children and adolescents

—*Dr. Russell Pate (1)*

This testimony made before the U.S. Senate in 2010 remains true today. Schools are a major public resource for promoting physical activity (PA) in youth. Key factors that make schools one of the most influential settings for PA promotion include:

I. In the fall of 2017, approximately 56 million U.S. children/adolescents were enrolled in public and private schools in which they attended school 8 to 9 hours most days per week (2).
A. Schools can provide equal access for all children regardless of demographic status to learn about and practice PA when they are young and develop habits for a lifetime (3).

© Springer Publishing Company DOI: 10.1891/9780826134592.0012

B. Schools can engage and encourage parents, often gatekeepers to children's out-of-school time activities, to participate in and learn from school-based PA interventions.

II. Evidence clearly links youth PA to academic achievement and brain health (4). PA participation has been shown to improve students' grades, school attendance, cognitive performance (e.g., memory, concentration), and classroom behaviors (e.g., on-task behavior) (5).

III. Schools are large employers in communities and often the central hub of communities.

   A. Worksite PA/wellness programs have a great potential to improve the overall health of school employees as well as provide workplace benefits (e.g., reduced healthcare costs and absenteeism; improved morale and productivity) (6).

   B. Physically active and health-conscious school staff can serve as role models for not only children/adolescents and coworkers within the school, but also parents and other community members (7).

   C. Utilizing the existing collaborative relations with multiple community sectors (e.g., public health, healthcare, business and industry, transportation), schools are uniquely positioned to provide opportunities to promote PA to all community residents (8).

IV. Schools can help mobilize PA opportunities before, during school, and after school because of available physical infrastructures (e.g., gyms, classrooms, playgrounds); organizational resources (e.g., established schedule for 9 months a year; staff/faculty content expertise and roles); policies and policy-making structures (e.g., PE class time requirements); and communication systems (e.g., daily announcements to students, letters sent home to parents). A whole-of-school approach, defined as utilizing the breadth of available PA opportunities at a school in a coordinated manner, is recommended for increasing PA during the school day and supporting all students in their quest of reaching 60 minutes or more of PA each day (3, 9).

■ Comprehensive School Physical Activity Program Model

The comprehensive school physical activity program (CSPAP) is the leading national model for planning and organizing whole-of-school PA interventions (9). Centered around the academic subject of *physical education (PE)* and its delivery of standards-based curricula and instruction focused on developing students' knowledge, skills, and dispositions for lifelong movement (10), the CSPAP model also includes *PA during school* opportunities (e.g., recess, classroom movement integration) and *PA before and after school* opportunities (e.g., active transportation) where *staff are involved* (e.g., employee wellness program) and *family and community are engaged* (e.g., fitness nights or homework) (9). The CSPAP model depicted in Figure 12.1 illustrates the collective possibilities of school PA interventions to foster at least 60 minutes of daily PA, of which 30 minutes or more should be accomplished during school hours (3). The five interactive components provide a strategic map for addressing the PE and PA aspect of the Whole School, Whole Community, Whole Child (WSCC) model via targeted points

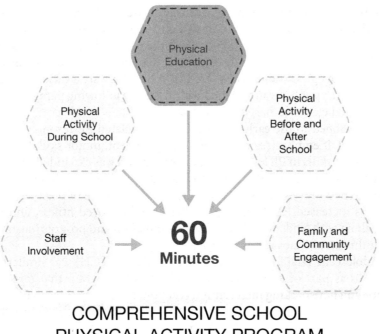

COMPREHENSIVE SCHOOL
PHYSICAL ACTIVITY PROGRAM

FIGURE 12.1 The CSPAP model, as graphically displayed by the University of Northern Colorado Active Schools Institute.
CSPAP, comprehensive school physical activity program.

of intervention for increasing PA in schools (9). In the following section, we review the most promising school-based PA interventions by single CSPAP component area and multicomponent areas.

■ PA Interventions That Work in Schools

PE Interventions

PE is a course of study in K-12 schools that "provides students with a planned, sequential, standards-based program of curricula and instruction designed to develop motor skills, knowledge, and behaviors for active living, physical fitness, sportsmanship, self-efficacy, and emotional intelligence" (10). Quality PE consists of sufficient instructional time to engage learners at each educational level (i.e., 150 minutes per week at the elementary level; 225 minutes per week at the secondary level), full inclusion of all students regardless of individual characteristics, and at least 50% of lesson time spent in moderate- to vigorous-intensity physical activity (MVPA) (10). PE is widely acknowledged as the cornerstone of a CSPAP (9, 10).

Sallis and McKenzie (11) coined the term "health-related physical education" to underline the distinct public health role for PE that included two primary objectives: (a) prepare youth for a lifetime of PA and (b) provide children with ample PA during classes. Within this approach, other traditional objectives of PE are still considered attainable but are not emphasized at the expense of health-enhancing PA engagement. In 2012, the authors revisited PE's role in public health and rephrased the approach "health-optimizing physical education" (HOPE) (12). Over the past three decades, scholars have conceptualized how PE can meaningfully contribute to public health goals using a variety of curricular and pedagogical frameworks (13, 14). While there are a variety of curricular resources that support a public health agenda within PE, the following paragraphs discuss two highly researched evidence-based resources.

SPARK was developed in the early 1990s as a health-related PE resource for the elementary school level. It emphasizes maximal PA engagement, motor skill development, and self-management skills in PE lessons. Later, the program was expanded to the middle school level and now includes early childhood and after-school components. It is one of the most researched PE resources available (15), with evidence of positive child-level outcomes such as increased PA during PE classes (16), improved fitness, and reduced adiposity (17), along with evidence of effective dissemination and program sustainability based upon a diffusion of innovations model (18).

Child and Adolescent Trial for Cardiovascular Health (CATCH) was similarly developed in the 1990s as part of a coordinated school health program that targeted diet, physical activity, and nonsmoking intervention components among third to fifth graders. The PE resource, designed for use by both PE specialists and classroom teachers, emphasized maximal MVPA during PE classes using effective instructional/management techniques and developmentally appropriate activities (19). Evidence has indicated that with ongoing professional development, teachers are able to increase MVPA during lessons to the recommended level of 50% (20), and positive effects are maintained for up to 5 years postintervention (21, 22).

Beyond curricular resources, there are also basic strategies used by teachers to maximize PA time during PE. Weaver et al. (23) summarize them quite effectively as the LET US Play principles: reduce time waiting in Lines, avoid Elimination games, keep Team sizes small, limit the number of Uninvolved students, and adjust Space, equipment, and rules to maximize participation. These basic strategies are presented in many foundational PE textbooks and are embedded within the curricular resources for teachers mentioned earlier. Overall, systematic reviews indicate that MVPA can be increased in PE using curricular and instructional interventions, with ongoing professional development emerging as a contributing element (24, 25). However, recent evidence suggests that programs continue to struggle to achieve the 50% MVPA benchmark, with elementary schools averaging approximately 45% MVPA and secondary schools averaging around 41% (26, 27). When coupling these modest proportions of MVPA with recent reports that only 22 U.S. states have time-specific requirements for PE, of which a small percentage meet or exceed the weekly PE minute recommendations at the elementary school level (37%) and secondary school level (20%), reiterates the importance of implementing PA interventions beyond PE (28).

During School Interventions

When considering incorporating PA during the school day, two primary intervention strategies have been studied: classroom movement integration and recess interventions.

Classroom Movement Integration

Classroom movement integration involves incorporating movement into the academic classroom in a variety of different capacities. Although the different strategies share a common goal, to reduce sedentary time throughout the school day, they vary with respect to the purpose of the movement. In general, movement integration activities seek to infuse PA into general education classrooms (3). At both the elementary and secondary school levels, teachers/schools can implement active transitions, energizers (also called brain breaks or activity breaks), and lessons that incorporate academic content with movement.

The research of classroom movement interventions have been comprehensively reviewed (29). Several recent publications describe the positive impact of classroom-based PA on several outcomes including PA levels (30, 31), academic achievement (32), and behavioral components such as improved concentration (33) and on-task behavior (34). Several associated studies have also considered the perceptions of teachers with respect to movement in the classroom. For example, Martin and Murtagh (30) discussed the importance of teacher satisfaction relative to increasing the probability of ongoing implementation. While teachers have positive dispositions toward PA in their classrooms, they report several competing pressures such as time and testing requirements that impact their ability to incorporate PA for their students throughout the school day (35, 36). Given the benefits of movement in the classroom, it is important to consider the perspectives of teachers and provide them with the necessary resources and tools to meaningfully incorporate PA in their classrooms.

Recess

Recess, lunch, and other break periods have also been identified as important opportunities for PA during the school day. At the elementary school level, recess can be enhanced by having age-appropriate equipment and adult recess supervisors who provide encouragement or activity ideas for students (37). At the middle and high school level, recess-like strategies can include daily schoolwide PA during morning announcements, drop-in PA sessions during lunch, and PA breaks during extended block periods (37).

Research suggests that environmental modifications to recess settings, such as creating "zones" for different activities, training recess supervisors, and providing equipment, have positive, but nonsignificant increases in PA during recess for elementary school children (38, 39). Conclusions of these studies have specifically identified the need for trained and effective recess supervisors and the consideration of school and student-level variables. Another strategy that has been less advocated, but has demonstrated positive effects on PA levels in adolescent girls, is peer-led programs that incorporate other students as motivational and emotional support for low active students (40). Additional recess intervention research can be accessed in a review (41).

Before School Interventions

Before-school PA programs are attractive because they have the added benefit of stimulating children's minds prior to the start of the school day (42), and they have the potential of contributing to the physical health of youth without sacrificing instructional time. Studies suggest that when children participate in PA before engaging in learning tasks, they tend to have better focus and perform better cognitively (43).

Research on the effectiveness of before-school PA interventions is still in its infancy, but two programs appear to hold the most promise. One program called Build Our Kids Success (BOKS) consists of 45-minute sessions 2 or 3 days per week, with a warm-up, aerobic activity, skill of the week, game time, and cool down. Session leaders utilize a formal curriculum with activity ideas and nutrition education content. Preliminary evidence indicates that elementary-aged children obtain approximately 20 minutes of MVPA during sessions (44) and can experience improvements in aerobic endurance and body composition with continued participation (45).

A second type of program, mileage clubs, consist of walking/running programs where children complete laps on a track, log their mileage, and earn incentives for reaching milestones (e.g., marathon distance). Commercial programs such as the 100 Mile Club are available, but many schools develop their own programs and systems for tracking mileage. Research suggests that children can accrue approximately 10 minutes of MVPA during 15 to 20 minute mileage club sessions (46) and tend to demonstrate better on-task behavior in the classroom after participation (47).

After School Interventions

After-school PA opportunities also offer health benefits without surrendering academic learning time. Traditional opportunities for after-school PA include childcare/enrichment programs, specialized PA clubs, intramural sports, and interscholastic sports.

Childcare/Enrichment Programs

Approximately 10 million children attend after-school childcare/enrichment programs in the United States (48). As such, the public health potential of promoting PA within these programs is substantial. According to the National AfterSchool Association (49), after-school programs are recommended to devote at least 30 minutes to PA each day, with 50% of that time spent in MVPA. Strategies for maximizing PA time during after-school programs include: (a) deliberately scheduling PA into daily routines (50), (b) having staff members engage with children (51, 52), and (c) following the LET US Play principles when facilitating activities/games (53). Structured curricula also exist to help program staff integrate PA into after-school programs. CATCH Kids Club, SPARK After-School, and Youth Fit for Life are a few programs that have been empirically tested, with mixed effects for PA participation in CATCH Kids Club (54, 55) and SPARK After-School interventions (56), and positive effects for fitness and voluntary PA participation in Youth Fit for Life (57).

Clubs

Specialized PA clubs tend to target certain segments of the population or focus on one particular sport. For example, GoGirlGo!, Girls on the Move, and Girls on the Run are all interventions designed to promote PA and life skills to sedentary girls after school. In parallel, the SCORES program is a PA club focused primarily on the sport of soccer. Empirical evidence indicates mixed results for promoting PA behaviors among youth (58, 59), with identified barriers to participation including lack of transportation, limited administrator support, and conflicting obligations, particularly in urban, high-poverty schools (60, 61).

Sports

Intramural and interscholastic sports are additional opportunities for children to accumulate PA after school. Intramural sports are typically open to all students, while interscholastic sports are offered to the most highly skilled athletes. Sport participation is associated with a myriad of benefits for children, including improved nutritional behaviors (62), reduced depression (63), and better academic achievement (64). A large-scale study in Canada found a positive association between the number of interscholastic sports offered in schools and self-reported participation among students (65). However, research has demonstrated that intramural sports have higher participation rates and allow for greater PA participation during sessions/practices (66); therefore, intramurals are recommended as an effective supplement to interscholastic sports.

Multicomponent School Interventions

There are fewer attempts to implement multicomponent PA interventions than single-component PA interventions (67). Aligned with the centerpiece of the CSPAP model, existing multicomponent PA interventions typically start with providing health-enhancing PE curricula, followed by the implementation of PA during school interventions via enhanced recess (e.g., structured activity zones, mobile PA equipment cart) or classroom movement integration (e.g., multiple 5-minute PA breaks), and PA after-school interventions (e.g., specialized PA club). Results indicate that PE +1 or +2 component interventions are modestly beneficial to children's objectively measured PA behaviors (e.g., 4–5 minutes more of MVPA per day or 1,000+ more step counts per day) and other student outcomes such as improvements in enjoyment, health-related physical fitness, classroom on-task behavior, cardiometabolic health markers (e.g., adiposity, cholesterol levels), and academic performance (68–70). Published multicomponent school PA interventions that also include family/community engagement or staff involvement interventions are rare, as is the evidence for the impact of a full five-component CSPAP model (96). However, reviews have indicated multicomponent school-based interventions are more effective at increasing children's PA behavior during school than single-component interventions (71, 72).

The main challenge of multicomponent PA interventions is that intervention efforts often occur in isolation across different segments of the school day. Applying long-standing principles from school health promotion models (e.g., social ecological model, WSCC model) (73, 74), the coordination of interconnected levels of influence are recommended for integrating multiple and, ultimately, impactful PA interventions throughout schools (3). The CSPAP conceptual framework depicted in Figure 12.1 addresses key facilitators and the importance of coordinators, often led by a trained CSPAP champion, for multicomponent PA interventions to operate in unison and meaningfully contribute to PA opportunities and behaviors at school (Figure 12.2) (75). For maximum benefit, multicomponent school PA interventions should apply carefully tailored *expansion* (i.e., adding new PA opportunities), *extension* (i.e., increasing time allocated to existing PA opportunities), and *enhancement* (i.e., augmenting existing PA opportunities with evidence-based practices) strategies (76).

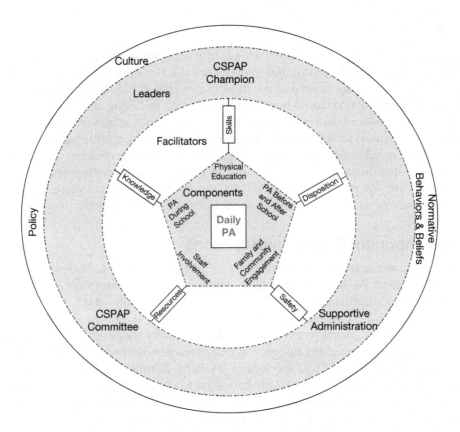

FIGURE 12.2 A conceptual framework for CSPAP research and practice based on a social ecological perspective.
CSPAP, comprehensive school physical activity program.

Source: Reprinted with permission from Carson RL, Castelli DM, Beighle A, et al. School-based physical activity promotion: a conceptual framework for research and practice. *Child Obes.* 2014;10(2):100–106. doi:10.1089/chi.2013.0134

▦ Current Issues in School PA Promotion

Emerging areas of science or practice that may inform the implementation of school-based PA interventions are presented in the following.

Professional Training Opportunities

Since presented as one of the Institute of Medicine's (IOM) (3) six recommendations for improving schoolwide PA, a growing number of professional training opportunities now exist for current and future school professionals to advance the implementation of CSPAP interventions. Most common, with modest effectiveness (77), is the continuing professional development of practicing teachers (mostly physical educators) to be trained as school-level CSPAP champions (i.e., Physical Activity Leader [PAL]). This form of training, currently known as the PAL learning system, typically starts with 1 day, in-person workshops that familiarize participants with CSPAP implementation steps (37) followed by yearlong mentorship and online resource support (78). Comparable CSPAP-related professional training is also occurring in university PE teacher education programs where undergraduate and graduate students are provided with CSPAP learning experiences ranging from coursework assignments and field experiences to research training (79). The shift in a broader focused, redesigned professional preparation curricula is referred to as Integrative Public Health-Aligned Physical Education (IPHPE), and the intended school-level consequences on daily school PA behaviors are not yet determined (14).

Technology Usage

Whether in the traditional classroom (e.g., computers, tablets, television, Internet videos, and applications) or in PE (e.g., heart rate monitors, accelerometers, pedometers, phone applications, smart watches, screen-based active video gaming [AVGs]), technology use is infiltrated into schools. Every year, public schools spend at least $3 billion on digital content for students, of which most is for digital instruction purposes (80). While technology has numerous benefits for schools (e.g., convenience [self-monitoring, goal setting], digital instruction), excessive screen time and sedentary behaviors are public health concerns tied to national goals to decrease the proportion of youth who exceed the daily 2-hour screen time recommendation in 2020 by 10% (81).

The paradox of limiting students' screen time while strengthening 21st century technology proficiencies may require innovative solutions. One promising technology for increasing school-based PA participation, albeit at light-to-moderate intensity levels, has been the integration of screen-based AVGs in schools (82). Factors inhibiting the success of AVG usage in schools include school policy for technology use, size of the gym or playground at the school, and teacher engagement with AVGs (83). Future research should continue to examine the possibilities of novel and emerging technology applications (e.g., social media platforms, mobile devices and apps, health wearables, virtual reality, global positing systems) to increase students' PA levels during the school day (84). Regularly updated information about new school PA technologies is available at thepegeek.com.

Standards and Policies

Local, regional, national, and international level-policy, recommendations, and standards have provided guidance on school-based PA promotion. The CSPAP framework (75) outlined earlier in this chapter emphasizes the position of policy with respect to impacting student PA levels. While many countries have developed national PA plans that highlight the importance of schools within a comprehensive strategy for increasing PA levels across the population (i.e., United States, Ireland, Canada), it is less clear how these plans translate into policies that directly impact PA opportunities for students in schools.

In the United States, schools that participate in federal Child Nutrition Programs have long been required to develop a school wellness policy (85). The school wellness policy must include several components connected to the WSCC model, including goals specifically targeting increased PA opportunities in schools. However, the extent to which these wellness policies are implemented varies based on factors such as perceived levels of support (86). The recently endorsed Every Student Succeeds Act (ESSA) also provides support for CSPAP implementation by including PE in the definition of a well-rounded education (87). However, the provisions associated with the implementation of ESSA recommendations are tasked to individual schools, and consequently, the support specifically targeting PE and PA interventions will likely vary based on local-level administrators' priorities.

Internationally, the *EU Action Plan on Childhood Obesity 2014-2020* (88) mentions the school several times and includes a goal to "*encourage PA*" and suggests the school as a venue to accomplish this. The World Health Organization (WHO) has long advocated for schools to be a venue for the promotion of PA in an attempt to combat childhood obesity within a behavior change model (89). However, similar to the issues discussed earlier that exist within the United States, the recommendations made by the WHO and the European Union (EU) leave implementation up to local stakeholders.

Several countries are now regularly participating in a global PA report card exercise that provides countries with "grades" associated with several different factors (90). Supported by the Active Healthy Kids Global Alliance, nearly four-dozen countries from six different continents participated in the most recent global matrix. When evaluating schools, 58% of the 38 countries who participated in the Global Matrix 2.0 in 2016 received good grades (A, B, or C) using the following indicators:

- Percentage of schools with active school policies
- Percentage of schools where the majority (≥80%) of students are taught by a PE specialist
- Percentage of schools where the majority (≥80%) of students are offered at least 150 minutes of PE per week
- Percentage of schools that offer PA opportunities (excluding PE) to the majority (≥80%) of their students
- Percentage of parents with children and youth who have access to PA opportunities at school in addition to PE
- Percentage of schools with students who have regular access to facilities and equipment that support PA

Unfortunately, the United States was one of the countries earning poor grades in school (D-) and overall PA (D-) (97). Given school-based PA recommendations are consistent across several different countries, international efforts may consider identifying ways to translate existing guidelines and recommendations into policies to support schools.

Cultural Considerations

Every child deserves an equal opportunity to be physically active regardless of race, ethnicity, sex, sexual orientation, gender identity, geographic location, family income status, and any other demographic factor. However, research has shown that disparities in rates of PA exist between low-, middle-, and high-income children (90). Theoretically, schools can provide equal access for all children to learn about and practice PA (3); however, noticeably few research attempts have compared the effects of school-based PA interventions on students from differing socioeconomic backgrounds. Studies that do exist provide strong evidence for short-term (up to 6 months), multicomponent, school-based interventions improving the PA and cholesterol levels of children and adolescents from low- and middle-income settings (69, 91). Similar results were found after a 2-year, controlled study, indicating a multicomponent school-based PA intervention can have superior effects on the PA participation among students from differing socioeconomic (low, middle, and high) backgrounds (92).

PE, as the cornerstone of the CSPAP model, has been recognized as an important subject for acknowledging the cultural issues that exist in school-based PA interventions. Culturally responsive PE has emerged as a viable approach for teachers to understand the community dynamics of their school, particularly in urban settings, in order to implement lessons that are culturally relevant to their school community (93). This curricular approach aims to foster students as culturally literate and critical consumers of sport and PA and has been implemented with modest success in high school PE classes (94). Complementary research has focused on understanding and improving PE teachers' cultural competency (95).

Summary

There is significant evidence for school-based PA promotion. CSPAP is a practical model for both researchers and practitioners to consider the effective implementation of PA in schools. Table 12.1 outlines key implementation strategies overviewed in the chapter that school stakeholders should consider to increase PA participation in schools. Despite these promising strategies, there remains several fruitful areas of inquiry including CSPAP education and training, technology usage for PA promotion in schools, community and family involvement in interventions, and the scalability and sustainability of school-based PA interventions. Researchers should consider developing partnerships with schools to pursue interventions that explore these inquiry areas, while school-based practitioners who are implementing PA interventions in their schools should advocate locally for their programs and connect with nearby universities for support. Schools hold great promise for building future generations of active healthy youth.

TABLE 12.1. Implementation strategies for CSPAP-based PA interventions

CSPAP COMPONENT	IMPLEMENTATION STRATEGIES FOR INCREASING PA AT SCHOOL
PE interventions	1. Provide recommended dose (150 min/wk at elementary school level; 225 min/wk at secondary level) of HOPE 2. Apply LET US Play principles to ensure that 50% of lesson time is spent in MVPA 3. Modify lessons to include students of all ability/fitness levels 4. Teach self-management skills that promote lifetime PA 5. Use evidence-based curricular resources (e.g., SPARK, CATCH)
During school interventions	1. Reduce sedentary time in the classroom using a variety of movement integration strategies (e.g., active transitions, activity breaks, academic integration) 2. Include movement opportunities in the daily school schedule (e.g., active morning routine, drop-in PA sessions, daily recess) 3. Maximize PA engagement during recess through designated activity zones, peer-led activities, developmentally appropriate equipment, and active supervision
Before-school interventions	1. Offer structured PA sessions (e.g., BOKS) before school hours 2. Encourage walking/running behaviors before school through mileage clubs

(continued)

TABLE 12.1. Implementation strategies for CSPAP-based PA interventions *(continued)*

CSPAP COMPONENT	IMPLEMENTATION STRATEGIES FOR INCREASING PA AT SCHOOL
After-school interventions	1. Deliberately schedule PA into daily routines of after-school enrichment programs 2. Encourage staff members to engage in PA with children 3. Adhere to LET US Play principles when facilitating activities/games to maximize MVPA 4. Facilitate specialized PA clubs tailored to the interests of students 5. Offer a variety of interscholastic and intramural sports
Multicomponent interventions	1. Start with implementing a quality PE program, before expanding to offering new or enhanced during school or before/after school PA interventions. 2. Coordinate using a triad of CSPAP leaders including a trained *school champion* (PAL), a *supportive school administrator*, and a school-level *CSPAP committee*.

NOTE: BOKS, Build Our Kids Success; CATCH, Child and Adolescent Trial for Cardiovascular Health; CSPAP, comprehensive school physical activity program; HOPE, health-optimizing physical education; MVPA, moderate- to vigorous-intensity physical activity; PA, physical activity; PAL, Physical Activity Leader; PE, physical education.

■ Case Example: Partnership to Create a Before-School PA Program

Located in a suburb of a large urban center in the southwest United States, Valley View High School is a large school with a diverse population that includes 62% ethnic minorities. Many of the student population of over 2,600 pupils arrive at school well before the 7:45 a.m. warning bell that starts the day as a result of being dropped off by busses, or parents who make long commutes to work. Seeing an opportunity, Tom, the PE teacher at the school, started opening the main gym on Friday morning for students who were in the school early. Realizing there was a demand, Tom reached out to the local university for help, and over the course of a semester, the university staff was able to start an elective course for PE majors to get experience developing and implementing components of a CSPAP.

The first group of preservice teachers who enrolled in this elective course started by taking what Tom was already doing and expanding it to include Tuesday and Thursday mornings and multiple PA spaces (i.e., the main gym, the auxiliary gym, an outdoor space, and a hallway space). They called the program *The Lair*, a nod to the school's wild animal mascot. The concept was simple: open the PA spaces, play current music, provide supervision, and put out equipment. Within 2 weeks of the program starting, attendance at *The Lair* was well over 100 students per morning. Students could come and go and use whatever equipment was available to play. Most chose to engage in informal pickup games, jump rope activities, or racquet sports; however, several dedicated students (mostly boys) laced up every morning in the main gym for an intense basketball scrimmage or in the auxiliary gym for indoor soccer. A small group of students would also meet in the back hallway for a relaxing yoga flow. One morning while observing the activities with university personnel, Tom remarked that the young people in the gym were mostly not ones he recognized—meaning that they were not the ones who excelled in PE or sport at the school. The majority of the regular attendees at *The Lair* arrived on the bus, some travelling from over 20 miles away and often from lower socioeconomic areas than the school's location. Some attendees told the preservice teachers that this was their only time to "play" because it was not safe to do so in their neighborhoods, or that their parents could not afford the fees associated with community sports leagues.

The partnership created between Valley View High School and the local university not only provided preservice PE teachers with experience developing and implementing a CSPAP, it also provided a valuable service to the school community and its students. Although Tom has now retired, 12 years on from implementation, this program is still thriving with continued support from the school's administration and the university faculty who initiated the partnership. The university elective course is now a required course, and the students who enroll each semester are also providing similar support to several other area schools.

Things to Consider

- A CSPAP is a multicomponent model for planning and organizing opportunities for students to be active 60 minutes or more during school days
- Schools are practical venues for PA promotion among young people
- School PA interventions should be facilitated by trained school PA professionals, ideally the PE teacher
- Schools should consider partnerships with community agencies and parents in an effort to increase the available PA opportunities for students
- Stakeholders should advocate for policy that will provide requirements and resources for school PA promotion

Acknowledgment

The authors thank Katie Hodgin for her assistance in preparing this chapter.

References

1. Pate RR. Hearing on "ESEA reauthorization: supporting student health. *physical education, and well-being*". 2010. Available at: https://www.help.senate.gov/imo/media/doc/Pate.pdf. Accessed April 18, 2018.
2. National Center for Education Statistics. Back to school statistics. Available at: https://nces. ed.gov/fastfacts/display.asp?id=372. Accessed April 18, 2018.
3. Institute of Medicine. *Educating the Student Body: Taking Physical Activity and Physical Education to School*. Washington, DC: National Academies Press; 2013.
4. Centers for Disease Control and Prevention. Health and academic achievement. Available at: https://www.cdc.gov/healthyyouth/health_and_academics/pdf/health-academic-achievement.pdf. 2014. Accessed April 18, 2018.
5. Castelli DM, Glowacki E, Barcelona JM, et al. *Active education: growing evidence on physical activity and academic performance*. 2015. Available at: https://activelivingresearch.org/sites/default/files/ALR_Brief_ActiveEducation_Jan2015.pdf. Accessed April 18, 2018.

6. Hutchinson AD, Wilson C. Improving nutrition and physical activity in the workplace: a meta-analysis of intervention studies. *Health Promot Int.* 2012;27(2):238–249. doi:10.1093/heapro/dar035

7. Partnership for Prevention. School-based physical education: working with schools to increase physical activity among children and adolescents in physical education classes: an action guide. April 2008. Available at: https://sparkpe.org/wp-content/uploads/2010/01/CDC_PE_Action_Guide.pdf. April 2018. Accessed April 18, 2018.

8. National Physical Activity Plan Alliance. National physical activity plan. Available at: http://physicalactivityplan.org/docs/2016NPAP_Finalforwebsite.pdf. Accessed April 18, 2018.

9. Centers for Disease Control and Prevention. Increasing physical education and physical activity: a framework for schools 2017. Available at: https://www.cdc.gov/healthyschools/physicalactivity/pdf/17_278143-A_PE-PA-Framework_508.pdf. 2017. Accessed November 22, 2018

10. Shape America. The essential components of physical education. 2015. Available at: https://www.shapeamerica.org//upload/theessentialcomponentsofphysicaleducation.pdf. Accessed April 18, 2018.

11. Sallis JF, McKenzie TL. Physical education's role in public health. *Res Q Exerc Sport.* 1991;62(2):124–137. doi:10.1080/02701367.1991.10608701

12. Sallis JF, McKenzie TL, Beets MW, et al. Physical education's role in public health. *Res Q Exerc Sport.* 2012;83(2):125–135. doi:10.1080/02701367.2012.10599842

13. Haerens L, Kirk D, Cardon G, et al. Toward the development of a pedagogical model for health-based physical education. *Quest.* 2011;63(3):321–338. doi:10.1080/00336297.2011.10483684

14. Webster CA, Stodden DF, Carson RL, et al. Integrative public health-aligned physical education and implications for the professional preparation of future teachers and teacher educators/researchers in the field. *Quest.* 2016;68(4):457–474. doi:10.1080/00336297.2016.1229628

15. McKenzie TL, Sallis JF, Rosengard P, et al. The SPARK programs: a public health model of physical education research and dissemination. *J Teach Phys Educ.* 2016;35(4):381–389. doi:10.1123/jtpe.2016-0100

16. McKenzie TL, Sallis JF, Kolody B, et al. Long-term effects of a physical education curriculum and staff development program: SPARK. *Res Q Exerc Sport.* 1997;68(4):280–291. doi:10.1080/02701367.1997.10608009

17. Sallis JF, McKenzie TL, Alcaraz JE, et al. The effects of a 2-year physical education program (SPARK) on physical activity and fitness in elementary school students. Sports, play and active recreation for kids. *Am J Public Health.* 1997;87(8):1328–1334. doi:10.2105/AJPH.87.8.1328

18. McKenzie TL, Sallis JF, Rosengard P. Beyond the stucco tower: design, development, and dissemination of the SPARK physical education programs. *Quest.* 2009;61(1):114–127. doi:10.1080/00336297.2009.10483606

19. McKenzie TL, Nader PR, Strikmiller PK, et al. School physical education: effect of the child and adolescent trial for cardiovascular health (CATCH). *Prev Med.* 1996;25(4):423–431. doi:10.1006/pmed.1996.0074

20. McKenzie TL, Stone EJ, Feldman HA, et al. Effects of the CATCH physical education intervention: teacher type and lesson location. *Am J Prev Med.* 2001;21(2):101–109. doi:10.1016/S0749-3797(01)00335-X

21. Kelder SH, Mitchell PD, McKenzie TL, et al. Long-term implementation of the CATCH physical education program. *Health Educ Behav.* 2003;30(4):463–475. doi:10.1177/1090198103253538

22. McKenzie TL, Li D, Derby CA, et al. Maintenance of effects of the CATCH physical education program: results from the catch-on study. *Health Educ Behav.* 2003;30(4):447–462. doi:10.1177/1090198103253535

23. Weaver RG, Webster C, Beets MW. LET US Play: maximizing physical activity in physical education. *Strategies.* 2013;26(6):33–37. doi:10.1080/08924562.2013.839518

24. Dudley D, Okely A, Pearson P, et al. A systematic review of the effectiveness of physical education and school sport interventions targeting physical activity, movement skills and enjoyment of physical activity. *Eur Phys Educ Rev*. 2011;17(3):353–378. doi:10.1177/1356336X11416734

25. Lonsdale C, Rosenkranz RR, Peralta LR, et al. A systematic review and meta-analysis of interventions designed to increase moderate-to-vigorous physical activity in school physical education lessons. *Prev Med*. 2013;56(2):152–161. doi:10.1016/j.ypmed.2012.12.004

26. Hollis JL, Williams AJ, Sutherland R, et al. A systematic review and meta-analysis of moderate-to-vigorous physical activity levels in elementary school physical education lessons. *Prev Med*. 2016;86:34–54. doi:10.1016/j.ypmed.2015.11.018

27. Hollis JL, Sutherland R, Williams AJ, et al. A systematic review and meta-analysis of moderate-to-vigorous physical activity levels in secondary school physical education lessons. *Int J Behav Nutr Phys Act*. 2017;14:1–26. doi:10.1186/S12966-017-0504-0

28. Kahan D, McKenzie TL. Energy expenditure estimates during school physical education: potential vs. reality? *Prev Med*. 2017;95:82–88. doi:10.1016/j.ypmed.2016.12.008

29. Erwin H, Fedewa A, Beighle A, et al. A quantitative review of physical activity, health, and learning outcomes associated with classroom-based physical activity interventions. *J Appl Sch Psychol*. 2012;28(1):14–36. doi:10.1080/15377903.2012.643755

30. Martin R, Murtagh EM. Preliminary findings of active classrooms: an intervention to increase physical activity levels of primary school children during class time. *Teach Teach Educ*. 2015;52:113–127. doi:10.1016/j.tate.2015.09.007

31. Goh TL, Hannon J, Webster CA, et al. Chapter 7. Effects of a classroom-based physical activity program on children's physical activity levels. *J Teach Phys Educ*. 2014;33(4):558–572. doi:10.1123/jtpe.2014-0068

32. Uhrich TA, Swalm RL. A pilot study of a possible effect from a motor task on reading performance. *Percept Mot Skills*. 2007;104(3):1035–1041. doi:10.2466/pms.104.3.1035-1041

33. Lowden K, Powney J, Davidson J, et al. *The Class Moves! Pilot in Scotland and Wales: An Evaluation*. Edinburgh: Scottish Council for Research in Education; 2001.

34. Mahar MT, Murphy SK, Rowe DA, et al. Effects of a classroom-based program on physical activity and on-task behavior. *Med Sci Sports Exerc*. 2006;38(12):2086–2094. doi:10.1249/01.mss.0000235359.16685.a3

35. McMullen J, Kulinna P, Cothran D. Chapter 5. Physical activity opportunities during the school day: classroom teachers' perceptions of using activity breaks in the classroom. *J Teach Phys Educ*. 2014;33(4):511–527. doi:10.1123/jtpe.2014-0062

36. Stylianou M, Kulinna PH, Naiman T. ' . . . because there's nobody who can just sit that long': teacher perceptions of classroom-based physical activity and related management issues. *Eur Phys Educ Rev*. 2016;22(3):390–408. doi:10.1177/1356336X15613968

37. Centers for Disease Control and Prevention. Comprehensive School Physical Activity Program (CSPAP). Available at: https://www.cdc.gov/healthyschools/physicalactivity/cspap.htm. Published September 25, 2015. Accessed April 18, 2018.

38. Huberty JL, Beets MW, Beighle A, et al. Effects of Ready for Recess, an environmental intervention, on physical activity in third- through sixth-grade children. *J Phys Act Health*. 2014;11(2):384–395. doi:10.1123/jpah.2012-0061

39. Ridgers ND, Stratton G, Fairclough SJ, et al. Children's physical activity levels during school recess: a quasi-experimental intervention study. *Int J Behav Nutr Phys Act*. 2007;4:19. doi:10.1186/1479-5868-4-19

40. Carlin A, Murphy MH, Gallagher AM. The WISH study: the effect of peer-led Walking In ScHools on school-time physical activity. *Proc Nutr Soc*. 2015;74(OCEA):E235. doi:10.1017/S0029665115002773

41. Ickes MJ, Erwin H, Beighle A. Systematic review of recess interventions to increase physical activity. *J Phys Act Health*. 2013;10(6):910–926. doi:10.1123/jpah.10.6.910

42. Ratey JJ, Hagerman E. *Spark: The Revolutionary New Science of Exercise and the Brain*. New York, NY: Little, Brown and Company; 2008.

43. Álvarez-Bueno C, Pesce C, Cavero-Redondo I, et al. Academic achievement and physical activity: a meta-analysis. *Pediatrics*. 2017;140(6):1–14. doi:10.1542/peds.2017-1498

44. Stellino M, Dauenhauer B. Before school physical activity programming: evidence for policy inclusion. Presented at the: Active Living Research Conference; 2015; San Diego, CA.
45. Westcott W, Puhala K, Colligan A, et al. Physiological effects of the BOKS before-school physical activity program for preadolescent youth. *J Exerc Sports Orthop.* 2015;2(2):1–7. doi:10.15226/2374-6904/2/2/00129
46. Stylianou M, van der Mars H, Kulinna PH, et al. Before-school running/walking club and student physical activity levels: an efficacy study. *Res Q Exerc Sport.* 2016;87(4):342–353. doi:10.1080/02701367.2016.1214665
47. Stylianou M, Kulinna PH, van der Mars H, et al. Before-school running/walking club: effects on student on-task behavior. *Prev Med Rep.* 2016;3:196–202. doi:10.1016/j.pmedr.2016.01.010
48. Afterschool Alliance. America after 3PM: afterschool programs in demand. Available at: http://afterschoolalliance.org/documents/AA3PM-2014/AA3PM_National_Report.pdf. Accessed April 18, 2018.
49. National Afterschool Association. National Afterschool HEPA Association Standards. 2011. Available at: https://naaweb.org/images/NAA_HEPA_Standards_new_look_2015.pdf. Accessed April 18, 2018.
50. Beets MW, Weaver RG, Turner-McGrievy G, et al. Making policy practice in afterschool programs: a randomized controlled trial on physical activity changes. *Am J Prev Med.* 2015;48(6):694–706. doi:10.1016/j.amepre.2015.01.012
51. Huberty JL, Beets MW, Beighle A, et al. Association of staff behaviors and afterschool program features to physical activity: findings from movin' after school. *J Phys Act Health.* 2013;10(3):423–429. doi:10.1123/jpah.10.3.423
52. Weaver RG, Beets MW, Turner-McGrievy G, et al. Effects of a competency-based professional development training on children's physical activity and staff physical activity promotion in summer day camps. *New Dir Youth Dev.* 2014(143):57–78. doi:10.1002/yd.20104
53. Brazendale K, Chandler JL, Beets MW, et al. Maximizing children's physical activity using the LET US Play principles. *Prev Med.* 2015;76:14–19. doi:10.1016/j.ypmed.2015.03.012
54. Dzewaltowski DA, Rosenkranz RR, Geller KS, et al. HOP'N after-school project: an obesity prevention randomized controlled trial. *Int J Behav Nutr Phys Act.* 2010;7:90–101. doi:10.1186/1479-5868-7-90
55. Slusser WM, Sharif MZ, Erausquin JT, et al. Improving overweight among at-risk minority youth: results of a pilot intervention in after-school programs. *J Health Care Poor Underserved.* 2013;24(2):12–24. doi:10.1353/hpu.2013.0111
56. Herrick H, Thompson H, Kinder J, et al. Use of SPARK to promote after-school physical activity. *J Sch Health.* 2012;82(10):457–461. doi:10.1111/j.1746-1561.2012.00722.x
57. Annesi JJ, Walsh SM, Greenwood BL, et al. Effects of the Youth Fit 4 Life physical activity/nutrition protocol on body mass index, fitness and targeted social cognitive theory variables in 9- to 12-year-olds during after-school care. *J Paediatr Child Health.* 2017;53(4):365–373. doi:10.1111/jpc.13447
58. Huberty J, Dinkel DM, Beets MW. Evaluation of GoGirlGo!; a practitioner based program to improve physical activity. *BMC Public Health.* 2014;14(1):1–21. doi:10.1186/1471-2458-14-118
59. Madsen K, Thompson H, Adkins A, et al. School-community partnerships: a cluster-randomized trial of an after-school soccer program. *JAMA Pediatr.* 2013;167(4):321–326. doi:10.1001/jamapediatrics.2013.1071
60. Garn AC, McCaughtry N, Kulik NL, et al. Successful after-school physical activity clubs in urban high schools: perspectives of adult leaders and student participants. *J Teach Phys Educ.* 2014;33(1):112–133. doi:10.1123/jtpe.2013-0006
61. Maljak K, Garn A, McCaughtry N, et al. Challenges in offering inner-city after-school physical activity clubs. *Am J Health Educ.* 2014;45(5):297–307. doi:10.1080/19325037.2014.934414
62. Pate RR, Trost SG, Levin S, et al. Sports participation and health-related behaviors among US youth. *Arch Pediatr Adolesc Med.* 2000;154(9):904–911. doi:10.1001/archpedi.154.9.904

63. Eime RM, Young JA, Harvey JT, et al. A systematic review of the psychological and social benefits of participation in sport for children and adolescents: informing development of a conceptual model of health through sport. *Int J Behav Nutr Phys Act*. 2013;10:98–118. doi:10.1186/1479-5868-10-98

64. Trudeau F, Shephard RJ. Physical education, school physical activity, school sports and academic performance. *Int J Behav Nutr Phys Act*. 2008;5:10. doi:10.1186/1479-5868-5-10

65. Nichol ME, Pickett W, Janssen I. Associations between school recreational environments and physical activity. *J Sch Health*. 2009;79(6):247–254. doi:10.1111/j.1746-1561.2009.00406.x

66. Bocarro JN, Kanters MA, Edwards MB, et al. Prioritizing school intramural and interscholastic programs based on observed physical activity. *Am J Health Promot*. 2014;28:S65–S71. doi:10.4278/ajhp.130430-QUAN-205

67. Russ LB, Webster CA, Beets MW, et al. Systematic review and meta-analysis of multi-component interventions through schools to increase physical activity. *J Phys Act Health*. 2015;12(10):1436–1446. doi:10.1123/jpah.2014-0244

68. Chen S, Gu X. Toward active living: comprehensive school physical activity program research and implications. *Quest*. 2018;70(2):191–212. doi:10.1080/00336297.2017.1365002

69. Burns RD, Brusseau TA, Hannon JC. Effect of Comprehensive School Physical Activity Programming on cardiometabolic health markers in children from low-income schools. *J Phys Act Health*. 2017;14(9):671–676. doi:10.1123/jpah.2016-0691

70. Centeio EE, Mccaughtry N, Moore W, et al. Building healthy communities: a comprehensive school health program to prevent chronic disease. *Med Sci Sports Exerc*. 2017;49(5S):1088. doi:10.1249/01.mss.0000519996.08196.2a

71. De Bourdeaudhuij I, Van Cauwenberghe E, Spittaels H, et al. School-based interventions promoting both physical activity and healthy eating in Europe: a systematic review within the HOPE project. *Obes Rev*. 2011;12(3):205–216. doi:10.1111/j.1467-789X.2009.00711.x

72. Kriemler S, Meyer U, Martin E, et al. Effect of school-based interventions on physical activity and fitness in children and adolescents: a review of reviews and systematic update. *Br J Sports Med*. 2011;45(11):923–930. doi:10.1136/bjsports-2011-090186

73. McLeroy KR, Bibeau D, Steckler A, et al. An ecological perspective on health promotion programs. *Health Educ Q*. 1988;15(4):351–377. doi:10.1177/109019818801500401

74. Association for Supervision and Curriculum Development. Whole school, whole community, whole child: a collaborative approach to learning and health. 2014. Available at: http://www.ascd.org/ASCD/pdf/siteASCD/publications/wholechild/wscc-a-collaborative-approach.pdf. Accessed April 18, 2018.

75. Carson RL, Castelli DM, Beighle A, et al. School-based physical activity promotion: a conceptual framework for research and practice. *Child Obes*. 2014;10(2):100–106. doi:10.1089/chi.2013.0134

76. Beets MW, Okely A, Weaver RG, et al. The theory of expanded, extended, and enhanced opportunities for youth physical activity promotion. *Int J Behav Nutr Phys Act*. 2016;13:120. doi:10.1186/s12966-016-0442-2

77. Carson RL, Castelli DM, Pulling Kuhn AC, et al. Impact of trained champions of comprehensive school physical activity programs on school physical activity offerings, youth physical activity and sedentary behaviors. *Prev Med*. 2014;69:S12–S19. doi:10.1016/j.ypmed.2014.08.025

78. SHAPE America. Physical activity leader learning system and training. Available at: https://www.shapeamerica.org/prodev/workshops/lmas/. Published 2018. Accessed April 18, 2018.

79. Carson RL, Castelli DM, Kulinna PH. CSPAP professional preparation: takeaways from pioneering physical education teacher education programs. *J Phys Educ Recreat Dance*. 2017;88(2):43–51. doi:10.1080/07303084.2017.1260986

80. Herold B. Technology in education: an overview—education week. Available at: https://www.edweek.org/ew/issues/technology-in-education/. Published February 5, 2016. Accessed April 18, 2018.

81. U.S. Department of Health and Human Services. *Physical activity | Healthy People*. 2020. Available at: https://www.healthypeople.gov/2020/topics-objectives/topic/physical-activity. Accessed April 18, 2018.

82. Norris E, Hamer M, Stamatakis E. Active video games in schools and effects on physical activity and health: a systematic review. *J Pediatr*. 2016;172:40–46.e5. doi:10.1016/j.jpeds.2016.02.001

83. Robertson J, Jepson R, Macvean A, et al. Understanding the importance of context: a qualitative study of a location-based exergame to enhance school childrens physical activity. *PLOS ONE*. 2016;11(8):e0160927. doi:10.1371/journal.pone.0160927

84. Gao Z, Zeng M, Mcdonough D, et al. Progress and possibilities for technology integration in CSPAP. In: *Comprehensive School Physical Activity Programs: Evidence-Based Research to Practice*. Champaign, IL: Human Kinetics. In press. Available at: https://scholar.google.com/scholar?hl=en&as_sdt=0,6&q=Gao+Z,+Pope+Zeng+N,+Mcdonough+D,+Lee+JE.+Progress+and+possibilities+for+technology+integration+in+CSPAP.+In%3A+Carson+RL,+Webster+CA,+eds.+Comprehensive+School+Physical+Activity+Programs%3A+Evidence-Based+Research+to+Practice.+Ch.+22.+Champaign,+IL%3A+Human+K. Accessed April 18, 2018.

85. Centers for Disease Control and Prevention. Putting local school wellness policies into action: stories from school districts and schools. Available at: https://www.cdc.gov/healthyschools/npao/pdf/SchoolWellnessInAction.pdf. Published 2014. Accessed April 19, 2018.

86. Hager ER, Rubio DS, Eidel GS, et al. Implementation of local wellness policies in schools: role of school systems, school health councils, and health disparities. *J Sch Health*. 2016;86(10):742–750. doi:10.1111/josh.12430

87. U.S. Department of Education L. S.1177—114th Congress (2015-2016): Every Student Succeeds Act. Available at: https://www.congress.gov/bill/114th-congress/senate-bill/1177. Published December 10, 2015. Accessed April 19, 2018.

88. European Commission EU. Action plan on childhood obesity 2014-2020. Available at: https://ec.europa.eu/health/sites/health/files/nutrition_physical_activity/docs/childhoodobesity_actionplan_2014_2020_en.pdf. Published February 24, 2014. Accessed April 19, 2018.

89. World Health. Organization. Report of the Commission on Ending Childhood Obesity—Implementation Plan: Executive Summary. Available at: http://apps.who.int/iris/bitstream/handle/10665/259349/WHO-NMH-PND-ECHO-17.1-eng.pdf?sequence=1. 2017. Accessed April 19, 2018.

90. Tremblay MS, Barnes JD, González SA, et al. Global Matrix 2.0: report card grades on the physical activity of children and youth comparing 38 countries. *J Phys Act Health*. 2016;13(11 suppl 2):S343–S366. doi:10.1123/jpah.2016-0594

91. Barbosa Filho VC, Minatto G, Mota J, et al. Promoting physical activity for children and adolescents in low- and middle-income countries: an umbrella systematic review: a review on promoting physical activity in LMIC. *Prev Med*. 2016;88:115–126. doi:10.1016/j.ypmed.2016.03.025

92. Vander Ploeg KA, Maximova K, McGavock J, et al. Do school-based physical activity interventions increase or reduce inequalities in health? *Soc Sci Med*. 2014;112:80–87. doi:10.1016/j.socscimed.2014.04.032

93. Flory SB, McCaughtry N. Culturally relevant physical education in urban schools. *Res Q Exerc Sport*. 2011;82(1):49–60. doi:10.1080/02701367.2011.10599721

94. Kinchin GD, O'Sullivan M. Incidences of student support for and resistance to a curricular innovation in high school physical education. *J Teach Phys Educ*. 2003;22(3):245–260. doi:10.1123/jtpe.22.3.245

95. Harrison L, Carson RL, Burden J. Physical education teachers' cultural competency. *J Teach Phys Educ*. 2010;29(2):184–198. doi:10.1123/jtpe.29.2.184

96. Braun HA, Kay CM, Cheung P, et al. Impact of an elementary school-based intervention on physical activity time and aerobic capacity, Georgia, 2013-2014. *Public Health Reports*. 2017;132(suppl 2):24S–32S. doi:10.1177/0033354917771970

97. National Physical Activity Plan Alliance. The 2018 United States Report Card on Physical Activity for Children and Youth. Washington, DC: National Physical Activity Plan Alliance. Available at: http://physicalactivityplan.org/projects/reportcard.html. 2018. Accessed November 22, 2018.

13

PHYSICAL ACTIVITY OPPORTUNITIES OUTSIDE OF SCHOOL

ANGIE L. CRADOCK

■ Physical Activity Opportunities Outside of School Time

While schools are essential settings for promoting physical activity, children and adolescents of school age spend most of their time each day in contexts outside of the school classroom. These time windows outside the school period allow for opportunities for moderate-to-vigorous physical activity (MVPA). Innovations in strategies to promote physical activity during the hours outside of school occur in the community setting where children and adolescents participate in programs and organized activities, during travel to and from school and other destinations, and in homes and with other family members. This chapter describes several opportunities for public health approaches to increase the physical activity levels of children in youth in contexts outside of school hours (see Figure 13.1).

© Springer Publishing Company DOI: 10.1891/9780826134592.0013

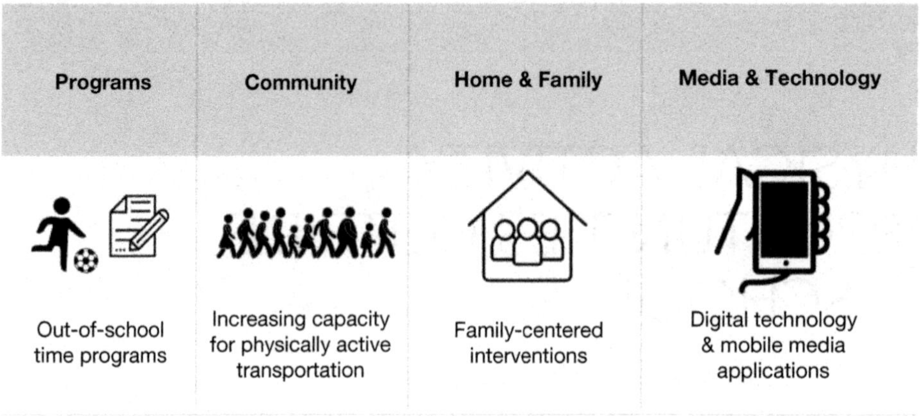

FIGURE 13.1 Key contexts for physical activity promotion outside of school.

Physical Activity in the Hours Outside of School

For both males and females, more than half (55%–57%) of their total daily time doing MVPA happens outside of regular school hours (1). The time of day during which children and adolescents engage in the most physical activity outside of school hours is the period directly after the school day. The physical activity that happens during the morning periods before the school day starts contributes in small proportion to total daily physical activity levels (1).

The percentage of total MVPA minutes accumulated in the different periods of the day outside of school are quite similar for children and adolescents, and for males and females. However, there are some significant differences to note. Nationally, boys aged 6 to 19 years accumulate more overall time in MVPA than girls of similar ages. Among girls, the amount of physical activity among adolescents aged 12 to 19 accumulated directly after school is roughly one third of that observed among girls aged 6 to 11, and half of that compared to boys of similar ages (Table 13.1). Among both males and females, adolescents are less active than children (1). Data capturing objectively measured physical activity over time collected from children as they aged suggest that between the ages of 9 and 15, there are significant increases in the amount of sedentary time accompanied by decreases in the amount of MVPA levels in the period after school. Furthermore, the decline in physical activity is higher among girls compared to boys and among children with overweight or obesity than among children without. Encouragingly, the most active boys at younger ages were three to four times more likely to be in the most active group as adolescents (2). It is clear that intervention strategies could promote maintenance of physical activity levels among all children in the periods outside of school hours.

Key Points

- Most physical activity happens during the periods outside of school.
- The physical activity in morning hours contributes a small percentage to overall daily physical activity.

TABLE 13.1. Minutes (percentage of total) of MVPA by time of day

	BEFORE SCHOOL	DURING SCHOOL	AFTER SCHOOL	EVENING
BOYS Age 6–11 y	**3.3** (4%)	**36.9** (43%)	**24.1** (28%)	**21.6** (25%)
Age 12–19 y	**2.7** (7%)	**17.7** (43%)	**11.3** (27%)	**9.7** (23%)
GIRLS Age 6–11 y	**2.5** (4%)	**28.3** (43%)	**18.4** (28%)	**16.8** (26%)
Age 12–19 y	**1.9** (8%)	**10.3** (45%)	**6.0** (26%)	**4.8** (21%)

NOTE: MVPA, moderate-to-vigorous physical activity.

SOURCE: Long MW, Sobol AM, Cradock AL, et al. School-day and overall physical activity among youth. *Am J Prev Med.* 2013;45(2):150-157. doi:10.1016/j.amepre.2013.03.011

- As children age, particularly girls, they become less active overall and less active in the periods after school.
- Strategies to increase physical activity overall and to prevent the age-related declines in physical activity outside of school are needed, particularly among girls.

Leveraging the Hours Outside of School

Mechanisms for Increasing Physical Activity

Conceptually, there are at least three different approaches practitioners and public health researchers might use to improve physical activity levels of children and adolescents in the periods outside of school. These are expanding opportunities, extending opportunities, and enhancing opportunities (3).

- Expanding opportunities—replacing time spent in light or sedentary activity with more active time.
- Extending opportunities—lengthening the time of existing physically active pursuits or programs.
- Enhancing opportunities—improving other aspects of existing opportunities for physical activity to make them more active.

Practitioners and researchers can use these approaches, either singly or in combination, in a variety of contexts and settings in which children and adolescents spend their time.

Contexts and Settings for Intervention

Key settings for interventions outside of school include organized out of school time programming, community interventions that encourage physically active travel, family-focused strategies, and interventions that address or build on media use.

Out of school programs

Nationally, a rising number of children are participating in after-school programs. Nearly 10.2 million children (18%) participated in an after-school program in 2014, an increase from 2009 (8.4 million; 15%) and 2004 (6.5 million; 11%). Program participation rates are highest in elementary grades, where 23% of elementary school students participate, and lowest in high school, where 12% of high school students participate (4). Effective strategies may include expanding programming opportunities to reach more children, increasing the length of physically active time in programs, or increasing the capacity of programs to ensure that existing time allocated to physical activity is sufficiently active (3). Implementation strategies that build more physical activity into the existing opportunities offered by many after-school programs can provide an avenue to reach many school-aged students.

Home and community-focused strategies

After the school day ends, 11.3 million children are without supervision between the hours of 3 and 6 p.m. (4). This early independence implies that efforts to increase physical activity might need to operate within a broader community context or focus on the time and activities that occur within a child's home or during the transition between home, school, and other community contexts. As they age, children and teens become increasingly independently mobile, making trips to and from different destinations, often using physically active modes. Greater independent mobility would draw attention to the need for interventions in the community setting that support the use of physically active transportation modes such as walking, bicycling, or using public transit. Using physically active transportation modes in the journey to and from school can prevent excess weight gain (5) and promote physical activity (6, 7).

Additionally, teenagers who may be less likely to participate in structured programs after school and those younger children in unsupervised care at home (4) might benefit from intervention strategies that replace (or capitalize on) time being spent using screen media and mobile devices (8, 9). Involving family and caregivers in providing additional supports and encouragements are newer strategies to enhance the physical activity levels of children.

Out of School Time Programs

■ *Out of school time programs are structured opportunities provided for school-age children and adolescents to participate in programming of different varieties.*

Current Status of Progress to Promote Physical Activity in Outside of School Time Programs

While opportunities to participate in an after-school program have increased since 2004, there is still considerable unmet demand. More than one third of parents with children not currently enrolled in a program say they would enroll if a program were available to them (4). Many out-of-school-time program opportunities are available through national organizations such as the Y of America and Boys and Girls Clubs of America, through funding from the U.S. Department of Education 21st Century Community Learning

Centers, and from other state and local partners (10). Programming in the hours outside of school can help children and adolescents become more physically active by adding physical activity options for those not enrolled, or by enhancing or extending existing physical activity opportunities (3).

In 2011, a coalition developed standards to promote healthy nutrition and physical activity practices in out-of-school-time programs. These standards—the National After-school Association Healthy Eating and Physical Activity (HEPA) standards—provide guidelines for program practices including information to address training, staff and family engagement, and program infrastructure and facilities. Some national after-school provider organizations have adopted some or all of these standards (11). However, other after-school programs may not yet be aware of these national best-practice recommendations for promoting healthy program physical activity opportunities. In other cases, programs may have significant challenges in the adoption and implementation of best-practice recommendations (12).

Key points

- There is considerable unmet demand for after-school programs—many parents report that they would send their children to programs if they were available.
- There are national best-practice recommendations for nutrition and physical activity practices in out-of-school-time programs.
- Some programs may not yet be aware of national guidelines for promoting physical activity during program hours.
- Strategies to promote implementation and adoption of best-practice guidelines for physical activity in after-school programs are needed.

Potential Challenges and Emerging Areas

In some cases, results from interventions aimed at increasing physical activity after school hours have been mixed (13–15). Some states, including North Carolina (16) and California, have developed policy or regulatory systems to support opportunities for HEPA in after-school programs (10). National organizations and partners are working to promote the awareness of best-practice guidelines (17), and collaborative interventions promoting the implementation of policy, systems, and programmatic changes to improve physical activity opportunities for children and adolescents in programs that operate outside of school hours have had some success (18–20). Promoting new opportunities for participation in programming that provides sufficient quality time for physical activity may be a cost-effective way to increase physical activity levels (21).

Several challenges exist in the implementation of best-practice guidelines including issues of compatibility of existing program requirements, rules or regulations that govern programs with best-practice standards, and ensuring sufficient resources for staffing, staff training, and professional development (10).

Future Directions

- *Policy and practice-based interventions that provide technical assistance, training, and support for program staff may be helpful in promoting increases in physical activity levels among children and adolescents participating in existing programs.*

■ *Promoting new opportunities for participation in programming that provides sufficient quality time for physical activity may be a cost-effective way to increase physical activity levels.*

Case studies of implementation and dissemination: out-of-school-time programs

Case Study 1: Dissemination and implementation of effective interventions promoting physical activity via collaboration with statewide associations of out-of-school-time providers in Massachusetts.

■ **Population addressed:** Between 2010 and 2012, a group of researchers worked with over 20 after-school sites in Boston as part of a group randomized controlled trial to evaluate whether the Out of School Nutrition and Physical Activity Initiative (OSNAP) collaborative learning approach improved nutrition, physical activity, and screen time practices and policies in participating programs (18). However, researchers were interested in how such initiatives to implement physical activity and nutrition primary prevention systems in after-school programs might be scaled in implementation to build capacity and foster sustainability within a network of statewide out-of-school-time program providers.

■ **Settings:** This collaboration included researchers and practitioners from a statewide organization of providers that offered early care and education, before and after school, and summer camp programs for school-aged children and adolescents.

■ **Design and outcomes:** Twenty-four programs operated by four regional agencies across the state of Massachusetts providing childcare and after-school programming for more than 1,500 children during the hours outside of school were invited to participate in a school-yearlong learning collaborative.

■ **Program implementation:** The intervention was designed to develop staff organizational capacity to deliver training and technical assistance at the local level using evidence-based training and implementation materials. At least two staff members in four regional out-of-school-time organizations were certified as OSNAP trainers through their participating in a full-day training conducted by program developers. Pairs of trained OSNAP trainers then implemented three OSNAP learning collaborative sessions each in four regions of Massachusetts during one school year. These learning collaborative sessions would bring together program staff from four or more local program sites to participate in a peer-to-peer exchange and organizational change program that included self-assessment, goal development, skill and knowledge development, and action planning consistent with the original research trial activities.

■ **Study design:** Researchers used a quasi-experimental, pre–post design, collecting baseline and follow-up self-assessments from program directors using a research-validated instrument to determine changes in key physical activity, nutrition, and screen time practices.

■ **Outcomes**: Following participation, program sites reported significant increases in the proportion of days that they provided all children with targeted amounts of MVPA (at least 30 minutes of moderate to vigorous activity each day, vigorous activities for 20 minutes at least three times per week), and limited use of any screen time for noneducational purposes. Additionally, after participating in OSNAP learning collaboratives, sites met significantly more OSNAP goals overall including physical activity, nutrition, and screen time goals. On average, sites reported meeting at least seven of the nine OSNAP goals daily and consistently reported providing water as a beverage at snack and ensuring program time did not include noneducational broadcast television or movies everyday.

■ **Challenges and successes:**
  ● Trainers spoke favorably about OSNAP content and compatability with organizational goals.
  ● Trainers reported wanting to include time for developing facilitation skills in their training sessions for becoming a learning collaborative facilitator.
  ● At the trainer and site levels, engagement and turnover were factors that may influence successful OSNAP implementation.

■ **Other considerations and future directions:** Project participants and researchers suggested that future train-the-trainer and learning collaborative meetings could benefit from team-building activities and greater breadth of team participation to ensure better sustainability in the face of organizational staff turnover.

Active Transportation, Community, and the Built Environment

■ *Active transportation encompasses transport modes like walking and bicycling that use human power to move from one place to the other.*

■ *Safe Routes to School is a program that engages schools, communities, students, and families to increase the rates at which students use active transportation modes.*

■ *Complete Streets is a movement including policies and practices that help communities design and create streets that enable safe access for everyone, including pedestrians, bicyclists, motorists, and transit riders.*

Current Status

Compared to passive forms of transportation such as riding in cars or on school buses, regular active transport via walking (6, 7) or bicycling (22) can contribute meaningful amounts of physical activity to the days of children and adolescents. While it is estimated that one half of school-aged students live within 2 miles of school, nationally only 11.7% of students in grades K-8 walk to school on a regular basis. Since 1969, when almost 48% of students walked or bicycled to school, our students have become regular passengers—45% ride to school in a personal vehicle (23). Studies simultaneously tracking the physical activity and geographic location of activities suggest that children and adolescents may accumulate up to two-fifths of their daily outdoor moderate–vigorous activity walking local streets (24), though patterns and location of activity may shift over time as the child ages. However, for students and caregivers to feel confident about walking or bicycling for transportation, appropriate infrastructure, encouragement, and traffic safety supports are critical.

Emerging Areas and Potential Challenges

Safe Routes to School, Complete Streets, and funding for active transportation

Nationally, just one-third (32.9%) of school districts report that they have programs that support or promote students walking or bicycling to or from school (25), and only 10 of 50 states have legislation and funding appropriations to support Safe Routes to School programs in their local communities (26, 27). State and community efforts to make it easier for individuals to walk and bicycle for general transportation are also meager. Only 5 of 50 states fund bicycle and pedestrian projects at levels recommended by active transportation experts, though 42% of states have adopted policies that are consistent with a Complete Streets model, ensuring that streets are built to accommodate all users including bicyclists and pedestrians (26). Additionally, projects, programs, and facilities that can promote walking and bicycling may also be less prevalent in rural communities (28). Readers interested in more information on physical activity interventions in rural communities may want to review Chapter 19.

Future Directions

- ■ Work on changes to state-level policy and practice can help support implementation of programs and environmental changes at the local level.

TABLE 13.2. Percentage of districts that support or promote transportation-related practices—SHPSS 2016.

PRACTICE	PERCENTAGE OF DISTRICTS	95% CONFIDENCE INTERVAL
Walking or biking to and from school	32.9	(28.8–37.3)
The use of public transportation for its students to travel to and from school[a]	13.4	(10.5–16.9)
The use of public transportation for its faculty and staff to travel to and from school[a]	4.1	(2.6–6.4)

NOTE: [a]An additional 67.4% of districts had no public transportation available.
SHPSS, School Health Policies and Practices Study.

SOURCE: Source: U.S. Department of Health and Human Services. *Results From the School Health Policies and Practices Study 2016*. Atlanta, GA: 2017.

- Work to expand the level of state Safe Routes to School program funding and supports in states or the local community.
- Work with local community and state partners to ensure that communities are planned for and accommodate all users via implementation of Complete Streets.

Family-Focused Interventions

Current Status

Recently, the Community Preventive Services Task Force recommended the use of family-based interventions to promote physical activity among children (29). The Task Force defines family-based interventions as those that combine activities that build family support and provide health education. The recommendations were based on a systematic review of studies conducted in multiple settings and with different family groupings (30, 31).

Family-focused intervention components included (29)

- Goal-setting tools and skills to monitor progress, which could include web-sites or other online or mobile content or prompts
- Positive reinforcement of health behaviors using rewards
- Role modeling of behaviors by family members or instructors
- Organized physical activity sessions

Potential Challenges and Emerging Areas

The family-focused intervention studies that were conducted in home-based settings versus through schools, clinics, or churches and used objectively assessed physical activity to measure outcomes included a small number of participants. This lack of evidence for large-scale implementation highlights potential difficulties that practitioners may find in scaling-up a time or resource-intensive family-centered intervention to reach greater numbers of families within a community or across multiple communities. In some cases, intervention activities were accomplished remotely using wearable physical activity monitoring devices and web-based materials and messaging. Strategies that make use of technology may improve the potential for large-scale interventions.

Future Directions

After review and syntheses of findings from multiple intervention studies focused on family-centered interventions to increase physical activity, the following suggestions emerged for future research and practice (30):

- Tailor family-focused interventions to the context in which they are delivered and the motivations and considerations of the specific family.
- Using both goal setting and reinforcement techniques might best increase motivation to improve physical activity.
- Education strategies alone are insufficient, but education may be useful in combination with other intervention approaches.
- A focus on other potential positive outcomes that coincide with physical activity (e.g., family time together, skill development) may work better than health-focused messages.

Screen Time, Media Use, and Mobile Technologies to Promote Physical Activity

- *Screen time can include behaviors such as watching or reading content, video chatting, playing games, or doing homework using a variety of media technologies like smartphones or tablets, television sets, computers and stationary consoles, or gaming devices.*
- *Games for health are electronic or digital games that are designed to influence a person's health or health-related behaviors.*
- *Exergames are games that use physical activity to move the game play forward.*
- *Apps are applications designed for mobile devices such as smartphones or tablets that can be used to target physical activity, sedentary behaviors, or other health outcomes.*

Current Status in Screen Media Use

While the total time children aged 0 to 8 spent using screen media (about 2 hours 15 minutes per day) has changed relatively little in the past 6 years, the ways that children are using screens has changed considerably. The majority of young children live in households with a mobile device (98%) and high-speed Internet access (96%). Forty-two percent (42%) of children aged 0 up to 8 own a tablet. In fact, while TV is still the most common screen use, a third of all screen time is mobile media use among 0- to 8-year-olds. Mobile media use is triple what researchers found in 2011 (8). Among older children and adolescents, the total time spent using screen media is considerably higher. While children aged 8 to 12 use screen media for over 4.5 hours per day, adolescents aged 13 to 18 spend about 6.6 hours per day using media during the hours outside of school, not including time spent on homework (9). Access to personal or household tablets or smartphones is common but differs by family income. Large portions of screen media time is spent using mobile devices, though watching content including TV/DVDs or videos contribute the largest to total screen media time (9).

Given the interest and time that children and adolescents spend with screen media, the use of screen technology to promote healthier levels of physical activity has received considerable attention in the fields of physical activity and health behavior research (32). Exergames are games that use physical movements or physical activity to advance the play of the game. Popular video games and video consoles have evolved in the past years to include exergames. However, research evidence from scientific studies is mixed with regard to the ability of exergames to meaningfully impact physical activity levels in both field-based and controlled laboratory settings. More research will be needed to determine how best to use exergames to promote meaningful increases in physical activity when used in a setting outside of a structured school or program environment (32–34) and whether their use is linked to long-term changes in physical activity (32).

Potential Challenges and Emerging Areas

Just like the frequency of use of mobile devices, digital technology for mobile devices has evolved considerably, bringing more commercial apps to market that are designed to alter physical activity and sedentary behaviors among child and adolescent populations. Mobile apps, those used on mobile devices such as smartphones and tablets, often in coordination with global positioning devices or wearable physical activity trackers, have been the subject of reviews of quality, features, and behavior change techniques (35) and efficacy of impact among adults and children (36, 37). However, with limited data on the effectiveness of such new applications, particularly among children and adolescents, more research will be needed to identify how best to design and disseminate such technology in a way to influence long-term or population-level changes in physical activity or sedentary behavior (35–37).

Future Directions

- *Identify features of exergames and apps that may facilitate sustained behavior change among different populations of children.*
- *Determine effective strategies to engage children and adolescents in taking up media-based technologies like exergames or mobile apps that can improve physical activity levels.*

Cultural considerations for interventions in different out-of-school-time contexts

Relevant research has identified several considerations that may be helpful to practitioners and researchers in order to enhance the cultural relevance of interventions to increase physical activity as they are adapted to a new setting or used among underrepresented populations (38).

- Solicit input from population members
- Link intervention content with participants' values
- Address language and literacy challenges
- Incorporate culturally relevant media figures
- Use forms of physical activity that are acceptable to the relevant population
- Mitigate culture- or population-specific barriers to participation or activity

Things to Consider

- The hours outside of school provide opportunities to promote additional physical activity among children of all ages.
- Because physical activity in the out-of-school time declines with age and is lower among girls than boys, there are essential strides to be made in expanding, extending, and enhancing existing options, particularly for adolescents.
- Many children and teens participate in after-school programs. Enhancing physical activity in these settings would have large population reach.
- Few children and teens regularly use active transportation to get to and from school. Walking or bicycling to and from school is associated with higher physical activity levels.
- Ensuring safe and convenient opportunities for active transportation can support students in getting more physical activity.
- Family-focused interventions that use family engagement and support to increase physical activity and media and mobile app-based strategies are emerging areas for promoting physical activity.

■ More research and evaluation on the uptake of family-focused and media and mobile app intervention strategies are needed to understand how best to expand these strategies in community settings for the most significant impact on physical activity among school-aged children and adolescents.

■ Resources

TOPIC AREA	RESOURCE SUMMARY AND LINKS
Out-of-school-time programs	■ NIOST (www.noist.org) has policy and research on the role of programs for child health and development ■ Afterschool Alliance (www.afterschoolalliance.org) provides information and resources for after-school programs and organizations ■ BOKS (www.bokskids.org) has resources and tools for implementing a before school program that provides opportunities for physical activity: ■ OSNAP (osnap.org) is a proven initiative that helps out-of-school-time programs improve practices and policies that promote increased physical activity:
Active transportation	■ Safe Routes to School National Partnership (www.saferoutespartnership.org) included comprehensive information and guides to implement Safe Routes to School programs and policies ■ Complete Streets (www.changelabsolutions.org/publications/laws-resolutions-cs) links to findings, model laws, and resolutions that can promote implementation ■ Complete Streets Coalition (smartgrowthamerica.org/program/nationalcomplete- streets-coalition) provides a comprehensive website and resources from Smart Growth America
Family-focused interventions	The Community Guide (www.thecommunityguide.org/findings/physical-activity-family-based-interventions) includes information on research, supporting materials, and implications for implementation of family-based interventions to increase physical activity among children
Technology and media	*Games for Health Journal* is a peer-reviewed journal dedicated to game research, technology, and applications.

NOTE: BOKS, Build Our Kids Success; NIOST, National Institute for Out of School Time; OSNAP, Out of School Nutrition and Physical Activity Initiative.

Acknowledgment

I would like to acknowledge Ms. Molly Knox for her support in conceiving the design and layout for the tables and figures appearing in this chapter.

References

1. Long MW, Sobol AM, Cradock AL, et al. School-day and overall physical activity among youth. *Am J Prev Med.* 2013;45(2):150–157. doi:10.1016/j.amepre.2013.03.011
2. Wickel EE, Belton S. School's out . . . now what? Objective estimates of afterschool sedentary time and physical activity from childhood to adolescence. *J Sci Med Sport.* 2016;19(8):654–658. doi:10.1016/j.jsams.2015.09.001
3. Beets MW, Okely A, Weaver RG, et al. The theory of expanded, extended, and enhanced opportunities for youth physical activity promotion. *Int J Behav Nutr Phys Act.* 2016;13:15. doi:10.1186/s12966-016-0442-2
4. Afterschool Alliance. *America After 3PM: Afterschool Programs in Demand.* Washington, DC: Afterschool Alliance; 2014.
5. Pabayo R, Gauvin L, Barnett TA, et al. Sustained active transportation is associated with a favorable body mass index trajectory across the early school years: findings from the Quebec Longitudinal Study of Child Development birth cohort. *Prev Med.* 2010;50:S59–S64. doi:10.1016/j.ypmed.2009.08.014
6. Cooper AR, Jago R, Southward EF, et al. Active travel and physical activity across the school transition: The PEACH project. *Med Sci Sports Exerc.* 2012;44(10):1890–1897. doi:10.1249/MSS.0b013e31825a3a1e
7. Huang WV, Wong SH, He G. Is a change to active travel to school an important source of physical activity for Chinese children? *Pediatr Exerc Sci.* 2017;29(1):161–168. doi:10.1123/pes.2016-0001
8. Common Sense Media. *The Common Sense Consensus: Media Use by Kids Age Zero to Eight.* San Francisco, CA: Common Sense Media. 2017.
9. Common Sense Media. *The Common Sense Consensus: Media Use by Tweens and Teens.* San Francisco, CA: Common Sense Media. 2015.
10. Wiecha J, Capogrossi K. *Using State Laws & Regulations to Promote Healthy Eating and Physical Activity in Afterschool Programs. Research.* Triangle Park, NC: RTI International. 2016.
11. Beets MW, Rooney L, Tilley F, et al. Evaluation of policies to promote physical activity in afterschool programs: are we meeting current benchmarks? *Prev Med.* 2010;51(3-4):299–301. doi:10.1016/j.ypmed.2010.07.006
12. Weaver RG, Moore JB, Turner-McGrievy B, et al. Identifying strategies programs adopt to meet healthy eating and physical activity standards in afterschool programs. *Health Educ Behav.* 2017;44(4):536–547. doi:10.1177/1090198116676252
13. Mears R, Jago R. Effectiveness of after-school interventions at increasing moderate-to-vigorous physical activity levels in 5-to 18-year olds: a systematic review and meta-analysis. *Br J Sports Med.* 2016;50:1315–1324. doi:10.1136/bjsports-2015-094976
14. Beets MW, Beighle A, Erwin HE, et al. After-school program impact on physical activity and fitness: a meta-analysis. *Am J Prev Med.* 2009;36(6):527–537. doi:10.1016/j.amepre.2009.01.033
15. Pate RR, O'Neill JR. After-school interventions to increase physical activity among youth. *Br J Sports Med.* 2009;43(1):14–18. doi:10.1136/bjsm.2008.055517
16. Moore JB, Schneider L, Lazorick S, et al. Rationale and development of the Move More North Carolina: recommended standards for after-school physical activity. *J Public Health Manag Pract.* 2010;16(4):359–366. doi:10.1097/PHH.0b013e3181ca2634
17. Wiecha JL, Beets MW, Colabianchi N, et al. Promoting physical activity in out-of-school-time programs: we built the bridge-can we walk over it? *Prev Med.* 2014;69:S114–S116. doi:10.1016/j.ypmed.2014.10.027

18. Cradock AL, Barrett JL, Giles CM, et al. Promoting physical activity with the Out of School Nutrition and Physical Activity (OSNAP) Initiative: a cluster-randomized controlled trial. *JAMA Pediatr.* 2016;170(2):155–162. doi:10.1001/jamapediatrics.2015.3406

19. Beets MW, Weaver RG, Turner-McGrievy G, et al. Making policy practice in afterschool programs: a randomized controlled trial on physical activity changes. *Am J Prev Med.* 2015;48(6):694–706. doi:10.1016/j.amepre.2015.01.012

20. Beets MW, Weaver RG, Turner-McGrievy G, et al. Are we there yet? Compliance with physical activity standards in YMCA afterschool programs. *Child Obes.* 2016;12(4):237–246. doi:10.1089/chi.2015.0223

21. Cradock AL, Barrett JL, Kenney EL, et al. Using cost-effectiveness analysis to prioritize policy and programmatic approaches to physical activity promotion and obesity prevention in childhood. *Prev Med.* 2017;95:S17–S27. doi:10.1016/j.ypmed.2016.10.017

22. Mendoza JA, Haaland W, Jacobs M, et al. Bicycle, trains, cycling, and physical activity: a pilot cluster RCT. *Am J Prev Med.* 2017;53(4):481–489. doi:10.1016/j.amepre.2017.05.001

23. McDonald NC, Brown AL, Marchetti LM, et al. U.S. school travel, 2009: an assessment of trends. *Am J Prev Med.* 2011;41(2):146–151. doi:10.1016/j.amepre.2011.04.006

24. McGrath LJ, Hopkins WG, Hinckson EA. Associations of objectively measured built-environment attributes with youth moderate-vigorous physical activity: a systematic review and meta-analysis. *Sports Med.* 2015;45(6):841–865. doi:10.1007/s40279-015-0301-3

25. U.S. Department of Health and Human Services. *Results From the School Health Policies and Practices Study, 2016.* Atlanta, GA; 2017.

26. Alliance NPAP. *The 2017 United States Report Card on Walking and Walkable Communities.* Columbia, SC; 2017.

27. Lieberman M, Pedroso M, Zimmerman S. *2016 State Report Cards on Support for Walking, Bicycling and Active Kids and Communities.* Oakland, CA: Safe Routes to School National Partnership; 2016.

28. Evenson KR, Aytur SA, Satinsky SB, et al. Planning for pedestrians and bicyclists: results from a statewide municipal survey. *J Phys Act Health.* 2011;8:S275–S284. doi:10.1123/jpah.8.s2.s275

29. The Community Preventive Services Task Force. *Task Force Findings: Physical Activity Family-Based Interventions.* Atlanta, GA: The Community Preventive Services Task Force. 2016.

30. Brown HE, Atkin AJ, Panter J, et al. Family-based interventions to increase physical activity in children: a systematic review, meta-analysis and realist synthesis. *Obes Rev.* 2016;17(4):345–360. doi:10.1111/obr.12362

31. Brown HE, Atkin AJ, Panter J, et al. Family-based interventions to increase physical activity in children: a systematic review, meta-analysis and realist synthesis (2016;17: 345) Erratum: *Obes Rev.* 2017;18(4):491–494. doi:10.1111/obr.12493

32. Baranowski T, Blumberg F, Buday R, et al. Games for health for children-current status and needed research. *Games Health J.* 2016;5(1):1–12. doi:10.1089/g4h.2015.0026

33. Gao Z, Chen S, Pasco D, et al. A meta-analysis of active video games on health outcomes among children and adolescents. *Obes Rev.* 2015;16(9):783–794. doi:10.1111/obr.12287

34. Gao Z, Chen S. Are field-based exergames useful in preventing childhood obesity? A systematic review. *Obes Rev.* 2014;15(8):676–691. doi:10.1111/obr.12164

35. Schoeppe S, Alley S, Rebar AL, et al. Apps to improve diet, physical activity and sedentary behaviour in children and adolescents: a review of quality, features and behaviour change techniques. *Int J Behav Nutr Phys Act.* 2017;14:83. doi:10.1186/s12966-017-0538-3

36. Schoeppe S, Alley S, Van Lippevelde W, et al. Efficacy of interventions that use apps to improve diet, physical activity and sedentary behaviour: a systematic review. *Int J Behav Nutr Phys Act.* 2016;13:127. doi:10.1186/s12966-016-0454-yy

37. Fedele DA, Cushing CC, Fritz A, et al. Mobile health interventions for improving health outcomes in youth: a meta-analysis. *JAMA Pediatr.* 2017;171(5):461–469. doi:10.1001/jamapediatrics.2017.0042

38. Conn V, Chan K, Banks J, et al. Cultural relevance of physical activity intervention research with underrepresented populations. *Int Q Community Health Educ.* 2013;34(4):391–414. doi:10.2190/IQ.34.4.g

PROMOTING PHYSICAL ACTIVITY IN PARKS AND RECREATION

MORGAN HUGHEY | BIANCA SHULAKER | ANDREW MOWEN | ANDREW T. KACZYNSKI

LEARNING OBJECTIVES

By the end of this chapter, the student should be able to

1. Describe the history of parks in the United States and how it affects the environment today.
2. Discuss the role of health in national, state, and local parks and recreation agencies.
3. Apply health in all policies to a local community issue.
4. Evaluate how a renovation to a park in your local community could enhance opportunities for physical activity (PA).
5. Compare different types of park-based PA programs and how they would work in the culture and context of your local community.

▓ Introduction

The relationships between park availability, park features, physical activity (PA), and positive health outcomes have been documented across the globe (1). Research has shown that living in closer proximity to parks and recreation facilities has positive health benefits for individuals across the life span including youth (2–4), adults (5, 6), and older adults (7, 8). While park proximity has demonstrated health benefits, the facilities, amenities, quality, and programming of public parks are also essential for attracting park users and promoting population-level PA (9). Parks and recreation professionals and researchers have emphasized the role of designing park spaces and park programs based on the needs of local communities. Using empirical and practice-based evidence, this chapter will present key ideas, strategies, and processes for improving PA through parks and recreation.

© Springer Publishing Company DOI: 10.1891/9780826134592.0014

Historical Perspective

Parks and recreation services include a diverse range of recreation facilities, trails, and green spaces as well as organized programs and events within these settings. These services are provided by governments, nonprofits, and private businesses at the local, state, and federal levels. The origins of the parks and recreation movement in the United States began in the late 19th century—primarily as a means to improve Americans' health (10). Parks and recreation spaces were touted as an antidote to the growing environmental and social concerns of an increasingly urbanized and industrialized nation. Pioneers who helped to advocate and establish parks and recreation services included such visionaries as Frederick Law Olmsted, Joseph Lee, Jane Addams, and John Muir, among many others (10). Over the past century and a half, parks and recreation have evolved to include over 108,000 outdoor parks and recreation facilities and over 65,000 indoor facilities that are within or close to nearly every city or town in the United States and supported primarily through public tax dollars (11). Numerous organized programs, tournaments, and events, either free or low cost, are provided at these places. What began as a service to reduce the impact of environmental degradation, address youth boredom and delinquency, and improve the morale and productivity of the workforce has expanded to address a much wider range of societal benefits (11).

Role of Health in National, State, and Local Parks and Recreation Agencies

The primary goal of many parks and recreation agencies is to provide infrastructure and programming that improves the quality of life within their communities. Indeed, an aging population, increasing rates of obesity, and diminished mental health status due to the demands of modern living suggest a strong role for health in parks and recreation today (11). National studies indicate that Americans view health and PA to be a top benefit of parks and recreation (12) and there is even evidence to suggest people view parks and recreation to be an essential part of the U.S. healthcare system (13). Beyond providing physical spaces for individuals to pursue healthful activities, public parks projects and programs can also afford opportunities for communities to gather socially as well as voice and address specific concerns. For instance, a community meeting to solicit input on the design or programming of a public park could reveal a reluctance to walk in the neighborhood due to traffic-related safety concerns, which may lead to increased collaboration across community sectors to initiate additional preventive health interventions.

Recreation practitioners are increasingly aware of the role parks play in promoting physical health. Correspondingly, explicit policy and intentional partnerships at various levels of governance and practice—from federal to local—not only signal that health outcomes should be a priority for parks practitioners, but they also encourage evidence-based and expert-informed designs and support the pursuit of evaluation of parks and their role in health promotion. Along with this increased awareness, there are an increasing number of policies, informational reports, and toolkits being created to assist with the implementation of this work.

At the federal level, calls to action, like the Surgeon General's Step It Up! Call to Action to Promote Walking and Walkable Communities (14), provide key points for local advocacy and interventions. Similarly, agencies such as the National Park Service have partnered with the Centers for Disease Control and Prevention to create workbooks and tool kits with specific tactics for embedding health considerations into parks-related decision making (15, 16). At the local level, the collaboration between parks and recreation and health departments can be influential at nearly every point in the park's design, development, and activation processes. For example, health departments might collect information about air quality, dangerous intersections, or brownfields that lead to intentional park siting and design decisions. Parks departments might also pursue different programs—from Walk With a Doc (17) to Parks Rx (18, 19) to arthritis-appropriate evidence-based interventions (20)—that facilitate PA through recreation.

In addition, the increased adoption of Health in All Policies (21) and the use of Health Impact Assessments (22) can indicate the desire to collaboratively address health concerns. Leveraging these types of policies can be an important catalyst for collaboration, as well as opening avenues to a wider variety of funding sources (23). Indeed, since the 1970s and in the wake of the more recent Great Recession of 2009, public dollars available for parks and recreation services have been shrinking, prompting parks and recreation agencies to explore alternative funding sources including user fees, private donations, sponsorships, and collaborative grants (24). Because of the reduced funding and resources available for public services, parks and recreation agencies are increasingly establishing partnerships with other community sectors (e.g., health, education, transportation) to figure out how to best leverage their strengths toward mutual desire to improve PA, health, and overall quality of life. For instance, New Jersey hospitals are using their community benefits requirements to fund park design, renovation, and maintenance (25). This practice is currently being more widely explored in numerous states. Overall, the focus on improving PA levels and health through parks and recreation can be felt at the local, state, and national levels.

BOX 14.1

Health in All Policies

Using collaborative approaches to improve and address complex health challenges by embedding health considerations into decision-making processes across a broad array of sectors. The *Health in All Policies: A Guide for State and Local Governments* was jointly developed by the Public Health Institute, California Department of Public Health, and the American Public Health Association (www.phi.org/uploads/files/Health_in_All_Policies-A_Guide_for_State_and_Local_Governments.pdf).

BOX 14.2

Health Impact Assessment

This is a process that helps evaluate potential health effects of a plan, project, or policy before development and implementation, providing practical recommendations to maximize positive benefits and minimize negative impacts. HIA tools can help communities, decision

(continued)

(*continued*)

makers, and practitioners make choices that improve public health through community design. (www.cdc.gov/healthyplaces/hia.htm).

HIA, Health Impact Assessment.

■ Current Issues in Promoting PA in Parks and Recreation

Park Renovations and Changes to the Built Environment

One key effort to promote improved health through parks and recreation is changing the infrastructure of public parks to support increased PA. The typical park design and development process consists of four phases: planning, design, construction, and post-construction activities (Figure 14.1), though this process can vary based on contextual differences. An example of intentional decisions made at each stage to embed health within the park development process is shown in Figure 14.2. This example involves the renovation of Balboa Park, a 25-acre public park in San Francisco, California, that occurred in collaboration with the Trust for Public Land.

There is an increasing amount of literature about the most effective ways to utilize parks as health interventions by increasing use and user PA levels. This includes siting parks in areas where communities currently lack access (or access to a variety of park sizes and features) or with consideration for the types of health concerns and interventions that would be effective for surrounding populations (5, 26, 27). Specific park features including trails or walking paths, green space or fitness zones, and quality (e.g., maintenance and aesthetics) have received investment through renovation and have been shown to be used for higher levels of PA (5, 28–31), although research around this topic is ongoing (32).

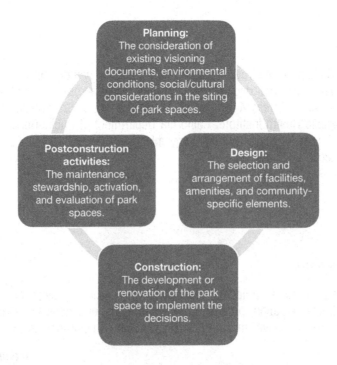

FIGURE 14.1 Typical park design and build process (Trust for Public Land).

Partnerships between organizations and community residents are central to the park design or renovation process. Many of the decisions in the Balboa Park renovation were arrived at through input from expert partners and community members (Figures 14.3 and 14.4). As an initial goal of the project was to create a public space that would support

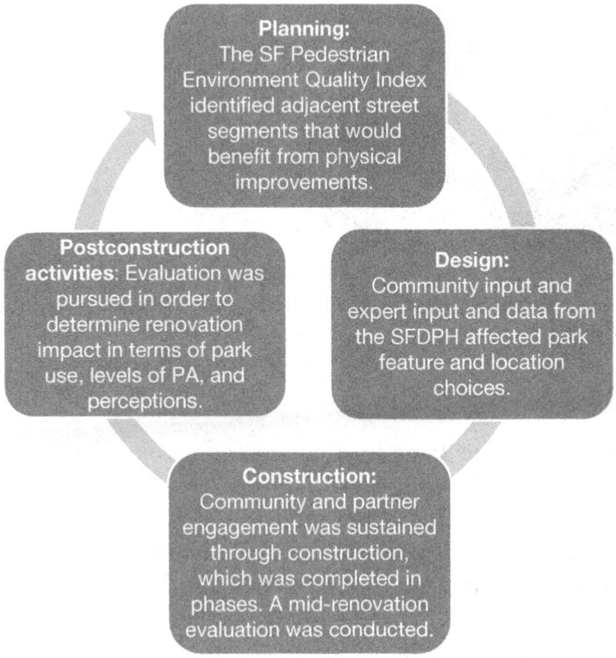

Planning:
The SF Pedestrian Environment Quality Index identified adjacent street segments that would benefit from physical improvements.

Postconstruction activities: Evaluation was pursued in order to determine renovation impact in terms of park use, levels of PA, and perceptions.

Design:
Community input and expert input and data from the SFDPH affected park feature and location choices.

Construction:
Community and partner engagement was sustained through construction, which was completed in phases. A mid-renovation evaluation was conducted.

FIGURE 14.2 Balboa Park, San Francisco example (Trust for Public Land).

PA, physical activity; SFDPH, San Francisco Department of Public Health.

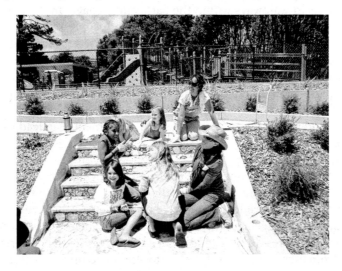

FIGURE 14.3 Friends and neighbors help create a mosaic piece on stairs in one of the playground areas at Balboa Park.

Trudy Garber/The Trust for Public Land, 2012

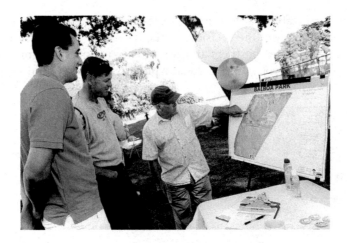

FIGURE 14.4 Community members providing feedback about park design renderings at the groundbreaking event at Balboa Park.

Pat Mazzera Photography, 2011.

participation in higher levels of PA, The Trust for Public Land (project lead) partnered with the San Francisco Department of Public Health's (SFDPH's) Program on Health, Equity and Sustainability, and the RAND Corporation (33). The SFDPH gave input about park designs, existing conditions, PA goals, and provided initial context data (e.g., San Francisco Indicator Project information and the Pedestrian Environment Quality Index) (34), and the RAND Corporation assisted with evaluation through surveys and observations pre-, mid-, and postconstruction.

Community input was essential for this project. For instance, based upon the aforementioned expert and community input, "real" accessibility was improved by upgrades to the intersections around the park, enhancing the entrances with supportive amenities such as benches, connections to walkways within the park, and signage. In the postrenovation survey of surrounding residents and park users, more people reported liking the proximity of the park, though the park itself had not been moved (30). Input from community members led to the renovation including the following features: adding active and a greater variety of play equipment, constructing multipurpose zones and fields, and changing the park layout to enable more visibility and improve perceptions of both safety and accessibility.

Community-wide park and recreation interventions and investments can lead to new or improved parks, trails, or features of those spaces. While these investments are laudable on the surface, undesired consequences for the neighboring communities such as increased congestion, user conflicts, and increased environmental gentrification should be considered (35). Environmental gentrification is the process whereby investments in green space serve to attract new residents and drive up property values, displacing low-income residents (35, 36). Park agencies, conservancies, and foundations are seeking ways to better engage community residents, giving them a voice in shaping park projects and protecting residents from increased property values to attempt to minimize potential negative effects. Some experts note that large-scale or significant urban park, recreation, and green space projects are destined for gentrification and suggest minor improvements that are "just green enough" to promote positive outcomes (including health) but not attract major real estate speculation (37).

Park-Based PA Programs

In addition to changes or development of park infrastructure, park-based programming and events are key ways to facilitate increased PA levels through recreation departments (38, 39). Park-based programming and events can provide structured or unstructured opportunities for PA for community members of all ages and backgrounds. Programming is also a potential mechanism to increase park use and PA levels in underutilized park spaces (40).

Structured park-based PA programs are organized activities that are typically led by staff-associated parks and recreation departments or other community agencies. Two key structured programs that are widespread in recreation departments are exercise programs and sports leagues. Increasingly, parks and recreation departments offer both indoor and outdoor group exercise classes including

- Fitness classes (e.g., boot camps, weight lifting, cross-training, running clubs)
- Aerobics/dance classes (e.g., zumba, pilates, barre)
- Yoga
- Tai Chi or Martial Arts
- Outdoor classes (e.g., fishing, paddleboarding, challenge courses)

The costs associated with exercise programs depend on the specific recreation agency and program. For example, New York City Parks offer a program called "Show Up and Shape Up" as a free, drop-in fitness program (41). Also, Charleston County Park and Recreation Commission in South Carolina provides a physician-referred, comprehensive fitness program (Move-IT!) to local residents as a fee-based program (42).

Many parks and recreation departments also offer sports leagues for youth, adults, and older adults to participate. Sports leagues are organized by recreation staff, including administrative details like securing the location, officials (e.g., umpires, referees), and scheduling. Sports that are offered typically depend on the interests and demand of the local community as well as the capacity of the parks and recreation department staff and facilities. Organized sports have demonstrated a positive impact on PA levels and overall development, particularly for children, and are widespread across the United States (43).

Parks and recreation departments can also offer unstructured PA programs where community members can participate in a program or activity at their own will. Fitness zones, or stationary fitness equipment, are a recent trend occurring in many parks and recreation facilities and have shown promise for increasing park-based PA (29). Fitness zones are structural changes to the parks but provide an opportunity for residents to be physically active at their own pace (29). Another example of unstructured PA programs offered through parks and recreation departments are scavenger hunts and geocaching. For example, LiveWell Greenville (livewellgreenville.org), a public health coalition in Greenville County, South Carolina, partnered with six local parks and recreation departments to develop a scavenger hunt across 20 selected parks called "Park Hop" aimed at increasing park use and PA among youth during summer (44). Recreation staff developed clues at each park, and coalition staff developed a paper and mobile app version of the scavenger hunt. Families and children could participate at their own pace during the summer and local organizations have sponsored PA-themed prizes to include in a drawing at the end of the program (44, 45). Other popular park-based events include races, educational classes, art in the park, and movie in the park. In summary, many existing park-based programs can provide opportunities for community members to visit recreation spaces and be physically active.

Trails and Greenways

Trails and greenways are often called "linear parks" and represent an important component of community recreation infrastructure and also often serve as a mechanism for active transportation in communities (46). Trails may vary in location (e.g., within a park or standalone trail), length, connectivity, surface (e.g., natural, paved), and amenities (e.g., parking, restrooms, benches). Trails are utilized for multiple modes of PA including walking, jogging, cycling, and rollerblading, and the presence or development of trails has shown associations with increased adult PA levels (46, 47). Rail trails have emerged as key projects in many cities across the United States where local planning and parks and recreation departments work to convert out–of-service rail lines to multiuse trails (48). Rail trails can provide connectivity between neighborhoods, schools, parks, and businesses and have also demonstrated a positive economic impact in many communities as they support small businesses and tourism (49, 50).

Trail development can happen at various levels in a local community (51). First, a trail may be constructed within a local park via recreation staff or in collaboration with local volunteers to provide an additional PA amenity within an existing park. Recreation departments may also work to identify new, standalone spaces that can serve as sites for a future trail. For a multimile greenway or rail-trail project, multiple departments within a municipality are often required to work together to develop a plan, secure funding, implement the project, and maintain the trail. A national nonprofit Rails to Trails Conservancy has developed trail-building basics and tool box as relevant planning tools for local communities to use (48).

Shared-Use Agreements

Efforts to enhance access to parks and recreation services do not always have to entail renovations, building new facilities, or creating new programs. Particularly in cities and suburban areas, there are existing facilities that could be more fully utilized if their owners collaborated and shared them with other community organizations for other purposes. These shared-use agreements (also including open use and community use) provide increased public access to existing facilities and are often allowed before or after hours of the facilities' primary use (52). The costs and risks of sharing the facility are often predefined through a series of agreed-upon terms and conditions. These agreements can be tailored to community organizational needs and could be based on either a formalized legal agreement or an informal agreement that shares the facility based on past practices (52).

A wide range of shared-use partners to enhance parks and recreation assets are possible including school districts, government entities, faith-based organizations, and private business/industry. Often, these facilities include schoolyards, tracks/fields, playgrounds, or community fitness facilities. Schools are one of the most common shared-use agreements, with research showing little to no increases in operational costs, although facility maintenance costs may be higher due to increased use (53). Shared-use research concludes these agreements provide "some evidence" of efficacy for enhanced PA access and behaviors through increased opportunities. Because they take advantage of preexisting infrastructure, shared-use agreements are a cost-efficient way to expand recreation programs and services (54, 55).

Despite this evidence, there are a number of barriers to consider regarding the development, adoption, and sustainability of shared-use agreements (56). First, elected officials and unit administrators must be committed to this type of use arrangement and work with local residents and current users to design shared-use spaces and policies to make sure that it can work for the primary users and secondary or shared-use visitors. With shared-use comes joint responsibility for maintenance and other costs, particularly if a shared-use facility needs upgrades in order to meet the needs of the primary and secondary users. Identifying mutual partner benefits and needs, building community support, formalizing the agreement, and monitoring impacts have been suggested as steps for improving shared-use effectiveness (55). When developing shared-use agreements, it is recommended to use participatory decision making to include a wide range of stakeholders—those who use and will use, those who live close to, and those who take care of these facilities should have a say in their design (57). Finally, it is important that communities take a systematic approach to identifying shared-use opportunities in the areas of greatest need—those places with poor access to parks and PA opportunities.

Community Engagement and Cultural Considerations

Community engagement is central to effective planning and public space design and development, programming, and partnerships, particularly when specifically addressing PA levels or improved health for local residents. Soliciting community input deepens the understanding of specific community values, needs, barriers, and preferences, all of which can inform park design and programming for community use and lead to the implementation of interventions to effectively influence behaviors.

Not only do participatory processes provide essential input about the physical design of park space, they build ownership of specific sites and instill a greater sense of belonging, which in turn can encourage greater use of those sites. Furthermore, engagement builds relationships between community members and builds social capital, which is associated with improved community health and well-being (58). Table 14.1 describes five commonly used community engagement methods (59).

TABLE 14.1. Commonly used community engagement methods to advance parks and recreation.

METHOD (60)	DESCRIPTION
Community meetings	Public meetings are a traditional method in planning and are typically designed to share information and solicit feedback. Participants are typically self-selected, but marketing and promotion of meetings can help reach new audiences.
Design charrettes	Used extensively in architecture-related fields, design charrettes are a type of meeting where participants sketch or share design ideas (60,61).

(continued)

TABLE 14.1. Commonly used community engagement methods to advance parks and recreation. *(continued)*

METHOD (60)	DESCRIPTION
Surveys	The type of information and scale are dependent upon the purpose and use of the data. Important to note are response rates and representation.
Hands-on creation	Contrasting from traditional practices where designs are created on paper, this approach involves the modeling of parks elements in a physical space to help determine the placement, size, and function of amenities and other park elements.
Festivals or other events	Festivals or other events can engage community members in more informal settings and lend flexibility in how new or varied audiences are reached. These can be held before renovations occur, as well as postconstruction to activate park spaces.

Community engagement is not "one size fits all." The methods selected can influence who takes part, and how many stakeholders participate. Using a combination of approaches gives different community members the opportunity to find the most appropriate method of involvement for them. Figure 14.5 highlights multiple parks and recreation community engagement methods from specific scenarios.

Table 14.2 shows important topics and key questions to ask before selecting methods and designing tools for community engagement.

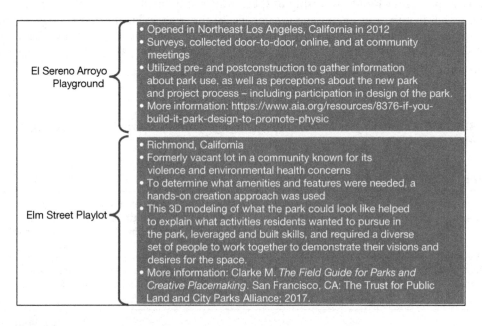

FIGURE 14.5 Parks and recreation community engagement examples .

TABLE 14.2. Key topics and questions to use when engaging communities.

TOPIC	QUESTIONS TO ASK
Define your geography and audience	■ Who do you seek to engage? ■ Are there key audiences that are currently underrepresented or have historically felt unwelcome in engagement efforts? ■ Are there barriers to participation? These can include limited access to tools (such as the Internet), constraints on capacity (such as working multiple jobs or not having access to child care), or other considerations (such as language barriers).
What are the dynamics of the geography and community you seek to engage?	■ Who makes decisions? Who is trusted in the community? ■ Are there other, existing efforts? What priorities have been identified through these efforts? ■ What is the history of the neighborhood and the relationships between the neighborhood and local government and parks and recreation department?

Parks and Environmental Justice

Environmental justice (EJ) is an increasingly important concern in the field of parks and recreation (54). EJ commonly refers to the idea that everyone has equal access to health-promoting resources and has the means and opportunity to participate in the processes that bring about that equality. Several studies have examined whether access to parks and recreation facilities are equitable across communities by income and race/ethnicity (62–65). For example, in examining 165 parks in Kansas City, Missouri, Vaughan et al. found that low-income census tracts contained more parks, but fewer parks with playgrounds and more quality concerns per park (66). Similarly, another study in El Paso, Texas, reported that high-income areas have fewer quality and safety concerns within or surrounding parks, and that areas with more foreign (non-U.S.) born residents had significantly greater park and neighborhood quality and safety concerns (67).

Because the availability, features, and quality of parks and recreation facilities can vary dramatically, tools are being developed to allow parks and recreation agencies, citizens, and other stakeholders to identify and remediate "park deserts" in communities. For example, The Trust for Public Land's ParkScore provides a rating for the 100 largest U.S. cities that takes into account park acreage, facilities and spending, and the percentage of the population living within a 10-minute walk of a park (parkscore/tpl.org). In addition, the Community Park Audit Tool (CPAT; activelivingresearch.org/community-park-audit-tool-cpat) was developed as a user-friendly method for evaluating the available facilities and amenities within and surrounding a park as well as their usability and condition (68). The CPAT is currently being developed into an app for mobile devices (eCPAT) that has been tested with youth (69, 70).

Measurement and Evaluation of PA in Parks and Recreation Settings

The increased use of rigorous research designs (e.g., multisite evaluations, more objective measurements of PA, and longitudinal analyses) are exciting developments that build an evidence base around PA interventions (3, 71). Measuring and evaluating the impact of parks and recreation facilities and programs on health behaviors and health outcomes, as well as other important social and economic indicators, is a key component of this discipline (72). Keeping pace with technological advancements and integrating them into data collection and analyses can be a daunting and potentially risky proposition for practitioners conducting community-based research. As one of the applications, those charged with monitoring and improving the use of parks for health promotion must consider which technological innovations can provide better park use data more accurately and for less cost. The System for Observing Play and Recreation in Communities (SOPARC) has proven to be a reliable and valid tool to assess park use and PA (73) and mobile SOPARC applications have helped to democratize its diffusion across many study sites and settings (74). A free, detailed workshop on the mobile SOPARC program can be found here via Active Living Research (activelivingresearch.org/systematic-observation-physical-activity-using-isoparc-ipad-application-research-and-practice-2015).

Technologies to assess park user behaviors that do not require SOPARC's human observation are now being touted and tested in a variety of park environmental and programmatic interventions. For example, the growth of mobile, wearable devices and technologies to capture human movement through Wi-Fi signals show promise for monitoring the effects of added park features, renovated parks, and organized PA programs (75, 76). Supporting environmental level changes in parks and recreation will continue to require sound empirical evidence captured by current measurement and evaluation techniques.

Case Study: Park Prescriptions: Doctors Doling Out Doses of Vitamin G

As public health and medical professionals seek innovative and scalable solutions to rising costs associated with a variety of mental and physical health issues, parks, trails, and other outdoor resources are increasingly being recognized as key components of the healthcare system. Not surprisingly, doctors are turning toward recommending visits to parks and natural areas as one element of patients' treatment and prevention plans (77–79). Indeed, as trusted sources of advice and information, counseling delivered by physicians has been shown to be an effective method for increasing PA (80, 81). Park prescriptions programs involve healthcare professionals instructing patients to visit local parks daily or weekly, sometimes in place of medication, and such initiatives are expanding in popularity across the country.

One of the earliest and most established park prescriptions programs is Park Rx America based originally in Washington, DC (www.parkrxamerica.org). Founded by Dr. Robert Zarr, a pediatrician who was concerned about growing problems such as attention deficit hyperactivity disorder (ADHD) and childhood obesity, the goal was to develop a system to connect primary care physicians with information about parks located close to their patients. To date, Park Rx America is the only park prescriptions program to link a searchable database of parks directly into electronic health records to make prescribing green exercise and relaxation simple and efficient for those who need it. Specifically, 342 parks in DC were rated for elements such as cleanliness, accessibility, level of activity, amenities, and safety, and a one-page summary was created that allows doctors to match each patient with a nearby park that fits with his or her interests and abilities (82). Efforts to formally evaluate and disseminate the Park Rx America program are ongoing, but a feasibility study found that providers were able to easily incorporate the intervention into the course of patient visits and that the percentage of parents reporting that their child had visited a park in the past year and who focused on PA regularly as a family increased significantly (82). As park prescriptions programs continue to expand, confidence is high that such initiatives might be just what the doctor ordered.

Case Study: Hoppin' to Health on the Greenville Health System Swamp Rabbit Trail

Trails and greenways have increased throughout many cities across the United States (46). Many greenways have been constructed along old rail line corridors and now provide a space for recreation and an alternative transportation option. One popular rail trail in the southeastern United States is the Greenville Health System Swamp Rabbit Trail (GHS SRT). The construction of the GHS SRT was a strategic partnership between officials at the City of Greenville, Greenville County, and Greenville Health System. The aims of the trail were to provide additional recreation and transportation options, stimulate economic activity, and promote health. In 2009, the original 9-mile core of the rail trail was constructed from Traveler's Rest, South Carolina, to downtown Greenville. Less than 10 years later, the trail has doubled in length for a total of 19.9 miles of multimodal trail systems that connect neighborhoods, parks, and local businesses (Figure 14.6) (83).

A multicomponent, multiyear evaluation study was conducted by Dr. Julian Reed at Furman University (83). Using direct observation methodology, intercept surveys, phone surveys, and focus groups, the evaluation study examined the demographic profile of trail users, PA types and levels, perceptions of the Swamp Rabbit Trail, and local business economic impact (83, 84). In 2013, a total number of 21,972 trail users were observed for 16 observation days, resulting in an estimated 503,236 trail users per year (2013); this represented a 20% increase from 2012 (83). The majority of trail users were male (60.1%), non-Hispanic White (90.3%), and were observed bicycling (75.2%) (83). Results from telephone surveys also showed that Greenville County residents that reported using the GHS SRT were more likely to be normal weight and to report better health compared to trail nonusers (85).

In addition to the positive evaluation results, the community adoption and engagement around the GHS SRT has been significant. While there was some uncertainty regarding the use of the trail at initial construction, residents and tourists have come to enjoy and appreciate the GHS SRT as a key community resource. One expression of this engagement is the naming of local businesses: the Swamp Rabbit Café & Grocery,

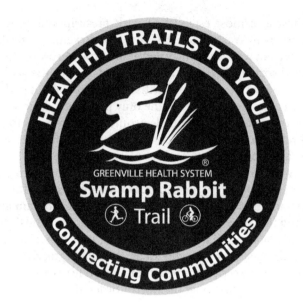

FIGURE 14.6   Logo of the GHS SRT.

GHS SRT, Greenville Health System Swamp Rabbit Trail.
Courtesy of Greenville County Parks, Recreation, and Tourism.

the Swamp Rabbit Brewery, and a rebranding of the local hockey team now called the Swamp Rabbits. A complete greenway plan for the entire county is in place, including connections to many of the smaller municipalities. A County Greenways director and Bikeville, a City of Greenville initiative to create a bike-friendly city, provide dedicated staffing to grow and develop the trails and biking networks in Greenville, South Carolina (Figure 14.7).

Case Study: Transformative Park Renovations That Cultivate Community Wellness: The Story of Boeddeker Park

San Francisco recently gained distinction as the first city in the nation where every resident lives within a 10-minute walk to a park. However, not every 10-minute walk, or the quality of each park, is the same. In the Tenderloin neighborhood where 3,500 children live within a 40-block area, there are very few green or open spaces, and existing spaces are often underutilized, unknown, or disconnected. This incredibly dense and impoverished neighborhood also has the highest incidences of homelessness, drug abuse, and mental illness in San Francisco, and one of the highest rates of violent crime. With high rates of heart disease and diabetes in the local population, it is imperative that spaces be available for active recreation and exercise.

At 0.97 acres, Boeddeker Park and Clubhouse is the largest public open space in the Tenderloin neighborhood. Although significant funds were spent on the construction of the original park, a multiyear gap of on-site programming and supervision led to deterioration of the space. As one of the few places local schools and after-school programs had to bring children to play, the park's inhospitable design and limited amenities generally discouraged use and raised safety concerns. Beginning in 2012, the City of San Francisco partnered with The Trust for Public Land to renovate Boeddeker Park.

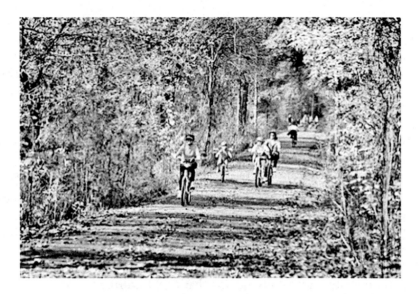

FIGURE 14.7 Image of the GHS SRT in 2013. GHS SRT, Greenville Health System Swamp Rabbit Trail.

Courtesy of Greenville County Parks, Recreation, and Tourism.

Major goals for this redevelopment project included providing usable and appropriate amenities, addressing inefficiencies and safety hazards of the existing park design, and improving health and wellness.

The Trust for Public Land worked extensively with City agencies, including San Francisco Recreation and Park and the SFDPH, community nonprofits, and community members to determine the designs for this space. A variety of community meetings in the neighborhood were held at different weekday and weekend times to accommodate residents with various employment, school, and family schedules. Food and beverages were served at all meetings, and translation services were available in Spanish, Vietnamese, Cantonese, and Russian. The design of the revitalized park—which reopened in December 2014—incorporates ideas generated in these community workshops and focus groups.

The renovated park includes outdoor fitness equipment, a walking path with accessible ramps, a large lawn, new play equipment, a full-size basketball court, and site furnishings, such as lighting, benches, tables, and bike racks. The location of target areas (such as the play area and lawn) were rearranged, new fencing and signage were installed, and most areas and landscaping were kept at or slightly above eye level from the street, making the space more visible and also more inviting. The dense population of seniors—an intentional outreach to these groups by holding meetings at local residential care and nursing homes—led to the incorporation of open areas for activities such as Tai Chi or walking groups.

Since the park's renovation began, three rounds of evaluation have been conducted. Before the renovation, most of the park was inaccessible for most of the day because gates were kept locked for afterschool use only. Many people also expressed strong feelings of discomfort and feeling unsafe, "like a prison." Postrenovation, more users were seen in the park, with the increase particularly high for children and seniors. Higher levels of PA were also observed among all age groups. Seventy-five percent of those surveyed also report that they do or would consider exercising in the park. Residents also reported that they liked the equipment, design, and proximity of the parks, and surveys revealed that 70% now feel the park is safe or very safe.

Through this work, several best practices and lessons learned have been identified:

- An effective park project should begin by identifying community concerns and vision. Often topics related to the social determinants of health are priorities for residents, as much as providing input about specific areas in the park space.

- Leadership from all stakeholder groups (residents and others served by the park, the city, community groups that could utilize the space, and health experts and providers) should be included from the onset of the project.

- Intended uses for the park, goals, and outcomes should be considered from the beginning of the project. This enables measurement and assessment of impact, as well as data to inform lessons for future projects.

Boeddeker is now an anchor space for the community, and providing opportunities for healthy choices continues to be a priority for the Tenderloin neighborhood. Furthermore, the demonstrated success and partnerships built through the Boeddeker Park project has catalyzed greater support and built capacity to tackle community health and well-being concerns and issues (Figures 14.8 and 14.9).

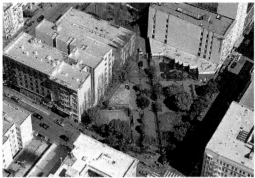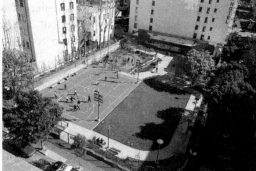

FIGURE 14.8 Aerial views of Boeddeker Park (A) before renovation (The Trust for Public Land, 2007) and (B) after renovation (Jeremy Beeton, 2015).

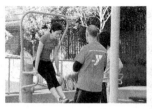
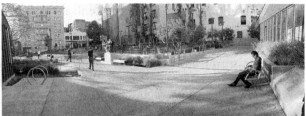
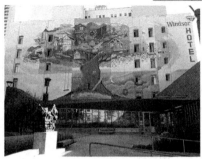
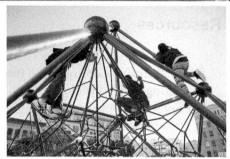

FIGURE 14.9 (A) A community member exercising in the Fitness Zone with a staff member from the YMCA supervising (Jeremy Beeton, 2015), (B) photo of Boeddeker Park and Clubhouse. Courtesy of WRNS Architectural firm (Matthew Millman, 2015), (C) a new mural painted on an adjacent building (Bianca Shulaker/The Trust for Public Land, 2017), and (D) local schoolchildren playing during the grand opening celebration of Boeddeker Park on December 10, 2014 (Quincy Stamper, 2014).

Summary

Early development of urban parks was geared toward improving the social, environmental, and physical well-being of individual community members and cities as a whole. Today, as communities continue to struggle with complex social, environmental, and health challenges such as urbanization, climate change, and impact of chronic disease illnesses, parks and recreation departments are key stakeholders in developing solutions to address such problems. Through recreation facilities, programs, and collaborative government and nongovernment initiatives, these key community spaces have the vast potential to impact population-level PA for individuals across the life span.

Things to Consider

- The primary goal of many parks and recreation agencies is to provide infrastructure and programming that improves the quality of life within their communities.
- Community-wide parks and recreation interventions and investments can lead to new or improved parks, trails, or features of those spaces.
- Park-based programming and events can provide structured or unstructured opportunities for PA for community members of all ages and backgrounds.

- Community engagement is central to effective planning and public space design and development, programming, and partnerships, particularly when specifically addressing PA levels or improved health for local residents.
- Measuring and evaluating the impact of parks and recreation facilities and programs on health behaviors and health outcomes, as well as other important social and economic indicators, is a key component of this discipline.

Resources

- Step It Up! The Surgeon General's Call to Action to Promote Walking and Walkable Communities: https://www.surgeongeneral.gov/library/calls/walking-and-walkable-communities/index.html
- Center for Disease Control and Prevention, Health Impact Assessment: https://www.cdc.gov/healthyplaces/hia.htm
- Center for Disease Control and Prevention, Healthy Community Design Checklist Toolkit: https://www.cdc.gov/healthyplaces/toolkit
- National Park Service and Center for Disease Control and Prevention, Parks, Trails, and Health Workbook: A Tool for Planners, Parks and Recreation Professionals, and Health Practitioners: https://www.nps.gov/public_health/hp/hphp/press/Parks_Trails_and_Health_Workbook_508_Accessible_PDF.pdf
- National Park Service and Centers for Disease Control and Prevention, Improving Public Health Through Public Parks and Trails: Eight Common Measures: https://npgallery.nps.gov/RTCA/GetAsset/f09e69fc-2696-45e8-b4d5-90e4cea5e689
- Rails to Trails Conservancy, Trail-Building Toolbox: https://www.railstotrails.org/build-trails/trail-building-toolbox
- Parkology, the online resource and community of experts and enthusiasts to improve access to close-to-home, quality parks: https://www.parkology.org/ParkHome

References

1. Sallis JF, Cerin E, Conway TL, et al. Physical activity in relation to urban environments in 14 cities worldwide: a cross-sectional study. *Lancet.* 2016;387(10034):2207–2217. doi:10.1016/S0140-6736(15)01284-2
2. Roemmich JN, Epstein LH, Raja S, et al. Association of access to parks and recreational facilities with the physical activity of young children. *Prev Med.* 2006;43(6):437–441. doi:10.1016/j.ypmed.2006.07.007
3. Wolch J, Jerrett M, Reynolds K, et al. Childhood obesity and proximity to urban parks and recreational resources: a longitudinal cohort study. *Health Place.* 2011;17(1):207–214. doi:10.1016/j.healthplace.2010.10.001
4. Hughey SM, Kaczynski AT, Child S, et al. Green and lean: is neighborhood park and playground availability associated with youth obesity? Variations by gender, socioeconomic status, and race/ethnicity. *Prev Med.* 2017;95(suppl):S101–S108. doi:10.1016/j.ypmed.2016.11.024

5. Kaczynski AT, Potwarka LR, Saelens BE. Association of park size, distance, and features with physical activity in neighborhood parks. *Am J Public Health*. 2008;98(8):1451–1456. doi:10.2105/AJPH.2007.129064

6. Sugiyama T, Cerin E, Owen N, et al. Perceived neighbourhood environmental attributes associated with adults' recreational walking: IPEN adult study in 12 countries. *Health Place*. 2014;28(suppl C):22–30. doi:10.1016/j.healthplace.2014.03.003

7. Cerin E, Nathan A, van Cauwenberg J, et al. The neighbourhood physical environment and active travel in older adults: a systematic review and meta-analysis. *Int J Behav Nutr Phys Act*. 2017;14:15. doi:10.1186/s12966-017-0471-5

8. Mowen A, Orsega-Smith E, Payne L, et al. The role of park proximity and social support in shaping park visitation, physical activity, and perceived health among older adults. *J Phys Act Health*. 2007;4(2):167–179. doi:10.1123/jpah.4.2.167

9. Bedimo-Rung AL, Mowen AJ, Cohen DA. The significance of parks to physical activity and public health: a conceptual model. *Am J Prev Med*. 2005;28(2 suppl 2):159–168. doi:10.1016/j.amepre.2004.10.024

10. Cranz G. *The Politics of Park Design. A History of Urban Parks in America* . Cambridge, MA: MIT Press; 1982.

11. Godbey G, Mowen A, Ashburn VA. *The Benefits of Physical Activity Provided by Park and Recreation Services: The Scientific Evidence*. Ashburn, VA: National Recreation and Park Association; 2010.

12. Mowen AJ, Graefe AR, Barrett AG, et al. *Americans' Broad-Based Support for Local Recreation and Park Services: Results From a Nationwide Study*. Ashburn, VA: National Recreation and Park Association; 2016.

13. Mowen AJ, Barrett AG, Graefe AR, et al. "Take in two parks and call me in the morning"—perception of parks as an essential component of our healthcare system. *Prev Med Rep*. 2017;6:63–65. doi:10.1016/j.pmedr.2017.02.006

14. Surgeon General. *Step It Up! The Surgeon General's Call to Action to Promote Walking and Walkable Communities*. Available at: https://www.surgeongeneral.gov/library/calls/walking-and-walkable-communities/index.html. Accessed September 16, 2017

15. Center for Disease Control and Prevention. Parks, trails, and health workbook. Available at: https://www.cdc.gov/healthyplaces/healthtopics/parks_trails_workbook.htm. Accessed September 16, 2017.

16. Merriam D, Bality A, Boehmer T. *Improving Public Health Through Public Parks and Trails: Eight Common Measures. Summary Report*. U.S. Department of Health and Human Services, Atlanta, GA: Centers for Disease Control and Prevention and U.S. Department of the Interior, National Park Service; 2017.

17. Walk With a Doc. Just a walk in the park. Available at: http://walkwithadoc.org/. Accessed September 12, 2017.

18. Park Rx. About: what are park prescriptions? Available at: http://parkrx.org/about. Accessed September 12, 2017.

19. Park Rx America. What is Park Rx America? Available at: https://parkrxamerica.org/about.php. Accessed September 12, 2017.

20. National Recreation and Park Association. Evidence-based interventions. Available at: http://www.nrpa.org/our-work/partnerships/initiatives/healthy-aging-in-parks/evidence-based-interventions/. Accessed September 12, 2017.

21. Rudolph L, Caplan J, Ben-Moshe K, et al. *Health in All Policies: A Guide for State and Local Governments*. Washington, DC and Oakland, CA: American Public Health Association and Public Health Institute; 2013.

22. Centers for Disease Control and Prevention. Parks and trails Health in All Policies toolkit. Available at: https://www.cdc.gov/healthyplaces/parks_trails/{#}toolkit. Accessed September 12, 2017.

23. Plan4Health. Health in All Policies resources. Available at: http://plan4health.us/health-in-all-policies-resources. Accessed September 12, 2017.

24. Pitas NAD. The relationship between self-rated health and use of parks and participation in recreation programs, United States, 1991 and 2015. *Prev Chronic Dis*. 2017;14:E02. doi:10.5888/pcd14.160441

25. Hacke R. *Improving Community Health by Strengthening Community Investment, Roles for Hospitals and Health Systems.* Cambridge, MA: Center for Community Investment; 2017.
26. Trust for Public Land. About ParkScore. Available at: http://parkscore.tpl.org/{#}sm.0001tyrxp8656dszqss1fhwk2re6i. Accessed September 12, 2017.
27. Elwell Bostrom H, Shulaker B, Rippon J, et al. Strategic and integrated planning for healthy, connected cities: Chattanooga case study. *Prev Med.* 2017;95(suppl):S115–S119. doi:10.1016/j.ypmed.2016.11.002
28. Gardsjord HS, Tveit MS, Nordh H. Promoting youth's physical activity through park design: linking theory and practice in a public health perspective. *Landsc Res.* 2014;39(1):70–81. doi:10.1080/01426397.2013.793764
29. Cohen DA, Marsh T, Williamson S, et al. Impact and cost-effectiveness of family fitness zones: a natural experiment in urban public parks. *Health Place.* 2012;18(1):39–45. doi:10.1016/j.healthplace.2011.09.008
30. Cohen DA, Han B, Nagel CJ, et al. The first national study of neighborhood parks. *Am J Prev Med.* 2016;51(4):419–426. doi:10.1016/j.amepre.2016.03.021
31. Cohen DA, Han B, Isacoff J, et al. Impact of park renovations on park use and park-based physical activity. *J Phys Act Health.* 2015;12(2):289–295. doi:10.1123/jpah.2013-0165
32. Koohsari MJ, Mavoa S, Villanueva K, et al. Public open space, physical activity, urban design and public health: concepts, methods and research agenda. *Health Place.* 2015;33:75–82. doi:10.1016/j.healthplace.2015.02.009
33. Shulaker BD, Isacoff JW, Cohen DA, et al. Partnerships for parks and physical activity. *Am J Health Promot.* 2014;28(3 suppl):S97–S99. doi:10.4278/ajhp.130430-ARB-215
34. The San Francisco Indicator Project. About the San Francisco Indicator Project. Available at: https://www.sfindicatorproject.org/about. Accessed September 12, 2017.
35. Eckerd A. Cleaning up without clearing out? A spatial assessment of environmental gentrification. *Urban Aff Rev.* 2011;47(1):31–59. doi:10.1177/1078087410379720
36. Checker M. Wiped out by the "Greenwave": environmental gentrification and the paradoxical politics of urban sustainability. *City Soc.* 2011;23(2):210–229. doi:10.1111/j.1548-744X.2011.01063.x
37. Wolch JR, Byrne J, Newell JP. Urban green space, public health, and environmental justice: the challenge of making cities 'just green enough'. *Landsc Urban Plan.* 2014;125:234–244. doi:10.1016/j.landurbplan.2014.01.017
38. National Recreation and Park Association. Park programming and better health. Available at: http://www.nrpa.org/our-work/three-pillars/health-wellness/parksandhealth/fact-sheets/park-programming-better-health/. Accessed September 16, 2017.
39. Cohen DA, McKenzie TL, Sehgal A, et al. Contribution of public parks to physical activity. *Am J Public Health.* 2007;97(3):509–514. doi:10.2105/AJPH.2005.072447
40. Tester J, Baker R. Making the playfields even: evaluating the impact of an environmental intervention on park use and physical activity. *Prev Med.* 2009;48(4):316–320. doi:10.1016/j.ypmed.2009.01.010
41. NYC Parks. Shape Up NYC. Available at: https://www.nycgovparks.org/programs/recreation/shape-up-nyc. Accessed September 19, 2017
42. Charleston County Parks and Recreation. Move IT! Fitness & wellness. Available at: https://ccprc.com/1710/Move-IT-Fitness-Wellness. Accessed September 19, 2017.
43. Holt NL. *Positive Youth Development Through Sport.* London, UK: Routledge; 2016.
44. Besenyi GM, Fair M, Hughey SM, et al. Park Hop: pilot evaluation of an inter-agency collaboration to promote park awareness, visitation, and physical activity in Greenville County, SC. doi:10.18666/JPRA-2015-V33-I4-6216
45. Fair ML. An initiative to facilitate park usage, discovery, and physical activity among children and adolescents in Greenville County South Carolina, 2014. *Prev Chronic Dis.* 2017;14:E14. doi:10.5888/pcd14.160043
46. Starnes HA, Troped PJ, Klenosky DB, et al. Trails and physical activity: a review. *J Phys Act Health.* 2011;8(8):1160–1174. doi:10.1123/jpah.8.8.1160
47. Fitzhugh EC, Bassett DR, Evans MF. Urban trails and physical activity: a natural experiment. *Am J Prev Med.* 2010;39(3):259–262. doi:10.1016/j.amepre.2010.05.010

48. Rails-to-Trails Conservancy. About Rails-to-Trails Conservancy. Available at: https://www. railstotrails.org/about. Accessed September 16, 2017.

49. Bowker JM, Bergstrom JC, Gill J. Estimating the economic value and impacts of recreational trails: a case study of the Virginia Creeper Rail Trail. *Tour Econ.* 2007;13(2):241–260. doi:10. 5367/000000007780823203

50. Wang G, Macera CA, Scudder-Soucie B, et al. A cost-benefit analysis of physical activity using bike/pedestrian trails. *Health Promot Pract.* 2005;6(2):174–179. doi:10.1177/ 1524839903260687

51. Heinrich KM, Lightner J, Oestman KB, et al. Efforts of a Kansas foundation to increase physical activity and improve health by funding community trails, 2012. *Prev Chronic Dis.* 2014;11:E208. doi:10.5888/pcd11.140356

52. County Health Rankings & Roadmaps. Shared use agreements. Available at: http://www. countyhealthrankings.org/policies/shared-use-agreements. Accessed September 12, 2017.

53. Kanters MA, Bocarro JN, Filardo M, et al. Shared use of school facilities with community organizations and afterschool physical activity program participation: a cost-benefit assessment. *J Sch Health.* 2014;84(5):302–309. doi:10.1111/josh.12148

54. Taylor WC, Floyd MF, Whitt-Glover MC, et al. Environmental justice: a framework for collaboration between the public health and parks and recreation fields to study disparities in physical activity. *J Phys Act Health.* 2007;4(suppl 1):S50–S63. doi:10.1123/jpah.4.s1.s50

55. Cooper T, Vincent JM. *Joint Use School Partnerships in California: Strategies to Enhance Schools and Communities.* Berkeley, CA: Center for Cities & Schools (CC&S), Public Health Law & Policy (PHLP), University of California-Berkeley; 2008.

56. Maddock J, Choy LB, Nett B, et al. Increasing access to places for physical activity through a joint use agreement: a case study in urban Honolulu. *Prev Chronic Dis.* 2008;5(3):A91. Available at https://www.cdc.gov/pcd/issues/2008/Jul/07_0117.htm

57. Harnik P, Mowen AJ. ParK-12 and beyond: converting schoolyards into community play space in crowded cities. In: *Implementing PA Strategies.* Champaign, IL: Human Kinetics; 2014:145–150.

58. Health Impact Assessments. UCLA School of Public Health. Available at: http://www. hiaguide.org/sectors-and-causal-pathways/pathways/social-capital. Accessed September 12, 2017.

59. The Trust for Public Land. Creative placemaking. Available at: https://www.tpl.org/our-work/creative-placemaking. Accessed September 12, 2017.

60. United States. Environmental Protection Agency. Public participation guide: charrettes. Available at: https://www.epa.gov/international-cooperation/public-participation-guide-charrettes. Published March 20, 2014. Accessed September 12, 2017.

61. Patton-López MM, Muñoz R, Polanco K, et al. Redesigning a neighborhood park to increase physical activity: a community-based participatory approach. *J Public Health Manag Pract.* 2015;21:S101. doi:10.1097/PHH.0000000000000206

62. Abercrombie LC, Sallis JF, Conway TL, et al. Income and racial disparities in access to public parks and private recreation facilities. *Am J Prev Med.* 2008;34(1):9–15. doi:10.1016/ j.amepre.2007.09.030

63. Engelberg JK, Conway TL, Geremia C, et al. Socioeconomic and race/ethnic disparities in observed park quality. *BMC Public Health.* 2016;16:395. doi:10.1186/s12889-016-3055-4

64. Hughey SM, Walsemann KM, Child S, et al. Using an environmental justice approach to examine the relationships between park availability and quality indicators, neighborhood disadvantage, and racial/ethnic composition. *Landsc Urban Plan.* 2016;148:159–169. doi:10. 1016/j.landurbplan.2015.12.016

65. Jones SA, Moore LV, Moore K, et al. Disparities in physical activity resource availability in six US regions. *Prev Med.* 2015;78:17–22. doi:10.1016/j.ypmed.2015.05.028

66. Vaughan KB, Kaczynski AT, Stanis SAW, et al. Exploring the distribution of park availability, features, and quality across Kansas City, Missouri by income and race/ethnicity: an environmental justice investigation. *Ann Behav Med.* 2013;45(1):28–38. doi:10.1007/s12160-012-9425-y

67. Kamel AA, Ford PB, Kaczynski AT. Disparities in park availability, features, and character-istics by social determinants of health within a U.S.-Mexico border urban area. *Prev Med.* 2014;69:S111–S113. doi:10.1016/j.ypmed.2014.10.001

68. Kaczynski AT, Wilhelm Stanis SA, Besenyi GM. Development and testing of a community stakeholder park audit tool. *Am J Prev Med.* 2012;42(3):242–249. doi:10.1016/j.amepre.2011.10.018

69. Besenyi GM, Diehl P, Schooley B, et al. Development and testing of mobile technology for community park improvements: validity and reliability of the eCPAT application with youth. *Transl Behav Med.* 2016;6(4):519–532. doi:10.1007/s13142-016-0405-9

70. Gallerani DG, Besenyi GM, Wilhelm Stanis SA, et al. "We actually care and we want to make the parks better": a qualitative study of youth experiences and perceptions after conducting park audits. *Prev Med.* 2017;95:S109–S114. doi:10.1016/j.ypmed.2016.08.043

71. Cohen DA, Han B, Derose KP, et al. Physical activity in parks: a randomized controlled trial using community engagement. *Am J Prev Med.* 2013;45(5):590–597. doi:10.1016/j.amepre.2013.06.015

72. Broyles ST, Mowen AJ, Theall KP, et al. Integrating social capital into a park-use and active-living framework. *Am J Prev Med.* 2011;40(5):522–529. doi:10.1016/j.amepre.2010.12.028

73. McKenzie TL, Cohen DA, Sehgal A, et al. System for Observing Play and Recreation in Com-munities (SOPARC): reliability and feasibility measures. *J Phys Act Health.* 2006;3(suppl 1):S208–S222. doi:10.1123/jpah.3.s1.s208

74. Santos MPM, Rech CR, Alberico CO, et al. Utility and reliability of an app for the system for observing play and recreation in communities (iSOPARC®). *Meas Phys Educ Exerc Sci.* 2016;20(2):93–98. doi:10.1080/1091367X.2015.1120733

75. Dunton GF, Almanza E, Jerrett M, et al. Neighborhood park use by children: use of accelerometry and global positioning systems. *Am J Prev Med.* 2014;46(2):136–142. doi:10.1016/j.amepre.2013.10.009

76. Almanza E, Jerrett M, Dunton G, et al. A study of community design, greenness, and physical activity in children using satellite, GPS and accelerometer data. *Health Place.* 2012;18(1):46–54. doi:10.1016/j.healthplace.2011.09.003

77. Messiah SE, Kardys J, Forster L. Reducing childhood obesity through pediatrician and park partnerships. *J Public Health Manag Pract.* 2017;23(4):356–359. doi:10.1097/PHH.0000000000000453

78. Seltenrich N. Just what the doctor ordered: using parks to improve children's health. *Environ Health Perspect.* 2015;123(10):A254–A259. doi:10.1289/ehp.123-A254

79. Razani N, Kohn MA, Wells NM, et al. Design and evaluation of a park prescription program for stress reduction and health promotion in low-income families: the Stay Healthy in Nature Everyday (SHINE) study protocol. *Contemp Clin Trials.* 2016;51:8–14. doi:10.1016/j.cct.2016.09.007

80. Calfas KJ, Long BJ, Sallis JF, et al. A controlled trial of physician counseling to promote the adoption of physical activity. *Prev Med.* 1996;25(3):225–233. doi:10.1006/pmed.1996.0050

81. Marcus BH, Goldstein MG, Jette A, et al. Training physicians to conduct physical activity counseling. *Prev Med.* 1997;26(3):382–388. doi:10.1006/pmed.1997.0158

82. Zarr R, Cottrell L, Merrill C. Park prescription (DC Park Rx): a new strategy to combat chronic disease in children. *J Phys Act Health.* 2017;14(1):1–2.

83. Reed JA. *Greenville Health System Swamp Rabbit Trail, Year 3 Findings.* 2014.

84. Price AE, Reed JA, Muthukrishnan S. Trail user demographics, physical activity behav-iors, and perceptions of a newly constructed greenway trail. *J Community Health.* 2012;37(5):949–956. doi:10.1007/s10900-011-9530-z

85. Hughey SM, Kaczynski AT, Clennin MN, et al. Pathways to health: association between trail use, weight status, and self-rated health among adults in Greenville County, South Carolina, 2014. *Prev Chronic Dis.* 2016;13:E168. doi:10.5888/pcd13.16019

PHYSICAL ACTIVITY AND THE FAMILY

JOSEPH A. SKELTON | CASEY FOSTER | KAELA YATES

LEARNING OBJECTIVES

By the end of this chapter, the student should be able to

1. Assess the effective components of family-based physical activity (PA) interventions.
2. Examine the differences among family types and how they may influence PA interventions.
3. Describe the role of parenting practices on PA interventions.
4. Compare and contrast different versions of parental modeling on PA behavior.
5. Differentiate components of successful family-based approaches to increasing PA.

◼ Introduction

There are several paradigms in which to envision exercise and physical activity (PA): strength versus aerobic training; competitive versus recreational sports and activities; group versus individual athletics; and planned versus unplanned activities. A paradigm that has not received significant attention is that of the family. For children, parents are the most proximal and significant influence on a child's well-being (1). Urie Bronfenbrenner's Social Ecological Model (2–4) postulates a child is greatly influenced by the family and surrounding environment—particularly the family being the buffer or mediator between the environment and the child. Conversely, adults will also be greatly influenced by the family system, attempting to schedule exercise around their children's schedules, spouse's preferences, and family activities. It is important to approach PA in children and adults within the context of the family. Therefore, a "deeper dive" to understand PA in the family is necessary, particularly to understand the contexts in which families can be physically active together, as well as how family members can support each other in establishing routines and habits resulting in an active lifestyle for individual family members. Consequently, PA and public health practitioners and researchers must take into account the family context when designing, implementing, or studying interventions and epidemiologic trends.

■ The Family is a System

The study of families can be incredibly complex, from focusing on parenting to overall family process and function. Hence, an entire academic discipline is focused on the study of families (Human Development and Family Studies) and a field of counseling specializes in helping them (Marriage and Family Therapy). One approach is to use an established model—Family Systems Theory (FST) (5, 6). Developed in the 1950s by psychiatrist Dr. Murray Bowen (7), FST postulates that people cannot be viewed as individuals alone, but must take into account their context, which for many people is their family, even if the definition of family is nontraditional (aka work colleagues, friends, communities). Families are interdependent and interconnected, made up of subsystems that collectively form an emotional unit. Table 15.1 highlights core tenets of FST. As it pertains to activity within the family, recognizing the interconnectedness is important, as activity levels will be influenced by, and will influence, others within the family system. The levels of a family system must be taken into account when considering intervening on PA (Table 15.1). A first level or first-order system change around PA involves the family's interactions with the environment. An example would be a family joining a gym. For this change to be made and have permanence, a second-order change must occur, such as budgeting for a gym membership, how family members communicate about PA, or organize their schedule to provide time to go to the gym. While this seems overly complicated for what is perceived to be a simple intervention to increase PA in a family, clinicians and public health professionals can appreciate the complexities of working with families, and better recognize challenges to increasing PA.

TABLE 15.1. Family systems theory

COMPONENTS OF INTERACTING SYSTEM OF THE FAMILY
■ Members are viewed as a whole—the family.
■ Elements of the system are interconnected.
■ The family interacts with the environment by a feedback loop.
■ The family system is goal oriented.
■ The family determines who are members, what the membership criteria is, sets boundaries for the flow of information, and establishes rules.
■ Families strive to maintain equilibrium, yet must adapt and change as needed.
■ Subsystems exist within the family system, and can influence the family as a whole.
■ Levels exist in the family system. 　● First order 　● Second order

Brown et al reviewed family-based PA interventions, finding them effective in increasing PA levels (8), and determined three components of effective family-based interventions:

1. PA interventions should be tailored to individual families, taking into account their cultural and ethnic backgrounds, individual and collective motivations, and schedules.

2. Interventions should combine appropriate goal-setting and reinforcement techniques. Educational strategies alone were not effective, but can be used when there is a knowledge- or resource deficit, in combination with other strategies. In line with FST, interventions can target the psychosocial environment of the family (see Box 15.1).

3. Utilizing the child as an agent of change is different than many obesity-related interventions in children that target parents exclusively (9, 10). An example would be a child participant being taught to encourage the parent to be active with him or her, doing activities mutually appealing to the child and parent. Other considerations are focusing on skills needed for PA, attention to self-esteem of the family members, and parents' accurate recognition of the child's present level of PA.

BOX 15.1

Effective family exercise and activity intervention

1. Tailored to the family
2. Utilize goal setting and reinforcement, not just education
3. Recognize the child as an agent of change

While this literature is encouraging, significant gaps remain, particularly investigating the broader family system, such as family-based intervention's success in increasing adult or sibling PA levels.

■ Parents and Parenting

In dissecting the family system, the parents' role in a family's PA is a key area for intervention, as parents serve as leaders and authority figures within families by setting schedules, agendas, and having the greatest influence on family dynamics, communication, and milieu. For some time, research into *parenting practices and behaviors* has informed the family studies and psychology literature, including how parenting influences child outcomes and how a child's willingness to be influenced mediates that impact (11). In childhood obesity research, parenting style is associated with child weight status (12). Much work has been done in parenting and feeding (13, 14), but not as much in PA and exercise. The framework for approaching parenting and health comes from developmental psychologist Diane Baumrind (15, 16), and later modified by others in the field (17), into parenting styles or types, using a two-by-two framework of demandingness and responsiveness of parenting (Table 15.2).

TABLE 15.2. Parenting styles typology

DIMENSIONS	RESPONSIVENESS		
Demandingness		High	Low
	High	Authoritative	Authoritarian
	Low	Permissive	Neglectful

Traditionally, a strict, controlling parent can best be understood as *authoritarian*, whereas a parent with appropriate levels of control, typically seen as providing structure and monitoring, while simultaneously being responsive to the child's needs, is *authoritative*, generally seen as the preferred and healthiest approach to parenting. Within obesity and feeding research, the authoritarian parent, exerting a high amount of control and restriction with feeding, is generally associated with the highest levels of obesity and dysfunctional eating patterns in children (12, 18). Generally, the same appears to pertain to parenting style and activity, though overall it is inconclusive and likely gender dependent (19, 20). Positive parenting practices, generally categorized as authoritative, were associated with increased PA in daughters/girls, though not as much in sons/boys. One study even found permissive parenting associated with higher amounts and intensity of activity in boys and girls (21). More investigation is needed to explore parent, child, and family PA.

Parental support of a child's PA is necessary and vital to maintaining healthy levels of activity, and is one of the primary influences of the child's activity-related behavior (22). Beets et al performed an extensive review of the literature and, by taking a narrative approach, they summarized the diverse literature in this area. As shown in Table 15.3, they determined four areas of parental social support of child PA, divided into two categories: tangible and intangible. Both support areas demonstrated positive association with PA in children. In line with FST, the literature outlining forms of parent social

TABLE 15.3. Parent social support for children's PA behaviors

TANGIBLE SUPPORT	INTANGIBLE SUPPORT
Instrumental: purchasing equipment, payment of participation fees, transportation to activities	Motivational: encouragement, praise, positive communication and reinforcement
Conditional: participating with children, attending sporting events, coaching, supervision	Informational: discussing benefits of PA, how to be active

NOTE: PA, physical activity.

SOURCE: Beets MW, Cardinal BJ, Alderman BL. Parental social support and the physical activity-related behaviors of youth: a review. *Health Educ Behav*. 2010;37(5):621–644. doi:10.1177/1090198110363884

support can greatly inform PA interventions in children and adolescents, providing clinicians and public health professionals guidelines in positively working with parents and caregivers to support their children's efforts to be physically active.

Parental modeling of PA has also been associated with child PA levels. A meta-analysis showed, similar to other topics of parents and activity, child gender influenced the effect of parents' role modeling behaviors (23). Fathers seemed to have an influence on their sons' PA levels more so than mothers did; neither parent appeared to have much influence on daughters' activity levels. While not fully understood, parents who set a good example for PA do appear to have a positive influence on their children.

> ■ *Children are influenced by the adults in their lives—parents should try to model active lifestyles.*

Spouses, Partners, and Significant Others

Families are diverse and unique, can involve multigenerations and extended relatives, or be as small as cohabitating partners, spouses, or significant others. The family system, even within a couple, can be complex, where the actions of one partner affect the other. Couples (romantic partners, spouses) tend to have very similar health habits and behaviors (24). The bulk of the literature pertaining to couples in regards to PA is found in weight loss research, which typically involves an exercise component, all supporting some advantage to including spouses in the intervention (25–28). Similar to differences seen in adolescents, Wing found differences in spouses by gender within a program for patients with diabetes: women did better in weight loss when their spouse was involved, whereas men did better in treatment alone (29). Specific to PA, there is less research, but it does support including partners in the intervention. Team-based approaches to increasing PA are successful; as part of a statewide campaign, if a team's activity level is high, then it raises individual activity levels (30). Men and women are more likely to make a positive health behavior change if their partner does. Specific to PA, the odds a person makes a healthy change is higher if the partner is also newly healthy, as compared to him or her being healthy at baseline (31), and overall PA level changes correlate between spouses (32). While the research is not extensive, there is evidence that targeting partners, spouses, and significant others to increase PA will increase the effectiveness of interventions, and should be considered an option.

Not All Families are the Same

Physical and Intellectual Disabilities

There are few studies on family-based PA in children of minority background or with physical or intellectual challenges. Shields et al, in a systematic review looking at data for PA among children with disabilities, discovered that many of the identified barriers (such as lack of knowledge and skills, parental behavior, inadequate facilities, lack of transportation, programs, and staff capacity) and facilitators (such as child's desire to be active, involvement of peers and family support, accessible facilities, skilled staff and information) are similar to those reported for children with typical development (33). Notably, children with disability were more likely to participate if activity included interaction, encouragement, and assistance with peers, friends, or siblings. One pilot program in New Zealand adapted a community-based healthy lifestyle program for children and families (Mind, Exercise, Nutrition, Do It! [MEND]; first developed in the United Kingdom), with the intention of targeting children and youth with intellectual disability and autism (34). The 10-week, school-based program consisted of 18 sessions, each of which included an hour of family PA, followed by an active session with students only while parents attended a nutritional or motivational segment for 1 hour. One of the first studies to examine PA and nutrition among this population, it was limited by a small sample size and no control group; however, it did find that parents reported fewer hospital visits and absences from school during the program study period and it represents an attempt to engage the family as a unit to promote PA among this high-risk population. Another study in children with cerebral palsy found parents of children identified more priority for daily activities, and that parents of older children had high priority for productivity as compared to the parents of younger children; discoveries that could help tailor interventions to best match the needs of the families they intend to help (35). When families of children with a physical disability were interviewed, Antle et al remarked that families commented often on the significance of PA for their children, sometimes seeing it as a means to achieving other goals such as self-discipline and self-confidence. This could be useful in designing, delivering, and evaluating activity interventions, as a person-centered outcome, self-confidence, and self-efficacy in exercise may be of greater importance to individuals than performance on aerobic testing (36).

Minority and Underserved Populations

In their review of family and environmental correlates of health behaviors in high-risk youth, Lawman and colleagues found support for the role of parenting and physical environment factors in PA (parental monitoring and social cohesion of the neighborhood) in children of low socioeconomic status (SES) or minority background (37). Cross-sectional data from a group of African American, Latino, and White girls included by Duncan et al as part of a longer multiyear study identified that girls with more physically active parents also reported greater parental support for PA (38). They proposed that increasing the PA of parents and their level of support of PA with community programs, which focus on involving parents and girls together, could have a beneficial impact on PA, particularly among minority populations. Taking a different approach of focusing on family functioning, a behavior-change intervention with Hispanic families, found by including the entire family and emphasizing skills that improve family functioning (communication, problem solving, relationships), the intervention achieved a high level of acceptance among the participants, which surprisingly resulted in facilitating family PA, reporting family walks, roller skating, dancing, taking the stairs, and enrolling children in sports (39). Similarly, Kuo et al studied African American adolescent girls, finding that greater family intimacy and support was associated with PA, with the thought that greater parent communication, monitoring, and warmth can affect a teenager's understanding of risky behaviors, with no real risk associated (40).

Children of Different Ages

A challenge in designing family-based activity interventions is having children of various ages within one family. One family-centered program based in two community centers in Boston, Massachusetts, called "Family Gym," created a model for a family gym program (see Box 15.2) (41). They targeted children 3 to 8 years old and their families, choosing play activities that were developmentally appropriate for the age of the children, with student volunteers to help guide the activities after the free/unstructured play time. They found that the developmental differences in physical ability and skills of the children compared to the adults had become a barrier to involvement and so they created *mini clinics* that focused on particular fitness skills that would target similar levels of exertion from adults and younger family members.

BOX 15.2

Examples of support for PA

Tangible: design activities so parents and adults can participate WITH children instead of just coaching or instructing.
  Intangible: motivate by being positive and encouraging, minimizing critical comments and language.

PA, physical activity.

Another potential model to address some of the aforementioned challenges with PA in the context of the family is "FAMILI" (family-centered action model of intervention layout and implementation). This model was designed to accommodate the ecologies of families and empower families in the process, knowing that preestablished interventions cannot be realistically expected to have equivalent efficacy and effectiveness over time in different ethnic groups and across settings (42). It encourages the use of theories of family development, the examination of factors affecting families, and the implementation of participatory methods to develop and evaluate family-centered interventions.

Conclusions From Previous Research

While there are still gaps in our understanding of families and PA, existing literature supports the understanding of families as unique, connected systems. The design and implementation of interventions to increase PA levels within these family systems should account for differences in racial/ethnic background, ages of children, and potential special needs of individuals within the family. Education alone is known to be not enough to motivate families to be more active, but efforts to utilize the children as agents of change within the family combined with appropriate goals setting and positive reinforcement can result in desired outcomes. Parents' role within the family is also of great importance, both as "heads of household" and as models of an active lifestyle. Interventions can take into account parenting skills and types, as parents who are overly strict and demanding will struggle in instituting change within the household, probably as much as parents that are overly permissive. Most importantly, parents can provide support to spouses, children, and the entire family to increase PA. More research is needed on how to motivate entire families, versus just a child or parent, regarding the best means in which to communicate within families about exercise, attractive avenues for increasing PA for families, and how best to design physical environments (neighborhoods, communities, homes) to support increased activity.

Case Studies

Family-Based Obesity Treatment, But Not Activity

Brenner FIT (Families In Training) is an interdisciplinary obesity treatment program with Brenner Children's Hospital, a part of Wake Forest Baptist Medical Center (43). Brenner FIT utilizes evidence-based approaches for the treatment of childhood obesity, including a behavioral approach to habit change. As with most programs, they strive to increase the time spent in PA and decrease the time spent in sedentary behaviors, using a combination of structured and unstructured activities (44). Structured activities could include encouragement to participate in sports, noncompetitive games, fitness centers, and gyms; unstructured activities include recreational activities like hiking, games, and, for younger children, free play. Obesity treatment programs increase time spent in PA through behavioral approaches, as well as providing opportunities for exercise through structured classes (45), aiming to overcome barriers to PA.

Brenner FIT employed a part-time physical therapist and full-time exercise specialist to work individually with children and parents. In addition to individual clinical appointments, in which they utilized motivational interviewing (see Box 15.3) (46) and exercise prescriptions to set activity-related goals (46), they organized group exercise activities during evenings and weekends, as well as providing day passes and discounted memberships to local fitness centers.

BOX 15.3

Components of family gym

Family engagement, recruitment and retention, university student engagement, resource coordination.

Clinically, they found little improvement in children's activity levels through these approaches. Separating children and parents during activity classes also seemed to limit the adoption of classes into the weekly routines of the family. Recognizing the family's influence on the child, they engaged their interdisciplinary team to improve their approach.

Brenner FIT had been researching family experiences in obesity treatment programs, finding children and adolescents desired and enjoyed spending time together as a family (47, 48). From this, the exercise specialists transitioned from formal child-focused classes and goal setting to family-focused activities that were enjoyable and play-based, accounting for preferences, child age, and ability of parents to participate. With the assistance of the interdisciplinary team, a process was put in place to adapt activities and games for use in clinic, geared toward instructing families to play within the home. Briefly, the clinicians would identify traditional games or sports children identified as enjoyable; this was accomplished through Internet searches of summer camp games and activities, as well as books, resource manuals, and surveying parents regarding games they remembered from their childhood. From this, the following steps were taken:

- Change the rules and structure of the game so adults and children of different ages and abilities could play

- Remove overly competitive aspects of the games so all could enjoy
- Adapt to home environments with minimal equipment and space requirements
- "Weatherproofing" so games can be played indoors and outdoors

The first games adapted were four-square and the basketball game HORSE, played with makeshift baskets. A larger space was created near the clinic site to allow the activity specialist to teach families these games; when necessary, hallways were used. Through trial and error, Brenner FIT found that family-based activity to be the most successful for all age children. Doing PA with the entire family helps everyone work together toward a common goal. Subsequent family-focused adaptations include

- *Play FIT*: Small group-based classes of three to six families in which they learn to play games together—parents, child, and siblings. Activity specialists, along with volunteers, role model play and activity with the families; the parents would then serve in this role at home. This is typically held in the late afternoon, minimizing time away from work for parents and absences from school for the children. Activities typically utilize limited equipment and are geared toward in-home implementation so families can enjoy being active without having to join a gym or drive to a park.
- *Family FIT*: Families attend a more exercise-focused class for kids 10 to 18 years old and their family. This class involves the entire family working together to be active. All exercises are done with a partner; this could be a sibling, parent, grandparent, or other member of the family. This helps include everyone and teaches each family member the correct way to do each exercise. Doing the exercises together allows children to see the parents, or adults, role model the routine and proper form for doing exercise.
- *Active Child Care:* In pediatric obesity treatment interventions of children younger than 12 years of age, parents are often the sole "agent of change" within the family (9, 10). These interventions have demonstrated parent-only treatment to be as effective as interventions that include children. Therefore, Brenner FIT will have the child meet with the activity specialist while the parent meets with other team members. During that time, the activity specialist will then engage the child in an activity or game. At the end of the clinic appointment, the activity specialist will return the child to his or her parent (often breathing hard and showing how much the child enjoyed the game or activity), and the activity specialist will provide an educational handout to the parent, which includes instructions on how to play the game at home with the child. The child's enjoyment of the game or activity will serve as positive reinforcement to the parent.

These changes in how to approach families wanting to increase PA have been very successful for the Brenner FIT program, with increased activity levels reported by the family, and in behavioral measures used in tracking family progress in clinic. The adoption of a family-based approach to activity, accounting for the child's enjoyment and the ability of family members to participate, can be useful approaches for others aiming to increase PA levels in children and families.

■ Summary

Increasing PA levels in children, adults/parents, and families has not been extensively studied, though much can be learned from theories of the family. Interventions designed to increase PA of children and adults could benefit by taking groups in the context of their family and understanding the complex systems and subsystems that can influence PA participation. Present best-practice examples account for these inherent complexities by targeting parents (modeling of PA, parenting style) and children (physical and intellectual considerations, developmental status) as agents of change. There are significant gaps in how public health practitioners can best impact family activity levels, either through designed interventions, such as family gyms or programming, or by extension through schools or using the child as an agent of change. Based on existing literature and best practice, professionals should consider family situations and dynamics when attempting to design, deliver, and evaluate PA interventions among children and/or adults.

■ Things to Consider

- ■ Family activity should be simple and not complex; this will increase the likelihood of families incorporating PA into their routine.
- ■ Start small with goals of increasing PA; families that are currently inactive are not going to increase their PA to recommended amounts all at one time.
- ■ Parents do not have to enroll their child in sports or a gym to provide PA for their child.
- ■ Have families decide what they would like to do for PA; what works for one family does not always work for another.
- ■ It is important to have knowledge of PA that can be done indoors and outdoors for families when weather is not ideal.

■ References

1. Schor EL. American Academy of Pediatrics Task Force on the Family. Family pediatrics: report of the task force on the family. *Pediatrics*. 2003;111(6 Pt 2):1541–1571.
2. Bronfenbrenner U. *The Ecology of Human Development: Experiments by Nature and Design*. Cambridge, MA: Harvard University; 1979.
3. Bronfenbrenner U. Ecology of the family as a context for human development: research perspectives. *Develop Psychol*. 1986;22:723–742. doi:10.1037/0012-1649.22.6.723
4. Bronfenbrenner U, Morris PA. The ecology of human developmental processes. In: Damon W, Eisenberg N, eds. *The Handbook of Child Psychology*. New York, NY: John Wiley & Sons; 1988:993–1027.
5. White JM, Klein DM, eds. The systems framework. In: *Family Theories*. 3rd ed. Thousand Oaks, CA: Sage; 2008:151–177.
6. Broderick CB. *Understanding Family Process: Basics of Family Systems Theory*. Newbury Park, CA: Sage; 1993.
7. Bowen M. The use of family theory in clinical practice. *Compr Psychiatry*. 1966;7(5): 345–374. doi:10.1016/S0010-440X(66)80065-2
8. Brown HE, Atkin AJ, Panter J, et al. Family-based interventions to increase physical activity in children: a systematic review, meta-analysis and realist synthesis. *Obes Rev*. 2016;17(4): 345–360. doi:10.1111/obr.12362

9. Golan M, Crow S. Targeting parents exclusively in the treatment of childhood obesity: long-term results. *Obes Res.* 2004;12(2):357–361. doi:10.1038/oby.2004.45

10. Golan M, Kaufman V, Shahar DR. Childhood obesity treatment: targeting parents exclusively v. parents and children. *Br J Nutr.* 2006;95(5):1008–1015. doi:10.1079/BJN20061757

11. Darling N, Steinberg L. Parenting style as context: an integrative model. *Psychol Bull.* 1993;113(3):487–496. doi:10.1037/0033-2909.113.3.487

12. Rhee KE, Lumeng JC, Appugliese DP, et al. Parenting styles and overweight status in first grade. *Pediatrics.* 2006;117(6):2047–2054. doi:10.1542/peds.2005-2259

13. Birch LL, Ventura AK. Preventing childhood obesity: what works? *Int J Obes (Lond).* 2009;33(suppl 1):S74–S81. doi:10.1038/ijo.2009.22

14. Savage JS, Fisher JO, Birch LL. Parental influence on eating behavior: conception to adolescence. *J Law Med Ethics.* 2007;35(1):22–34. doi:10.1111/j.1748-720X.2007.00111.x

15. Baumrind D. Current patterns of parental authority. *Dev Psychol.* 1971;4:101–103. doi:10.1037/h0030372

16. Baumrind D. Effects of authoritative control on child behavior. *Child Dev.* 1966;37:887–907. doi:10.2307/1126611

17. Maccoby E, Martin J. Socialization in the context of the family: parent-child interaction. In: Hetherington E, ed. *Handbook of Child Psychology: Socialization, Personality and Social Development.* New York, NY: Wiley; 1983:1–101.

18. Rhee K. Childhood overweight and the relationship between parent behaviors, parenting style, and family functioning. *Ann Am Acad Pol Soc Sci.* 2008;615:11–37. doi:10.1177/0002716207308400

19. Schmitz KH, Lytle LA, Phillips GA, et al. Psychosocial correlates of physical activity and sedentary leisure habits in young adolescents: the Teens Eating for Energy and Nutrition at School study. *Prev Med.* 2002;34(2):266–278. doi:10.1006/pmed.2001.0982

20. Vollmer RL, Mobley AR. Parenting styles, feeding styles, and their influence on child obesogenic behaviors and body weight. A review. *Appetite.* 2013;71:232–241. doi:10.1016/j.appet.2013.08.015

21. Jago R, Davison KK, Brockman R, et al. Parenting styles, parenting practices, and physical activity in 10- to 11-year olds. *Prev Med.* 2011;52(1):44–47. doi:10.1016/j.ypmed.2010.11.001

22. Beets MW, Cardinal BJ, Alderman BL. Parental social support and the physical activity-related behaviors of youth: a review. *Health Educ Behav.* 2010;37(5):621–644. doi:10.1177/1090198110363884

23. Yao CA, Rhodes RE. Parental correlates in child and adolescent physical activity: a meta-analysis. *Int J Behav Nutr Phys Act.* 2015;12:10. doi:10.1186/s12966-015-0163-y

24. Arden-Close E, McGrath N. Health behaviour change interventions for couples: a systematic review. *Br J Health Psychol.* 2017;22(2):215–237. doi:10.1111/bjhp.12227

25. Wing RR, Jeffery RW. Benefits of recruiting participants with friends and increasing social support for weight loss and maintenance. *J Consult Clin Psychol.* 1999;67(1):132–138. doi:10.1037/0022-006X.67.1.132

26. Gorin AA, Wing RR, Fava JL, et al. Weight loss treatment influences untreated spouses and the home environment: evidence of a ripple effect. *Int J Obes (Lond).* 2008;32(11):1678–1684. doi:10.1038/ijo.2008.150

27. Gorin A, Phelan S, Tate D, et al. Involving support partners in obesity treatment. *J Consult Clin Psychol.* 2005;73(2):341–343. doi:10.1037/0022-006X.73.2.341

28. Kumanyika SK, Wadden TA, Shults J, et al. Trial of family and friend support for weight loss in African American adults. *Arch Intern Med.* 2009;169(19):1795–1804. doi:10.1001/archinternmed.2009.337

29. Wing RR, Marcus MD, Epstein LH, et al. A "family-based" approach to the treatment of obese type II diabetic patients. *J Consult Clin Psychol.* 1991;59(1):156–162. doi:10.1037/0022-006X.59.1.156

30. Leahey TM, Crane MM, Pinto AM, et al. Effect of teammates on changes in physical activity in a statewide campaign. *Prev Med.* 2010;51(1):45–49. doi:10.1016/j.ypmed.2010.04.004

31. Jackson SE, Steptoe A, Wardle J. The influence of partner's behavior on health behavior change: the English Longitudinal Study of Ageing. *JAMA Intern Med.* 2015;175(3):385–392. doi:10.1001/jamainternmed.2014.7554

32. Cobb LK, Godino JG, Selvin E, et al. Spousal influence on physical activity in middle-aged and older adults: the ARIC study. *Am J Epidemiol.* 2016;183(5):444–451. doi:10.1093/aje/kwv104

33. Shields N, Synnot AJ, Barr M. Perceived barriers and facilitators to physical activity for children with disability: a systematic review. *Br J Sports Med.* 2012;46(14):989–997. doi:10.1136/bjsports-2011-090236

34. Hinckson EA, Dickinson A, Water T, et al. Physical activity, dietary habits and overall health in overweight and obese children and youth with intellectual disability or autism. *Res Dev Disabil.* 2013;34(4):1170–1178. doi:10.1016/j.ridd.2012.12.006

35. Chiarello LA, Palisano RJ, Maggs JM, et al. Family priorities for activity and participation of children and youth with cerebral palsy. *Phys Ther.* 2010;90(9):1254–1264. doi:10.2522/ptj.20090388

36. Antle BJ, Mills W, Steele C, et al. An exploratory study of parents' approaches to health promotion in families of adolescents with physical disabilities. *Child Care Health Dev.* 2008;34(2):185–193. doi:10.1111/j.1365-2214.2007.00782.x

37. Lawman HG, Wilson DK. A review of family and environmental correlates of health behaviors in high-risk youth. *Obesity (Silver Spring).* 2012;20(6):1142–1157. doi:10.1038/oby.2011.376

38. Duncan SC, Strycker LA, Chaumeton NR. Personal, family, and peer correlates of general and sport physical activity among African American, Latino, and White girls. *J Health Dispar Res Pract.* 2015;8(2):12–28.

39. Cason-Wilkerson R, Goldberg S, Albright K, et al. Factors influencing healthy lifestyle changes: a qualitative look at low-income families engaged in treatment for overweight children. *Child Obes.* 2015;11(2):170–176. doi:10.1089/chi.2014.0147

40. Kuo J, Voorhees CC, Haythornthwaite JA, et al. Associations between family support, family intimacy, and neighborhood violence and physical activity in urban adolescent girls. *Am J Public Health.* 2007;97(1):101–103. doi:10.2105/AJPH.2005.072348

41. Castaneda-Sceppa C, Hoffman JA, Thomas J, et al. Family gym: a model to promote physical activity for families with young children. *J Health Care Poor Underserved.* 2014;25(3):1101–1107. doi:10.1353/hpu.2014.0120

42. Davison KK, Lawson HA, Coatsworth JD. The Family-centered Action Model of Intervention Layout and Implementation (FAMILI): the example of childhood obesity. *Health Promot Pract.* 2012;13(4):454–461. doi:10.1177/1524839910377966

43. Skelton JA, Irby M, Beech BM. Bridging the gap between family-based treatment and family-based research in childhood obesity. *Child Obes.* 2011;7(4):323–326. doi:10.1089/chi.2011.0400.prog

44. Barlow SE. Expert committee recommendations regarding the prevention, assessment, and treatment of child and adolescent overweight and obesity: summary report. *Pediatrics.* 2007;120(suppl 4):S164–192. doi:10.1542/peds.2007-2329C

45. Savoye M, Shaw M, Dziura J, et al. Effects of a weight management program on body composition and metabolic parameters in overweight children: a randomized controlled trial. *JAMA.* 2007;297(24):2697–2704. doi:10.1001/jama.297.24.2697

46. Miller WR, Rollnick S. *Motivational Interviewing: Preparing People for Change.* 2nd ed. New York, NY: The Guilford Press; 2002.

47. Skelton JA, Martin S, Irby MB. Satisfaction and attrition in paediatric weight management. *Clin Obes.* 2016;6(2):143–153. doi:10.1111/cob.12138

48. Bishop J, Irby MB, Skelton JA. Family perceptions of a family-based pediatric obesity treatment program. *ICAN.* 2015;7(5):278–286.

BEST PRACTICES FOR ENSURING A HEALTHY AND ACTIVE LIFESTYLE IN OLDER ADULTS

MARCIA G. ORY | BARBARA RESNICK | MARK STOUTENBERG | AYA YOSHIKAWA | MATTHEW LEE SMITH

LEARNING OBJECTIVES

By the end of this chapter, the student should be able to

1. Describe factors of the aging population that might influence physical activity interventions.
2. Examine the physical activity guidelines for older adults and discern special circumstances for recommendations related to this population.
3. Assess the role of screening in physical activity interventions for older adults.
4. Examine the principles for designing physical activity interventions for older adults.
5. Assess the evidence on effective components of physical activity interventions for older adults.

▦ Introduction

This chapter will address the selection, implementation, and evaluation of physical activity interventions for older adults. As background, we will introduce basic principles of aging and public health, review the U.S. national guidelines for physical activity for older adults, and document what is historically known about physical activity patterns across the life course for different populations. A common theme across this chapter will be the importance of promoting physical activity at every age and avoiding stereotypic views about the abilities or interests of older adults. We discuss current issues in terms of what is known about factors influencing or impeding physical activity and best-practice principles for motivating older adults to be more physically active. The discussion will include challenges older adults face about knowing how to become more active and offer recommendations about how health providers, aging service providers, and exercise specialists can work together to set expectations for older adults and provide timely and accurate resource information.

Examples of best-practice tools and evidence-based interventions will be provided, along with factors to consider when choosing, implementing, and evaluating different interventions that are both scalable and sustainable. In addition to actual interventions, the value of national movements such as *Exercise is Medicine (EIM)* will be highlighted. These examples illustrate that there are many pathways to becoming more physically active and that the best pathway will depend upon a match between the older adult's preferences and capacities and the availability of evidence-based interventions and trained professionals/lay leaders to meet the older adult's needs for physical activity. We conclude with a discussion about the importance of evidence-based interventions for older adults and how planning and evaluation can be informed by public health frameworks such as the RE-AIM model. Finally, resources are provided for individuals interested in working to increase physical activity among older adults.

■ Basic Principles of Aging

The past several decades have brought attention to, and a better understanding of, aging in the United States as well as globally (1–3). Declining fertility and mortality rates across the world have made aging a global phenomenon, sparking unprecedented change in views toward older adults. In the United States, the older adult population is expected to double from 46 million today to nearly 100 million by 2060 (4, 5). Several seminal principles of aging (6) can help guide how society will respond to this "gray tsunami" in general and also provide specific guidance about appropriate interventions for increasing physical activity across the life course. These are

- The older population is not *homogeneous*. In fact, there is often more variability among older people than younger cohorts. It is important to differentiate among the young-old (those 65–74 years of age), the old (those 75–84 years of age), and the oldest old (those 85 and older) in terms of gender, race/ethnicity, education, and geographic residency.

- Aging is a *lifelong process*. Aging does not begin at a certain age such as 65, but rather is a product of lifelong experiences, interacting with biology and genetics. Consider aging as a biopsychosocial phenomenon and process that progressively occurs from birth to death.

- Aging is influenced by *social context*. Each aging cohort is unique and is influenced by social conditions. For example, being born in the early 1900s when the average life expectancy was less than 50 years is much different from living in a society where the average life expectancy is almost double and there are many different roles and supports for older adults.

- Aging is *not immutable* but subject to intervention. We are learning that aging is a dynamic process instead of something that is static and prede-termined. Medical interventions once thought to be restricted to younger populations are now being successfully implemented among older popula-tions. We are moving beyond the stereotypic view that older adults are set in their ways and do not want to, or cannot, change their lifestyle behaviors.

A key theme relevant to physical activity and aging is that there are many pathways to becoming more physically active (see Box 16.1). The best pathway will depend upon a match between older adults' preferences and capacities and the availability of evidence-based interventions and trained professionals/lay leaders to meet older adults' needs for physical activity.

Physical Activity Guidelines for Older Adults

BOX 16.1

Differentiating Physical Activity and Exercise

Physical activity is movement that is carried out by the skeletal muscles that requires energy. In other words, any movement one does is actually physical activity. Physical activities are generally considered to be low intensity. Low-intensity activity can include a casual walk, a stretch session, a beginners' yoga class or tai chi, bike riding, or using a cross trainer (e.g., an elliptical) at an easy pace. Routine activities such as bringing in the groceries, housework, gardening, going up and down stairs, and walking also count as low-intensity physical activity.

Exercise, however, is planned, structured, repetitive, and intentional movement intended to improve or maintain physical fitness. Exercise is a subcategory of physical activity. Some examples of these exercises are swimming, cycling, running, and sports such as golf and tennis. Exercise has also been referred to as moderate- or vigorous-intensity physical activity. Moderate-intensity activity includes walking at a moderate or brisk pace of 3 to 4.5 miles per hour on a level surface inside or outside. This speed is the equivalent of taking 200 steps in a minute. Alternatively, biking 5 to 9 miles per hour or doing continuous dancing are other types of moderate-intensity exercise. Vigorous-intensity exercise involves walking 5 miles per hour or faster, jogging or running, mountain or rock climbing, skating, biking faster than 10 miles per hour, taking an aerobics class, or doing aerobic dancing.

Research provides significant evidence that **ALL** physical activity positively contributes to overall health and well-being.

Based on scientific evidence, the U.S. Department of Health and Human Services first published national physical activity guidelines in 2008 and updated in 2018 (7). The physical activity guidelines are generally the same for adults and older adults, with the expectation that physical inactivity is a major risk factor for people of all ages. The guidelines indicate

- Regular physical activity is essential for healthy aging. Adults ages 65 years and older gain substantial health benefits from regular physical activity, and these benefits continue to occur throughout their lives.
- Promoting physical activity for older adults is especially important because this population is the least physically active of any age group.
- For adults aged 65 years and older who are fit and have no limiting chronic conditions, the guidelines are the same as those for all adults.

There is recognition that special circumstances might exist for some older adults, and the guidelines further indicate

- When older adults cannot do 150 minutes of moderate-intensity aerobic activity a week because of chronic conditions, they should be as physically active as their abilities and conditions allow.
- Older adults should do specific activities that maintain or improve balance if they are at risk of falling.
- Older adults should determine their level of effort for physical activity relative to their level of fitness.
- Older adults with chronic conditions should understand whether and how their conditions affect their ability to do regular physical activity safely.

Physical Activity Patterns Over the Life Course

Despite the recognition that physical activity is important for persons across the life course, and especially for older adults to prevent or better manage age-related chronic conditions, older adults are among the least active segment of the American population. National statistics (8, 9) repeatedly illustrate how age is related to meeting physical activity guidelines.

Screening for Physical Activity Interventions

Traditionally, older adults were deliberately excluded from physical activity interventions due to their age and concerns about their increased risk of physical harm. This can be attributed to many factors such as a failure to recognize the importance of continued physical activity for older adults, a concern that physical activity was "dangerous" for older adults, or the lack of trained professionals to guide older adults into being more active (10). Due to safety concerns, older adults were often "screened" before they could join research studies or community exercise programs. There is often a stepped approach to screening. Two practical preliminary screening tools are frequently recommended: the Revised Physical Activity Readiness Questionnaire (PAR-Q) (11) and the AHA/ACSM Health/Fitness Facility Preparticipation Screening Questionnaire (12). Based on results of screening, the older adult may be encouraged to see his or her primary healthcare provider, and/or have the healthcare provider approve participation in an exercise program by signing the screening form. Characteristically, these guidelines trigger medical consultation before the initiation of an exercise program for anyone age 50 and older, or those with a chronic illness such as cardiovascular disease, diabetes, or arthritis. Designed as a safety feature, these guidelines inadvertently act as a barrier to program participation for those without a primary care physician, insurance, transportation, time to go to the physician, and so forth.

Further, the screening guidelines and implementation checklists differentiate between vigorous versus moderate activity. In practice, however, there is confusion about what constitutes light versus moderate versus vigorous activity. The screenings may also be used to stratify individuals at risk and establish the need for more extensive follow-up medical testing. There is also widespread concern about liability issues associated with commencement of a regular program of physical activity. Uncertainties will generally result in more aggressive versus less-intensive screening and testing.

In particular, the PAR-Q often screened older adults who typically have at least one chronic condition out of exercise programs (11). The idea that older adults needed to get permission from their doctors to be physically active reinforced the perception that "exercise" was dangerous, and discouraged many older adults from beginning even light- or moderate-intensity programs. Moreover, and ironically, exercise is prescribed for optimal management of chronic conditions that were perceived as reasons for exclusion (13–15). This has changed some over time, due in part to the spread of the public health message that incorporating physical activity into everyday life (e.g., through active transportation, using the stairs, housework, or carrying grocery bags) is necessary for making a population change in health outcomes. In line with this new perspective of physical activity as an important part of an older adult's life, a national working group of experts in physical activity and aging was formed (16). Their charge was to consider how to best screen older adults for physical activity programs and recommend appropriate activity for different functional level or disease types (see Box 16.2).

BOX 16.2

For the EASY

Getting started
It is always a good idea to start at a level that is easy for you and to build up slowly. See the attached safety tips.

While it is generally not necessary to see a healthcare provider before beginning everyday physical activities that are of light or moderate intensity, we encourage you to talk with your healthcare provider about your health and exercise as part of your regular visits.

Answering the six easy questions

EASY QUESTIONS (circle response)

1. Do you have pains, tightness, or pressure in your chest during physical activity (walking, climbing stairs, household chores, similar activities)?	Yes	No
2. Do you currently experience dizziness or light-headedness?	Yes	No
3. Have you ever been told you have high blood pressure?	Yes	No
4. Do you have pain, stiffness, or swelling that limits or prevents you from doing what you want or need to do?	Yes	No
5. Do you fall, feel unsteady, or use an assistive device while standing or walking?	Yes	No
6. Is there a health reason not mentioned why you would be concerned about starting an exercise program?	Yes	No

(continued)

(*continued*)

If you answer No to all of the EASY questions, follow these four steps to begin or continue your exercise program:

1. Choose enjoyable activities that fit into your everyday routine.
2. Set a goal of being active 30 minutes daily most days of the week (it is best to work toward this goal slowly).
3. Review the safety tips in this packet.
4. Request a free copy of the NIA Exercise Guide by calling 1-800-222-2225 or go to www.easyforyou.info for additional exercise options.

If you answered Yes to any of the EASY questions, use the recommendations sheet for engaging in physical activity safely with your condition. It is always a good idea to review the safety hints and be aware of what the experts say are the most appropriate activities for any specific condition. For each question, we provide a link for further information. Talk with your healthcare provider about your physical activity program during your regular visits.

Safety Tips
Follow these EASY safety tips for when to start and stop physical activities.

Safety Tips to Always Consider Prior to and During Physical Activity
- Always wear comfortable, loose-fitting clothing and appropriate shoes for your activity.
- Warm-up: Perform a low- to moderate-intensity warm-up for 5 to 10 minutes.
- Drink water before, during, and after physical activity.
- When outdoors, evaluate your surroundings for safety traffic, pavement, weather, and strangers.
- Wear clothes made of fabrics that absorb sweat and remove it from your skin.
- Never wear rubber or plastic suits. These could hold the sweat on your skin and make your body overheat.
- Wear sunscreen when you are outdoors.

Safety Tips for When to STOP Physical Activity
Stop activity right away if you

- Have pain or pressure in your chest, neck, shoulder, or arm.
- Feel dizzy or sick.
- Break out in a cold sweat.
- Have muscle cramps.
- Feel acute (not just achy) pain in your joints, feet, ankles, or legs.
- Slow down if you have trouble breathing. You should be able to talk while exercising without gasping for breath.

EASY, Exercise Assessment and Screening for You.

Toward this end, the working group developed a new screening instrument, the Exercise Assessment and Screening for You (EASY) (17). The goal was to provide healthcare providers and older adults with an easy-to-use web-based tool that matches underlying health problems with a physical activity program known to be safe and beneficial for individuals with the underlying health problem. For example, it provides several physical activity options for older adults with arthritis. This tool builds upon prior work in the area of screening for physical activity among older adults and makes accessible for providers and older adults a wide variety of professionally sanctioned physical activity options that meet the needs of older adults across a wide range of ability levels and health conditions. It has been used successfully in many different populations and settings (18).

The EASY screening tool addresses many of the weaknesses in the currently available screening processes because it incorporates an interactive system to guide the older individual or healthcare provider through a series of six questions. The purpose of these questions is to identify any health problems the individual may have that might impact the type of physical activity that he or she should perform, and to highlight those that might best benefit his or her clinical problems. The recommended interventions are from respected professional organizations. In addition, the older adult completing the EASY is encouraged to use the comprehensive listing of Safety Tips before, during, and after physical activity.

Since the introduction of the EASY, there have been changes made to traditional screening algorithms to prevent screening out older adults, all of whom can benefit from being more physically active. One example is the new American College of Sports Medicine (ACSM) prescreening algorithm, which relies on (a) current exercise participation; (b) history and symptoms of cardiovascular, metabolic, or renal disease; and (c) desired exercise intensity to determine referral status (19). Such algorithms are less likely to require preexercise medical consultation (10).

Factors Facilitating or Impeding Physical Activty for Older Adults

Studies have examined social, behavioral, and environmental factors associated with activity patterns across the life course (20–22). Sociodemographic factors are consistently associated with physical activity levels; for example, those who are older, poorer, less educated, and living in rural settings are less likely to meet physical activity guidelines (23, 24). Health and psychosocial factors such as fear of falling, motivation, perceived efficacy for engaging in physical activity, and social support are also related to physical activity (25–30).

There is an emergent literature about the role of environmental factors (with neighborhood features such as safety, street design, and presence of places for physical activity) being key determinants to older adults' physical activity patterns (31–34). For older adults, well-maintained sidewalks and benches for resting are particularly important for accommodating age-related balance and strength changes (35). In addition, it has been reported that environmental facilitators of physical activity in the community include (a) being able to park outside one's house; (b) having access to pleasant parks; (c) being close to shopping areas and restaurants; and (d) having ramps, wide-open areas for walking, crosswalks, and resting places for outdoor walking (36–38).

Another major factor has been the confusion regarding lack of clarity on how to translate guidelines into practice. For example, traditionally health professionals did not typically ask patients about their physical activity levels, or, when asked to recommend physical activity, they were often unclear about specific strategies or places for meeting the national guidelines. Some communities are creating resource directories so both health professionals and older adults will know where they can safely exercise and/or join physical activity programs (39). Additionally, there is often a lack of coordination between community and clinical settings, resulting in an imbalance in supply and demand for community-based interventions. A recommended solution is having dedicated programming so that evidence-based interventions are consistently offered and routinely updated in the community and health professionals will feel comfortable routinely referring their patients to such interventions (40, 41).

■ Principles for Designing Physical Activity Interventions for Older Adults

The emerging value of planned physical activity interventions for older adults stimulated the development of a set of best practices that includes the following suggestions (42):

- The ideal intervention, in terms of health benefits, is a multidimensional activity program that includes endurance, strength, balance, and flexibility training.
- Physical activity interventions for older adults should incorporate principles of behavior change such as social support, self-efficacy, active choices, health contracts, assurances of safety, and positive reinforcement to enhance adherence.
- Risk management is an important consideration but should not exclude individuals from engaging in physical activity. Physical activity can be achieved by beginning at low intensity and gradually increasing to moderate physical activity.
- Community-based interventions should provide informational materials to older adults and healthcare providers about programs and ways in which to increase the time spent in physical activity safely and have an emergency procedure plan.
- Engagement in physical activity should be monitored to guide progression and enhance motivation.

■ Emergence of Evidence-Based Interventions

There are now many evidence-based interventions promoting physical activity among older adults (1, 43, 44), eliminating the need to create new intervention approaches from scratch. Selecting an evidence-based intervention helps guarantee maximal health benefit for older adults. Evidence-based interventions are those that have been tested and shown positive outcomes, have results published in a peer-reviewed journal, are standardized with an implementation manual so the intervention can be delivered consistently over time, and have a structure for training and monitoring over time (45).

It is important to know where to find an inventory of evidence-based physical activity interventions and how to select the best one for your purposes. The evidence2program website is a resource for both selecting and implementing evidence-based interventions (46). Additionally, the National Council on Aging maintains a listing of interventions that have achieved the Administration for Community Living's highest level for evidence-based programs (47). This listing describes intervention goals, target audience, intervention description, delivery staff, training requirements, and intervention costs—all key criteria that should be considered when selecting an evidence-based intervention. For example, one should consider whether a specific intervention can be easily adopted by the organization and whether it will appeal to the intended audience. The Centers for Disease Control and Prevention (CDC) also maintains a compendium of evidence-based interventions for falls prevention (48). Most of the identified interventions include physical activity strategies for improving balance and strength, key factors in reducing the risks of falling.

Examples of Best Practices

Here we present four different best practices in more detail so that the reader can visualize a range of interventions. These examples reflect a behavioral-based physical activity intervention (Active for Life®), a multimodal lifestyle intervention with a supervised physical activity component (Texercise Select), a function-focused approach for frail older adults (Function Focused Care), and a health systems approach (Exercise is Medicine).

Active for Life®

ACTIVE FOR LIFE®, a Robert Wood Johnson Foundation-funded National Program Office (2001–2009), was one of the first national initiatives to test the feasibility of translating evidence-based interventions to increase physical activity for midlife and older adults (49). Drawing on similar behavioral change principles, two interventions were selected reflecting two different channels of delivery. Active Living Every Day used facilitated group-based problem-solving methods to integrate physical activity into everyday living. Active Choices emphasized participating in individually selected activities facilitated with ongoing, brief telephone and mail follow-up delivered to the home. Using a pre–post, quasi-experimental design, nine community-based communities across the country were recruited to implement the Active for Life intervention they felt best met the needs of their target population. Findings from over 5,000 participants showed the successful translation of these interventions with positive increases in moderate- to vigorous-intensity physical activity (50).

The greatest success was the ability of the translated interventions to reach larger and more diverse populations than typically seen in highly controlled efficacy studies, while yielding outcomes with comparable effect sizes. This success was attributed, in part, to the sites working with the original program developers to adapt the program to different populations and settings without sacrificing adherence to essential intervention components such as goal setting. Of key importance was considering the social and cultural context, and incorporating examples of physical activity barriers and solutions that would resonate in different populations (51).

The Active for Life® National Program Office also examined factors related to intervention sustainability, providing technical assistance to sites on developing and implementing sustainability plans from the very start (52). Most of the sites were able to sustain the intervention over time in some fashion. A major lesson learned was the importance of having program champions and aligning the physical activity interventions with the organizational mission. An unexpected, but welcomed, consequence of this effort was the national recognition of these two interventions as effective evidence-based interventions by the Administration for Community Living, the agency responsible for providing health promotion services to older adults (47). As a consequence, both Active Living Every Day and Active Choices have been more broadly disseminated throughout the aging services network. These interventions had positive outcomes, demonstrating the power of social cognitive approaches for motivating older adults to be more physically active. However, the Active for Life® interventions were limited by being single modality behavioral interventions focused on group discussions, and not offering participants the opportunity to engage in actual physical activity during the programmatic sessions. This pointed to the need for a next generation of evidence-based programs combining both behavioral skill building and physical activity programming.

Texercise Select

Multimodal interventions health promotion/disease prevention interventions are seen as most effective (1, 6). Texercise Select is a unique evidence-based lifestyle enhancement intervention with a strong physical activity component (28). Instead of being developed and tested by research investigators, it began in the 1990s as Texercise Classic, a practice-based physical activity intervention generated through state government sponsorship (53). It had wide appeal being targeted to community-dwelling Texans 45 and older. As a result, the intervention has already achieved considerable reach throughout the state, especially among those 60 and older. However, because of its unstructured nature there was no evidence whether Texercise Classic was effective in modifying behaviors to achieve desired outcomes and health improvements. Hence, it was revamped starting in 2012 to provide the standardization necessary to be able to feel confident that the intervention was being delivered consistently, and to examine its impact in a systematic manner.

As reconfigured, Texercise Select is now a highly interactive, 90-minute, 20-session program that meets twice weekly for 10 weeks (53). Materials, such as handbooks, DVDs, and workshop incentives, are provided to participants by the Texas Health and Human Services Commission. Each session has a scripted educational component focused on a nutritional or physical activity topic as well as guided interactive discussion sessions. All of the materials are available in English, as well as Spanish, allowing the workshop to be delivered in either language. The training materials also assist the program leaders in being sensitive to the cultural beliefs regarding preferred physical activity as well as foods of Texans from different minority or ethnic backgrounds.

As a multimodal intervention, Texercise Select includes 30 to 50 minutes of physical activity that consists of a warm-up and exercises focused on strength, balance, and flexibility. Program leaders decide in advance of each session which exercises they will do for the lower and upper body, such as leg extensions or bicep curls. Participants are encouraged to also exercise outside of the class to begin building self-efficacy for maintaining physical activity habits after the class ends. An initial pre–post, single-group design study revealed that participation in the Texercise Select program resulted in significant improvements in physical activity (54, 55). A second more rigorous study utilizing a pre–post, quasi-experimental design confirmed the positive physical activity impacts for older adults (28).

The greatest strength of Texercise Select is that it is embedded in a state agency and receives ongoing infrastructure support that maintains a positive cost-benefit ratio for those wanting to implement the intervention (56). Partnering with the Healthy South Texas initiative (57) has enabled further dissemination to the Texas–Mexico border where the intervention has been met with much initial enthusiasm in low-income

Latino populations, demonstrating its universal appeal across different populations and settings. However, with broader dissemination, there is always the concern that there may be intervention drift over time and that the intervention will no longer be delivered as originally developed and tested. The development of a new online training system will be instrumental in training class facilitators throughout the state and maintaining intervention consistency. A final key to the success of Texercise Select is having a structured intervention that is also flexible with interactive sessions that appeal to all different ethnic groups and income levels.

Function-Focused Care

Frail older adults, particularly those living in long-term care settings, are sedentary and experience functional decline beyond what is expected from disease progression. This decline is multifactorial and due to resident, caregiver, and setting-related factors. Caregiving staff tend to limit residents' activities because they fear residents might fall and/or the staff might be reprimanded by the agency for not getting care tasks done quickly (58). Limited physical activity increases residents' risk for falls, pain, pressure ulcers, and hospitalizations (59–61) as well as decreases quality of life (62–65).

To prevent functional decline, a four-step theory-based approach, function-focused care (FFC), was developed. FFC is a philosophy of care that teaches direct care workers to evaluate older adults' underlying capability with regard to function and physical activity and optimize their participation in all activities (66). Examples of FFC interactions include (a) modeling behavior for residents (e.g., oral care; eating); (b) providing verbal cues during dressing; (c) walking a resident to the dining room rather than transporting via wheelchair; (d) doing resistance exercises with residents prior to meals; and (e) providing recreational physical activity (e.g., Physical Activity Bingo).

A review article evaluating the impact of FFC (67) concluded that it was beneficial for residents. Benefits included improving or maintaining function as well as mood and behavior. There was no evidence that FFC increased resident falls or adverse events (68, 69). Moreover, implementing FFC decreased transfers to the hospital for nonfall-related events (67, 69).

Disseminating and implementing evidence-based care approaches such as FFC across any healthcare system occurs slowly and is challenging (69–72). To facilitate dissemination and implementation of FFC, an evidence integration triangle (EIT) model was incorporated (73, 74). This combines a participatory implementation process that includes all stakeholders, uses practical progress measures, and incorporates key components of an effective intervention. As part of implementation of FFC, direct care workers are taught to use social cognitive approaches to overcome many of the resident-level challenges. Examples include modeling behavior and providing verbal encouragement to motivate individuals, decrease fear, overcome cultural expectations, and manage cognitive and behavioral challenges (Table 16.1) (66–69).

Prior to implementation of FFC, the stakeholder team and a nurse facilitator (who has an understanding of FFC and believes in the benefits of function and physical activity for older adults and is an in-house champion) should be identified. The nurse facilitator and in-house champion work together with staff and meet monthly with the stakeholder team to implement the following four-step process: (a) environment and policy assessments; (b) education of staff; (c) establishing resident FFC service/care plans or goals; and (d) mentoring and motivating. During monthly visits (approximately 1–2 hours each),

TABLE 16.1. Techniques to motivate older adults to engage in physical activity across a variety of clinical challenge

CLINICAL CHALLENGE	INTERVENTION
Delirium	Evaluate for the underlying cause of delirium and remove causative factor(s)[a] Implement preventive interventions which are consistent with evaluation and management of all intrapersonal factors in this table
Impaired cognitive status	Set simple goals Multiple cues (verbal, written) Role modeling—show individuals what to do versus telling them what to do and do it with them Inform and work with proxy/caregivers on patient goals
Pain	Coordinate pain management with healthcare provider as appropriate Use pharmacological and nonpharmacological interventions prior to physical activity Nonpharmacological management includes ice, heat, music, positioning, massage, and herbals
Fear of falling or getting hurt	Discuss fear Review ways to prevent falls Initiate graded exposure plan[b] Build confidence with activity
Depression	Discuss pharmacological management with healthcare provider as appropriate Encourage physical activity to decrease depression Recommend counseling as appropriate
Nutritional status	Assure regular meals are available Monitor individual for sufficient fluid and calorie intake and provide high-protein supplements as appropriate
Daytime somnolence	Review medications as possible cause Work with healthcare team to alter medication management to decrease daytime somnolence Optimize nighttime sleep via appropriate sleep hygiene, personal preferences, and appropriate medication use
Fatigue	Schedule rest periods prior to or after physical activity as per individual preference Be flexible with physical activities so that the patient can rest first and then perform the activity Reinforce that physical activity can decrease fatigue
Shortness of breath	Determine if shortness of breath is a new symptom or worse than previously noted. Establish if the individual needs supplemental oxygen to perform physical activities Provide time for the individual to rest between steps in completion of the activity Teach pursed lip breathing

(continued)

TABLE 16.1. Techniques to motivate older adults to engage in physical activity across a variety of clinical challenge *(continued)*

CLINICAL CHALLENGE	INTERVENTION
Low self-efficacy	Strengthen the individual's beliefs in his/her ability to perform the physical activity by getting the individual to do at least one part of it (e.g., walk for 1 minute) Teach the individual about the benefits of physical activity and the negative impact of being sedentary Support, encourage, and reward the individual for participating in any amount of physical activity Recognize and reinforce positive outcomes associated with physical activity (e.g., a decrease in blood pressure, weight loss) Explore with the individual what STOPS him or her from engaging in physical activity and help the individual eliminate the barrier (e.g., fear of getting hurt, not enough time) Provide the individual with role models similar to him- or herself that engage in physical activity Provide the individual with an activity program that will be of benefit to him or her. Provide cues to perform that activity (e.g., a calendar or poster) Alter the physical environment to facilitate physical activity (e.g., arrange furniture so that there are clear pathways for walking)

the nurse facilitator explores challenges, celebrates successes, and gives feedback to the stakeholder team based on changes made in the environment, policies, and service plans and observed care interactions.

Exercise Is Medicine

As discussed in chapter 11, EIM is a global health initiative that seeks to integrate physical activity as a standard of care in health systems by engaging the entire healthcare team in assessing patient physical activity levels, providing brief counseling and/or a written prescription, and referring patients to physical activity resources within the health systems, the local community, or to self-directed resources (i.e., independent walking programs, physical activity apps). EIM can be modified to fit the needs of specific health systems, communities, and patient populations.

In Taiwan, the New Taipei Ministry of Health has adopted components of EIM as part of their Fit for Age program. First, physicians throughout Taiwan undergo a daylong training workshop that provides them with a foundation related to the benefits of physical activity, safety screening for older adults, physical activity assessment and prescription, referring patients to community resources, and implementing behavior change strategies with their patients. When older adult patients attend an appointment with participating Fit for Age physicians, they undergo a frailty screening test based on criteria developed by Fried and colleagues (75). Patients determined to be "frail" or "pre-frail" are then eligible for referral to community-based physical activity interventions. These interventions are led by exercise and allied health professionals and are then reimbursed by the New Taipei Ministry of Health. However, to be eligible to receive reimbursement, intervention leaders must successfully complete a daylong workshop that provides in-depth training about serving as an extended member of the healthcare team, implementing health behavior change into their physical activity interventions, and working with older adults with chronic diseases.

Another example of the use of the EIM approach in older adults comes from a partnership between researchers at the University of Washington, Sound Generations, and local Seattle area YMCAs. In this project, physical therapists are trained to conduct basic physical activity assessments with older adult patients attending their clinics for any number of musculoskeletal conditions. As patients successfully rehabilitate their injuries, the physical therapists refer them to local YMCAs. As part of this partnership, local YMCAs agreed to adopt Enhance®Fitness (76), a low-cost, evidence-based, group exercise intervention that helps older adults at all levels of fitness become more active, energized, and empowered to sustain independent lives. Enhance®Fitness is a practice-based intervention that has been endorsed by the CDC arthritis program. Exercise professionals at the YMCA receive specialized training to successfully and safely offer the Enhance®Fitness program to patients referred by the physical therapists. Key themes related to the adoption of Enhance®Fitness programs at the YMCAs include alignment with the mission of the YMCA, obtaining support across different levels of the organization, securing initial and ongoing financial support, and the presence of champions within the YMCA to promote the intervention (77).

■ Summary

Summary of Need for and Use of Evidence-Based Physical Activity Interventions for Older Adults

Many health fields including medicine, nursing, and public health have endorsed the trend toward practice-based evidence (78). Additionally, population-based groups such as the aging services network are starting to take up the evidence-based mantle as they strive to meet the needs of their burgeoning client population (1, 79). In a time of rapidly escalating healthcare costs coupled with tight fiscal resources, evidence-based interventions for older adults are seen as particularly cost-effective for improving the health and well-being of our aging population. As discussed in Chapter 20, cost-effectiveness of a physical activity intervention is a critically important outcome for many stakeholders and therefore needs to be considered when designing and measuring interventions. In fact, the Administration for Community Living, the federal agency responsible for supporting health promotion and disease prevention programs for older Americans, requires that interventions meet a high standard of evidence before they are eligible for federal reimbursement through title 3D funding (80). Over the past 10 years, a series of national initiatives have been implemented to promote the dissemination and implementation of evidence-based interventions for helping older adults manage their chronic conditions, prevent falls, and reduce their caregiving stresses (1). The best practices presented in this chapter are examples of some of the most widely disseminated interventions for increasing physical activity for adults with varying degrees of chronic conditions and frailties, and from different sociocultural backgrounds. Linking clinical referrals to community interventions remains a public health challenge. Fortunately, there are positive signs within the aging services network with area agencies on aging recognizing the need for their programs to be coordinated with healthcare delivery systems and the EIM movement that explicitly links clinical and exercise professionals.

Application of RE-AIM Model

As the evidence-based movement matures in the aging services network, there is increased recognition of the importance of systematic intervention planning and evaluation. The RE-AIM model has been adopted as one framework for helping program planners and administrators understand program successes and challenges (81). The RE-AIM mnemonic stands for basic components needed to ensure high-quality research and practice. It provides a guide for assessing the extent to which any evidence-based program achieves its recruitment and intended population goals (REACH), desired program outcomes (EFFECTIVENESS), adherence to treatment fidelity and protocols (IMPLEMENTATION), organizational ability to adopt (ADOPTION), and sustain both individual and program benefits (MAINTENANCE). The advantage of this model over others is in its simplicity as well as flexibility to address many different types of interventions for improving physical activity in older adults (Table 16.2) (82, 83).

Current Gaps and Future Directions

There has been much progress over the past decade in understanding risk factors for physical inactivity over the life course and the importance of staying as active as possible regardless of one's age. Yet, older adults remain one of the least physically active segments of the population. This chapter identifies the potential benefit of evidence-based interventions. The issue is not knowing what to do, but having the will to do

TABLE 16.2. For RE-AIM

DIMENSION	EXAMPLES OF INDICATORS OF ACHIEVEMENT
Reach refers to the proportion of representativeness of the population targeted by the innovation.	Recruitment of settings or participants
Effectiveness refers to the extent to which the intervention improved outcomes of participants.	Evidence of change in the environment, policies you are trying to change or change in participant behavior
Adoption refers to the proportion of organizations or settings that adopt the innovation.	Setting's willingness to work with the interventionists on the activity; evidence that the participants are coming to physical activity classes
Implementation refers to evidence that the intervention was implemented as intended.	Evidence that the participants were exposed to the physical activity classes or that they go to a walking group daily
Maintenance refers to long-term adherence to the intervention and transition of the intervention into routine participation in physical activity.	Evidence of adherence beyond a 6-month period of time

what is needed. There needs to be a transformation in what society expects of its older population—the new normal should be being physically active throughout one's life and not the exception (6). Fundamental changes will be needed at many levels. Family members will need to provide support for older people being more physically active and encourage age and chronic disease appropriate activities. Health professionals will need to be aware of, and recommend, appropriate physical activity interventions to older adults. Communities will need to design safe and convenient places for older adults to walk and engage in other popular physical activities such as gardening. Only working together can we ensure healthy aging be the new normal.

■ Things to Consider

- All older adults should be encouraged to engage in a multidimensional activity program that includes endurance, strength, balance, and flexibility training.
- To enhance adherence, physical activity interventions for older adults should incorporate principles of behavior change and address motivational issues such as social support, self-efficacy, active choices, health contracts, assurances of safety, and positive reinforcement.
- Physical activity programs should be matched to the underlying ability of the older individual, the older adult's preferences, and the availability of evidence-based programs and trained leaders.
- Decreasing risk of adverse events associated with exercise is an important consideration; however, it should not be a reason to exclude any older adult from engaging in physical activity. While appropriate forms of physical activity are encouraged for adults of all ages based on their physical and cognitive functioning, interventions must emphasize safety and have an emergency procedure plan.
- All sectors interacting with older adults should promote participation in community-based physical activity programs. There are a variety of evidence-based programs to choose from, which eliminates the need to create new intervention approaches from scratch.
- Program scalability and sustainability are important issues that emphasize the importance of providing informational materials to older adults and healthcare providers so they can learn more about available programs (logistics and anticipated benefits) and ways to safely enjoy physical activity.

■ Resources

Please refer to the following websites for excellent materials from vetted international, national, state, and local sites.

- ACSM Issues Position Stand on Exercise and Older Adults
  http://www.acsm.org/about-acsm/media-room/news-releases/2009/07/20/acsm-issues-position-stand-on-exercise-and-older-adults
- Active for Life®
  https://activeforlife.info

- Active Living Research
  https://www.activelivingresearch.org
- AHA/ACSM Health/Fitness Facility Preparticipation Screening Questionnaire
  http://www.wm.edu/offices/wellness/campusrec/documents/
  fitnessquestionnaire.pdf
- CDC Compendium of Effective Fall Interventions
  https://www.cdc.gov/homeandrecreationalsafety/falls/compendium.html
- CDC Healthy Aging in Action
  https://www.cdc.gov/aging/pdf/healthy-aging-in-action508.pdf
- CDC STEADI (Stopping Elderly Accidents, Deaths, & Injuries) Toolkit
  https://www.cdc.gov/steadi/index.html
- Center for Population Health & Aging
  https://sph.tamhsc.edu/research/centers/pha.html
- Evidence2programs
  http://evidencetoprograms.com
- Exercise is Medicine®
  http://www.exerciseismedicine.org
- Federal Interagency Forum on Aging-Related Statistics
  https://agingstats.gov
- Function Focused Care
  http://www.functionfocusedcare.org
- MyHealthFinder (TAMU)
  https://sph-healthynow.tamhsc.edu
- National Council on Aging—Offering Evidence-Based Programs
  https://www.ncoa.org/center-for-healthy-aging/basics-of-evidence-based-
  programs
- NIA Go4LIFe
  https://go4life.nia.nih.gov
- Physical Activity Guidelines
  https://health.gov/paguidelines
- Profile of older adults
  https://www.acl.gov/sites/default/files/Aging%20and%20Disability%20in%20
  America/2016-Profile.pdf
- RE-AIM
  http://www.re-aim.org
- Revised Physical Activity Readiness Questionnaire (PAR-Q+)
  http://eparmedx.com/wp-content/uploads/2013/03/January2017PARQPlus
  Updated.pdf
- Texercise
  https://hhs.texas.gov/services/health/food-fitness/texercise
- WHO World Report on Aging and Health
  http://apps.who.int/iris/bitstream/handle/10665/186463/9789240694811_eng.
  pdf?sequence=1

■ Acknowledgments

We thank the American College of Sports Medicine, Exercise is Medicine, and Older Adult Committee for their insights into physical activity and aging issues and best practices for remaining active throughout life.

■ References

1. Ory MG, Smith ML, eds. Evidence-based programming for older adults. In: *Frontiers in Public Health*. 2015. Available at: https://www.frontiersin.org/research-topics/2551/evidence-based-programming-for-older-adults.
2. World Health Organization, World Report on Ageing and Health. 2015. Available at: http://apps.who.int/iris/bitstream/handle/10665/186463/9789240694811_eng.pdf; jsessionid=69403B91727B8E84A16A11181EA7CDDD?sequence=1. Accessed November 13, 2018.
3. U.S. Department of Health and Human Services & WHO. Global Health and Aging. October 2011. Available at: https://www.nia.nih.gov/sites/default/files/2017-06/global_health_aging.pdf. Accessed November 13, 2018
4. Mather M, Jacobsen LA, Pollar KM. *Aging in the United States*. Washington, DC: Population Reference Bureau; 2015;70(2):2–4.
5. Mather M. *Fact sheet: aging in the United States*. Washington, DC: Population Reference Bureau; 2016. Available at: https://www.prb.org/aging-unitedstates-fact-sheet. Accessed November 13, 2018.
6. Ory M, Smith ML. What if healthy aging is the 'new normal'? *Int J Environ Res Public Health*. 2017;14(11):1389. doi:10.3390/ijerph14111389
7. U.S. Department of Health and Human Services. Physical activity guidelines for Americans. 2nd Edition. 2018. Available at: https://health.gov/paguidelines/second-edition/pdf/Physical_Activity_Guidelines_2nd_edition.pdf. Accessed November 13, 2018.
8. Centers for Disease Control and Prevention. Behavioral risk factor surveillance system. 2018. Available at: https://www.cdc.gov/brfss/. Accessed November 13, 2018.
9. Centers for Disease Control and Prevention. Early release of selected estimates based on data from the National Health Interview Survey, January–June 2016. 2016. Available at: https://www.cdc.gov/nchs/data/nhis/earlyrelease/earlyrelease201611_07.pdf. Accessed November 13, 2018.
10. Whitfield GP, Riebe D, Magal M, et al. Applying the ACSM preparticipation screening algorithm to U.S. adults: National Health and Nutrition Examination Survey 2001-2004. *Med Sci Sports Exerc*. 2017;49(10):2056–2063. doi:10.1249/MSS.0000000000001331
11. Thomas S, Reading J, Shephard RJ. Revision of the physical activity readiness questionnaire (PAR-Q). *Can J Sport Sci*. 1992;17(4):338–345.
12. AHA/ACSM Health/Fitness Facility Preparticipation Screening Questionnaire. https://www.twu.edu/media/documents/pioneer-performance-clinic/AHA-ACSM-Risk-Screening-ADA.pdf. Accessed November 18, 2018.
13. Weston KS, Wisloff U, Coombes JS. High-intensity interval training in patients with lifestyle-induced cardiometabolic disease: a systematic review and meta-analysis. *Br J Sports Med*. 2014;48(16):1227–1234. doi:10.1136/bjsports-2013-092576
14. Desveaux L, Beauchamp M, Goldstein R, et al. Community-based exercise programs as a strategy to optimize function in chronic disease: a systematic review. *Med Care*. 2014;52(3):216–226. doi:10.1097/MLR.0000000000000065
15. Herring MP, Puetz TW, O'Connor PJ, et al. Effect of exercise training on depressive symptoms among patients with a chronic illness: a systematic review and meta-analysis of randomized controlled trials. *Arch Gen Intern Med*. 2012;172(2):101–111. doi:10.1001/archinternmed.2011.696
16. Crum R. Older adults can get moving: new screening tool tailors activities to individual needs. 2010. Available at: https://www.rwjf.org/en/library/research/2010/09/older-adults-can-get-moving-.html. Accessed November 13, 2018.

17. Resnick B, Ory MG, Hora K, et al. A proposal for a new screening paradigm and tool called Exercise Assessment and Screening for You (EASY). *J Aging Phys Act.* 2008;16(2):215–233. doi:10.1123/japa.16.2.215
18. Smith ML, Ory MG, Ahn S, et al. Older adults' participation in a community-based falls prevention exercise program: relationships between the EASY tool, program attendance, and health outcomes. *Gerontologist.* 2011;51(6):809–821. doi:10.1093/geront/gnr084
19. Riebe D, Franklin BA, Thompson PD, et al. Updating ACSM's recommendations for exercise preparticipation health screening. *Med Sci Sports Exerc.* 2015;47(11):2473–2479. doi:10.1249/MSS.0000000000000664
20. Bauman AE, Reis RS, Sallis JF, et al. Correlates of physical activity: why are some people physically active and others not? *Lancet.* 2012;380(9838):258–271. doi:10.1016/S0140-6736(12)60735-1
21. Sun F, Norman IJ, While AE. Physical activity in older people: a systematic review. *BMC Public Health.* 2013;13:449. doi:10.1186/1471-2458-13-449
22. Trost SG, Owen N, Bauman AE, et al. Correlates of adults' participation in physical activity: review and update. *Med Sci Sports Exerc.* 2002;34(12):1996–2001. doi:10.1097/00005768-200212000-00020
23. Dunlop DD, Song J, Arnston EK, et al. Sedentary time in US older adults associated with disability in activities of daily living independent of physical activity. *J Phys Act Health.* 2015;12(1):93–101. doi:10.1123/jpah.2013-0311
24. Sallis JF, Owen N, Fisher E, eds. Ecological models of health behavior. In: *Health Behavior: Theory, Research, and Practice.* 5th ed. San Francisco, CA: Jossey-Bass; 2015:43–64.
25. Cortis C, Puggina A, Pesce C, et al. Psychological determinants of physical activity across the life course: a "DEterminants of DIet and Physical Activity" (DEDIPAC) umbrella systematic literature review. *PLOS ONE.* 2017;12(8):e0182709. doi:10.1371/journal.pone.0182709
26. Fleig L, Ashe MC, Voss C, et al. Environmental and psychosocial correlates of objectively measured physical activity among older adults. *Health Psychol.* 2016;35(12):1364–1372. doi:10.1037/hea0000403
27. Greaney ML, Lees FD, Blissmer BJ, et al. Psychosocial factors associated with physical activity in older adults. *Annu Rev Gerontol Geriatr.* 2016;36(1):273–291. doi:10.1891/0198-8794.36.273
28. Ory MG, Lee S, Han G, et al. Effectiveness of a lifestyle intervention on social support, self-efficacy, and physical activity among older adults: evaluation of Texercise select. *Int J Environ Res Public Health.* 2018;15(2):E234. doi:10.3390/ijerph15020234
29. Resnick B, Boltz M. Incorporating function and physical activity across all settings. *Annu Rev Gerontol Geriatr.* 2016;36(1):293–321. doi:10.1891/0198-8794.36.293
30. Resnick B, Nigg C. Testing a theoretical model of exercise behavior for older adults. *Nurs Res.* 2003;52(2):80–88. doi:10.1097/00006199-200303000-00004
31. Brownson RC, Baker EA, Housemann RA, et al. Environmental and policy determinants of physical activity in the United States. *Am J Public Health.* 2001;91(12):1995–2003. doi:10.2105/AJPH.91.12.1995
32. Chaudhury H, Campo M, Michael Y, et al. Neighbourhood environment and physical activity in older adults. *Soc Sci Med (1982).* 2016;149:104–113. doi:10.1016/j.socscimed.2015.12.011
33. Eisenberg Y, Vanderbom KA, Vasudevan V. Does the built environment moderate the relationship between having a disability and lower levels of physical activity? A systematic review. *Prev Med.* 2017;95S:S75–S84. doi:10.1016/j.ypmed.2016.07.019
34. Moran M, Van Cauwenberg J, Hercky-Linnewiel R, et al. Understanding the relationships between the physical environment and physical activity in older adults: a systematic review of qualitative studies. *Int J Behav Nutr Phys Act.* 2014;11:79. doi:10.1186/1479-5868-11-79
35. Satariano W, Ory M, Lee C. Planned and built environments. In: Prohaska T, Anderson L, Binstock R, eds. *Public Health in an Aging Society.* Baltimore, MD: Johns Hopkins Press; 2012:323–352.

36. Zhou P, Grady SC, Chen G. How the built environment affects change in older people's physical activity: a mixed-methods approach using longitudinal health survey data in urban China. *Soc Sci Med (1982)*. 2017;192:74–84. doi:10.1016/j.socscimed.2017.09.032

37. Chen YJ, Matsuoka RH, Tsai KC. Spatial measurement of mobility barriers: improving the environment of community-dwelling older adults in Taiwan. *J Aging Phys Act*. 2015;23(2):286–297. doi:10.1123/japa.2014-0004

38. Rosenberg DE, Huang DL, Simonovich SD, et al. Outdoor built environment barriers and facilitators to activity among midlife and older adults with mobility disabilities. *Gerontologist*. 2013;53(2):268–279. doi:10.1093/geront/gns119

39. Vollmer Dahlke D, Ory M. Health applications use and potential for older adults, overview of. In: Pachana NA, ed. *Encyclopedia of Geropsychology*. Singapore: Springer Singapore; 2015:1–9.

40. Smith ML, Towne SD, Motlagh AS, Jr. Programs and place: risk and asset mapping for fall prevention. *Front Public Health*. 2017;5:28. doi:10.3389/fpubh.2017.00028

41. Lee S, Towne SDJ, Smith ML, et al. Determinants and effects of repeated evidence-based program participation among older adults. Poster presented at: American Academy of Health Behavior Annual Conference; 2017; San Antonio, TX.

42. Cress ME, Buchner DM, Prohaska T, et al. Best practices for physical activity programs and behavior counseling in older adult populations. *Eur Rev Aging Phys Act*. 2006;3(1):34–42. doi:10.1007/s11556-006-0003-9

43. Ory MG, Towne SD, Stevens AB, et al. Implementing and disseminating exercise programs for older adult populations. In: Sullivan G, Pomidor A, eds. *Exercise for Aging Adults: A Guide for Practitioners*. New York, NY: Springer Publishing; 2015.

44. Shubert TE, Smith ML, Goto L, et al. Otago exercise program in the United States: comparison of 2 implementation models. *Phys Ther*. 2017;97(2):187–197. doi:10.2522/ptj.20160236

45. Altpeter M, Bryant L, Schneider E, et al. Evidence-based health practice: knowing and using what works for older adults. *Home Health Care Serv Q*. 2006;25(1-2):1–11. doi:10.1300/J027v25n01_01

46. Stevens AB, Coleman SB, McGhee R, et al. EvidenceToPrograms.com: a toolkit to support evidence-based programming for seniors. *Front Public Health*. 2015;3:18. doi:10.3389/fpubh.2015.00018

47. National Council on Aging. Highest tier evidence-based health promotion/disease prevention programs. n.d.. Available at: https://www.ncoa.org/resources/ebpchart. Accessed November 13, 2018.

48. Stevens J, Burns E. A CDC compendium of effective fall interventions: what works for community-dwelling older adults. 2015. Available at: https://www.cdc.gov/homeandrecreationalsafety/pdf/falls/cdc_falls_compendium-2015-a.pdf. Accessed April 2, 2018.

49. Wilcox S, Dowda M, Griffin SF, et al. Results of the first year of Active for Life: translation of 2 evidence-based physical activity programs for older adults into community settings. *Am J Public Health Res*. 2006;96(7):1201–1209. doi:10.2105/AJPH.2005.074690

50. Baruth M, Wilcox S, Wegley S, et al. Changes in physical functioning in the active living every day program of the Active for Life Initiative(R). *Int J Behav Med*. 2011;18(3):199–208. doi:10.1007/s12529-010-9108-7

51. Mier N, Ory MG, Toobert D, et al. A qualitative case study examining intervention tailoring for minorities. *Am J Health Behav*. 2010;34(6):822–832. doi:10.5993/AJHB.34.6.16

52. Estabrooks PA, Smith-Ray RL, Dzewaltowski DA, et al. Sustainability of evidence-based community-based physical activity programs for older adults: lessons from Active for Life. *Transl Behav Med*. 2011;1(2):208–215. doi:10.1007/s13142-011-0039-x

53. Ory MG, Smith ML, Howell D, et al. The conversion of a practice-based lifestyle enhancement program into a formalized, testable program: from Texercise classic to Texercise select. *Front Public Health*. 2014;2:291.

54. Ory MG, Smith ML, Jiang L, et al. Texercise effectiveness: impacts on physical functioning and quality of life. *J Aging Phys Act*. 2015;23(4):622–629. doi:10.1123/japa.2014-0072

55. Smith ML, Ory MG, Jiang L, et al. Texercise select effectiveness: an examination of physical activity and nutrition outcomes. *Transl Behav Med*. 2015;5(4):433–442. doi:10.1007/s13142-014-0299-3

56. Akanni OO, Smith ML, Ory MG. Cost-effectiveness of a community exercise and nutrition program for older adults: Texercise select. *Int J Environ Res Public Health*. 2017;14(5):E545. doi:10.3390/ijerph14050545

57. Texas A&M Healthy South Texas. Annual Report 2016. 2016. Available at: http://agrilife.org/healthytexas/files/2017/03/HSTX_32886_0217_annual_report_SINGLES-1.pdf. Accessed April 2, 2018.

58. Chung G. *Quality of Care in Nursing Homes from the Perspective of Nursing Assistants*. Los Angeles, CA: Social Welfare, University of California; 2009.

59. Galik E, Resnick B, Lerner N, et al. Function focused care for assisted living residents with dementia. *Gerontologist*. 2015;55(suppl 1):S13–S26. doi:10.1093/geront/gnu173

60. Nazir A, Mueller C, Perkins A, et al. Falls and nursing home residents with cognitive impairment: new insights into quality measures and interventions. *J Am Med Dir Assoc*. 2012;13(9):819.e811–816. doi:10.1016/j.jamda.2012.07.018

61. Resnick B, Galik E, Gruber-Baldini A, et al. Testing the effect of function-focused care in assisted living. *J Am Geriatr Soc*. 2011;59(12):2233–2240. doi:10.1111/j.1532-5415.2011.03699.x

62. Kim SJ, Park EC, Kim S, et al. The association between quality of care and quality of life in long-stay nursing home residents with preserved cognition. *J Am Med Dir Assoc*. 2014;15(3):220–225. doi:10.1016/j.jamda.2013.10.012

63. Lapane KL, Quilliam BJ, Chow W, et al. The association between pain and measures of well-being among nursing home residents. *J Am Med Dir Assoc*. 2012;13(4):344–349. doi:10.1016/j.jamda.2011.01.007

64. Morrison RS, Magaziner J, Gilbert M, et al. Relationship between pain and opioid analgesics on the development of delirium following hip fracture. *J Gerontol A Biol Sci Med Sci*. 2003;58(1):76–81. doi:10.1093/gerona/58.1.M76

65. Rao AK, Chou A, Bursley B, et al. Systematic review of the effects of exercise on activities of daily living in people with Alzheimer's disease. *Am J Occup Ther*. 2014;68(1):50–56. doi:10.5014/ajot.2014.009035

66. Resnick B, Galik E, Boltz M, et al. *Implementing Restorative Care Nursing in All Setting*. New York, NY: Springer Publishing; 2011.

67. Gruber-Baldini AL, Resnick B, Hebel JR, et al. Adverse events associated with the Res-Care Intervention. *J Am Med Dir Assoc*. 2011;12(8):584–589. doi:10.1016/j.jamda.2010.05.011

68. Resnick B, Galik E, Boltz M. Function focused care approaches: literature review of progress and future possibilities. *J Am Med Dir Assoc*. 2013;14(5):313–318. doi:10.1016/j.jamda.2012.10.019

69. Beck C, Heacock P, Mercer SO, et al. Sustaining a best-care practice in a nursing home. *J Healthc Qual*. 2005;27(4):5–16. doi:10.1111/j.1945-1474.2005.tb00563.x

70. Glasgow RE, Toobert DJ, Hampson SE, et al. Implementation, generalization and long-term results of the "choosing well" diabetes self-management intervention. *Patient Educ Couns*. 2002;48(2):115–122. doi:10.1016/S0738-3991(02)00025-3

71. Parrish MM, O'Malley K, Adams RI, et al. Implementation of the care transitions intervention: sustainability and lessons learned. *Prof Case Manag*. 2009;14(6):282–293. doi:10.1097/NCM.0b013e3181c3d380

72. Schnelle JF, Alessi CA, Simmons SF, et al. Translating clinical research into practice: a randomized controlled trial of exercise and incontinence care with nursing home residents. *J Am Geriatr Soc*. 2002;50(9):1476–1483. doi:10.1046/j.1532-5415.2002.50401.x

73. Glasgow RE. What does it mean to be pragmatic? Pragmatic methods, measures, and models to facilitate research translation. *Health Educ Behav*. 2013;40(3):257–265. doi:10.1177/1090198113486805

74. Glasgow RE, Green LW, Taylor MV, et al. An evidence integration triangle for aligning science with policy and practice. *Am J Prev Med*. 2012;42(6):646–654. doi:10.1016/j.amepre.2012.02.016

75. Fried LP, Tangen CM, Walston J, et al. Frailty in older adults: evidence for a phenotype. *J Gerontol A Biol Sci Med Sci.* 2001;56(3):M146–156. doi:10.1093/gerona/56.3.M146
76. Petrescu-Prahova MG, Eagen TJ, Fishleder SL, et al. Enhance®Fitness dissemination and implementation: 2010-2015: a scoping review. *Am J Prev Med.* 2017;52(3S3):S295–S299.
77. Belza B, Petrescu-Prahova M, Kohn M, et al. Adoption of evidence-based health promotion programs: perspectives of early adopters of Enhance®Fitness in YMCA-affiliated sites. *Front Public Health.* 2014;2:164. doi:10.3389/fpubh.2014.00164
78. Brownson RC, Baker EA, Leet TL, et al. *Evidence-Based Public Health.* New York, NY: Oxford University Press; 2002.
79. Boutaugh ML, Jenkins SM, Kulinski KP, et al. Closing the disparity gap: the work of the Administration on Aging. *Generations.* 2015;38(4):107–118.
80. Administration for Community Living. Health promotion. 2018. Available at: https://www.acl.gov/programs/health-wellness/disease-prevention. Accessed November 13, 2018.
81. Marcia GO, Mary A, Basia B, et al. Perceptions about community applications of RE-AIM in the promotion of evidence-based programs for older adults. *Eval Health Prof.* 2014;38(1): 15–20.
82. Belza B, Toobert DJ, Glasgow RE. RE-AIM for program planning: overview and application. n.d.. Available at: https://www.ncoa.org/wp-content/uploads/IssueBrief_ReAim_Final-2.pdf. Accessed November 13, 2018
83. Harden SM, Smith ML, Ory MG, et al. RE-AIM in clinical, community, and corporate settings: perspectives, strategies, and recommendations to enhance public health impact. *Front Public Health.* 2018;6:71. doi:10.3389/fpubh.2018.00071

PHYSICAL ACTIVITY PRACTICES FOR INDIVIDUALS WITH DISABILITIES

KILEY J. TYLER

LEARNING OBJECTIVES

By the end of this chapter, students should be able to

1. Define disability as it relates to the design and implementation of physical activity (PA) interventions.
2. Describe PA recommendations for children and adults with disabilities.
3. Describe accommodations that may be required to ensure inclusivity for PA interventions serving individuals with intellectual disabilities (IDs).
4. Describe accommodations that may be required to ensure inclusivity for PA interventions serving individuals with physical disabilities (PDs).
5. Design an intervention to promote PA among individuals with IDs and/or PDs.

■ Defining Disability and Understanding Critical Background Information Before Designing and Delivering Interventions

The World Health Organization (WHO) defines *disability* as "an umbrella term for impairments, activity limitations, and participation restrictions," indicating that it is the interaction between a person's ability and his or her environment that determines the extent of disability (1, 2). In this way, disability describes the health condition hindered by the environment in which the person lives, in this case how the person performs physical activity (PA). While historically, the definition of disability was person centered and focused on the impairment (i.e., problem with body function and structure), perspectives on disability have changed, and disability is now viewed in terms of a dynamic interaction between the features of a person's body and the features of the environment (2).

© Springer Publishing Company DOI: 10.1891/9780826134592.0017

The diversity of disability can be described according to the *International Classification of Functioning, Disability and Health (ICF)*. The *ICF* is a classification system that takes components of functioning and disability (i.e., body functions and structures, activities, and participation) in conjunction with contextual factors (i.e., personal and environmental factors) to classify disability. A more traditional approach to understanding disability and classifying people, and one that continues to be widely used in PA research, involves a focus on the type of disability and/or the condition itself. Understanding the common physical, behavioral, and cognitive characteristics associated with a condition, for example, cerebral palsy or Down syndrome, may assist practitioners and researchers in planning and adapting their efforts to meet the PA needs of a person with a given disabling condition. This approach does have limitations since disability is very heterogeneous and people within the same classification are very diverse; however, most of the PA research involving people with disabilities has used this traditional approach to classification. As such, the following sections will present information on PA for people with disabilities using two overarching disability types: intellectual disability (ID) and physical disability (PD).

Intellectual Disability

ID is characterized by significant limitation and/or impairment in intellectual functioning (e.g., learning, problem solving, and judgment) and adaptive behavior (e.g., communication and activities of daily living) that originates before age 18 (3). Common disability subtypes encompassed under the term ID are autism spectrum disorder, Down syndrome, learning disability, and attention deficit hyperactivity disorder. The PA behavior of both adults and children with ID varies, given the diversity of both individual and environmental characteristics present during PA engagement. It is well established that participation in PA provides health-related benefits including reduced risk of chronic conditions such as diabetes, high blood pressure, high cholesterol, cancer, and obesity (4). There are also unique benefits for people with ID, including improved functional independence (5); reduced stereotypical behaviors such as hand flapping, spinning, and displaying awkward figure or hand mannerisms common in children with autism spectrum disorder (6–8); improved motor skill function; skill- and health-related physical fitness (9); psychosocial domains (10, 11); and reduced depression and anxiety (12). While a paucity of research exists concerning the PA behavior of both adults and children with ID, studies comparing the PA levels of people with ID to people without ID indicate that those with ID are significantly less active (13, 14). Box 17.1 highlights what is known about the PA of adults and children with ID.

BOX 17.1

PA Fast Facts for Adults and Children with ID

PA Fast Facts for Adults Aged 18 Years and Older With ID (12–17)

PA status: On average, only 13%–47% of adults with ID meet PA recommendations

PA mode: The most commonly reported PAs engaged in by adults with ID are walking, cycling, housework, and dancing

---

(continued)

(continued)

> **PA facilitators:** Music, community participation, social engagement, PA enjoyment, caregiver support, individualized PA opportunities
> **PA barriers:** Lack of transportation, money, time, and PA opportunities; poor caregiver support; weather conditions
> PA Fast Facts for Children Aged 6–17 Years With ID (18–24)
> > **PA status:** Children with ID do not meet PA guidelines; less PA than children without ID
> > **PA behavior pattern:** Spontaneous and intermittent, with participation declining with age
> > **PA facilitators:** Preferred PA mode; peer and parental support; reduced levels of depression, anxiety, and self-efficacy (one's belief in his or her ability to participate successfully in PA)
> > **PA barriers:** Poor social skills, feelings of tiredness and boredom, safety and bullying concerns, lack of peer and parental support, time spent watching TV or playing video games, lack of transportation
>
> ID, intellectual disability; PA, physical activity.

Physical Disability

A PD is a limitation on a person's physical, functioning, mobility, dexterity, or stamina. PD is an overarching term that typically includes subtypes such as fibromyalgia, spinal cord injury, multiple sclerosis, and cerebral palsy. While individual characteristics vary among people with PD, use of limbs and ability to ambulate influence the type of PA that is most suitable. More importantly, as seen in Box 17.2, environmental accessibility has been identified as a significant factor of participation in PA for adults and children with PD.

BOX 17.2

PA Fast Facts for Adults and Children with PD

PA Fast Facts for Adults With PD Aged 18 Years and Older (25–28)
> **PA/health status:** Of adults with PD, 57% are considered inactive, and 54% experience a secondary (sometimes chronic) condition such as diabetes, cancer, stroke, and/or heart disease
> **PA facilitators:** Social engagement, knowledgeable PA staff, accessible PA programming, inclusive PA environment, autonomy in PA mode
> **PA barriers:** Depression and anxiety; lack of money, poor environmental accessibility, and lack of social support

PA Fast Facts for Children With PD Aged 6–17 Years (29–33)
> **PA status:** Inconclusive; however, less PA than children without PD
> **PA behavior pattern:** Spontaneous and intermittent, with participation declining with age
> **PA facilitators:** Self-efficacy (e.g., PA performance ability, athletic competence), peer and parent social support, gross motor function, cognitive function, activity preference/enjoyment, access to adaptive PA equipment, family recreational orientation (e.g., parents physically active and believing that PA is important)
> **PA barriers:** Lack of environmental accessibility (e.g., programming, equipment, and transportation), lack of knowledge about how and where to be physically active

PA, physical activity; PD, physical disability.

The level of PA in people with both ID and PD is significantly lower than in those without either ID or PD (25, 34–38), which poses a risk for poor overall health. To address these health disparities, the *Physical Activity Guidelines Advisory Committee (PAGAC) Report* (39) provides specific PA recommendations for adults and children with both ID and PD.

Adults With Disabilities

The PAGAC outlines current PA recommendations for the achievement of health outcomes in adults with disabilities (39). While research has yet to establish exercise dose (i.e., frequency, duration, and mode in relation to specific health outcome improvement) as it pertains to the ability level of adults with disabilities, general guidelines are provided. The National Center on Physical Activity and Disability (NCHPAD) has expanded on PAGAC's guidelines to consider the many barriers adults with disabilities face when engaging in PA across various environments. While the guidelines are comparable to those recommended for adults without disabilities, flexibilities in PA duration, mode, and intensity are provided. NCHPAD (www.nchpad.org) is a free resource that provides information on the most up-to-date scientific literature and is user-friendly for people with disabilities, caregivers, health practitioners, and researchers (40). Box 17.3 shows the current PA guidelines for adults with disabilities per NCHPAD's frequency, intensity, time, and type (F.I.T.T.) principles.

BOX 17.3

NCHPAD F.I.T.T. Principles for Adults with Disabilities Aged 18 Years and Older

Frequency: Two to three times a week
Intensity: Moderate to vigorous PA
Time: 30 minutes per day to 150 minutes per week
Type: Any variation of aerobic and muscle strengthening, activities of daily living, aquatic exercise, walking, and cycling
What we know: Time spent in PA decreases risk for chronic disease, improves mental health, and improves independence
What we need to find out: Exact dose of PA as it relates to ability level

F.I.T.T., frequency, intensity, time, and type; NCHPAD, National Center on Physical Activity and Disability; PA, physical activity.

Children With Disabilities

Population-specific exercise guidelines for children with disabilities can be obtained by using evidence-based resources such as NCHPAD. NCHPAD provides developmentally appropriate, inclusive, up-to-date exercise guidelines for children with disabilities in video, audio, and narrative format. Current exercise guidelines revolve around developmentally appropriate frequency, duration, intensity, and mode adaptations, in addition to using inclusive exercise promotion formats typically seen in adapted physical education classrooms. Box 17.4 shows the current PA guidelines for children with both ID and PD per NCHPAD's F.I.T.T. principles.

BOX 17.4

NCHPAD F.I.T.T. Principles for Children with Disabilities Aged 6–17 Years

Characteristics of PA behavior: Population specific, developmentally and ability level dependent, intermittent and spontaneous PA behavior patterns
Intensity: Light to moderate to vigorous PA
Frequency/duration: 60 minutes per day or more if possible
Mode: Aerobic (e.g., dancing, cycling), muscle strengthening (e.g., using playground equipment, lifting weights), and bone strengthening (e.g., jumping, running)
What we know: Time spent in PA complements positive physical and mental health and social well-being, and reduces the risk of chronic disease
What we need to find out: Exact dose of PA as it relates to ability level

F.I.T.T., frequency, intensity, time, and type; NCHPAD, National Center on Physical Activity and Disability; PA, physical activity.

Special Considerations for Designing and Delivering PA Interventions among People with Disabilities

PA interventions for people with disabilities are theorized in WHO's *International Classification of Functioning of Disability and Health's (ICF's)* (2001) conceptualization of disability. Thus, when intervening for PA behavior, whether for children or adults, one should recognize that PA behavior, much like any human behavior, is shaped through the context of a dynamic interaction between the person and his or her environment. This perspective is often described as a *biopsychosocial* approach and is presented by the *ICF* as a model to describe and understand health-related states of people with disabilities (Figure 17.1).

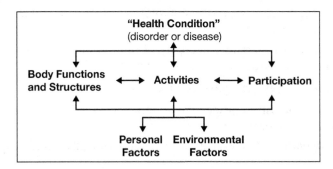

FIGURE 17.1 ICF model. ICF, *International Classification of Functioning, Disability and Health.*
Source: Reprinted with permission of World Health Organization.

An intervention for PA is intended to enable the person with disability to participate fully in PA behavior across a variety of environments, modes, and intensities, and for sufficient durations. Successful PA interventions for people with disabilities involve modification of the physical and/or social environment so that the needs of the person are met. PA interventions can be delivered using a multitude of PA modes (e.g., swimming, group exercise class, recess, walking, climbing), frequencies (e.g., 3–5 days per week), and intensities (e.g., low, moderate, and vigorous). People with disabilities can participate in PA in a variety of settings (e.g., schools, day-care centers, homes, recreation facilities, parks), but inaccessibility to a facility is a frequently reported barrier. As such, PA interventions for people with disabilities must address modifiable barriers such as inaccessible aspects of the physical environment (e.g., parking access; wheelchair access in restrooms, ramps, and elevators; and ease of wheelchair use on sidewalks and paths) or barriers embedded in a facility's policies or procedures (18, 26).

Reasons for implementing PA interventions in people with disabilities can be categorized into two primary categories: (a) enabling improved PA behavior and (b) enabling improved health-related outcomes such as physical fitness, mobility, balance, overall well-being, depression, anxiety, immune response, and improved enjoyment or happiness (35, 41).

Two examples of successful interventions for both adults and children with disabilities are summarized here:

1. **Combined Exercise Program (42)**

   ■ *Intervention goal:* Improvement of exercise economy and exercise capacity

   ■ *Intervention population:* Adults with Down syndrome

   ■ *Intervention setting:* University facility

   ■ *Intervention design:* 12-week combined exercise training consisting of endurance training 3 days per week for 30 minutes, resistance training 2 days per week, and small-group exercise sessions using heart rate training and circuit modes of exercise 3 days per week

   ■ *Intervention outcomes:* Walking economy (e.g., increased efficiency of walking) and peak oxygen consumption (e.g., improved cardiovascular function)

   ■ *Intervention strengths:* Easy replication of intervention design and facility in the community

   ■ *Intervention challenges:* Potential necessity of one-on-one participant-to-trainer monitoring throughout the intervention

2. **"Team Up for Fitness" Exercise Training Program (43)**

   ■ *Intervention goal:* Inclusive engagement of adolescents with disabilities in an effective exercise program

   ■ *Intervention population:* Adolescents with ID and typically developing peer partners

   ■ *Intervention setting:* Community-based recreational facility (YMCA)

   ■ *Intervention design:* 15-week, 2 days per week, 1-hour exercise sessions consisting of aerobic, anaerobic, and flexibility training. Reciprocal support provided by partnering an adolescent with disability and an adolescent without disability

■ *Intervention outcomes:* Improvement of health-related physical fitness components by engagement in both aerobic and anaerobic exercise

■ *Intervention strengths:* Outcomes improved by reciprocal peer-tutoring design, intervention, community-based setting, and personalized exercise programs provided to each participant

■ *Intervention challenges:* Sustainability of the program in the community

Intervention research and evaluation are important for informing best practice. Exercise interventions for adults with disabilities have improved in quality and quantity during the past 20 years (35). Even though there is still a need for improved PA levels in adults and children with disabilities, exercise intervention research as it pertains to people with disabilities is still in its infancy stage (44). Nevertheless, the research conducted thus far has demonstrated that exercise interventions are useful in increasing the time both children and adults with disabilities spend in PA, in addition to the improvement of various population-specific health outcomes (10, 35, 37). However, it has yet to be determined whether the improvement of postintervention PA behavior can be sustained (35, 44).

Exercise interventions for both adults and children are implemented to increase the time spent in PA or improve functional or health-related outcomes such as improved gross motor function, aerobic capacity, and social skills, among others (35, 44–47). Current research has indicated that the time taken for the majority of exercise interventions for adults with disabilities ranges from 3 to 4 months in duration, and these exercises are delivered using aerobic, strength, or sports modalities (35, 45). Opportunities for further exercise intervention research as it pertains to adults and children with disabilities should focus attention on robust research designs (e.g., randomized controlled trials or quasi-experimental designs), population-specific health outcomes (e.g., on-task behavior, stereotypical behaviors, anxiety), and increasing study sample sizes, in addition to exploring ways to sustain intervention-improved PA levels after the intervention ends (44, 46, 47).

Summary

In summary, disability describes a dynamic interaction between the features of a person's body and the features of the environment (2). Disability is in fact diverse, yet is often referenced as two overarching disability types: ID and PD. Research indicates that the majority of adults and children with disabilities engage in less PA than people without disabilities; however, PA levels can be improved with intervention. Common facilitators of PA in adults with disabilities consist of community/social engagement, autonomy in PA mode, and enjoyment in the activity (18–28), whereas in children, peer and parental support, self-efficacy (e.g., PA performance ability, athletic competence), and access to adapted PA equipment are key facilitators of PA (18, 19–24, 29–33). Successful exercise interventions tailored for people with disabilities often employ PA facilitators and/or modify PA barriers (i.e., transportation, environmental inaccessibility, lack of social support, etc.) by adapting the environment to meet the person's needs. Public health practitioners and researchers alike can implement this strategy by utilizing the resources presented in this chapter.

▓ Things to Consider

- ▪ People with disabilities participate in PA across many different settings such as fitness and recreation facilities. Although physical inaccessibility is a common barrier to the PA participation of people with disabilities, fitness and recreation center staff, and/or owners, can assure accessibility through the use of Accessibility Instruments Measuring Fitness and Recreation Environments (AIMFREE). AIMFREE is a series of questionnaire measures that assess the accessibility of recreation and fitness facilities. You can learn more about AIMFREE on the NCHPAD website (40).

- ▪ Aquatic exercise is a safe and effective form of exercise for people with disabilities. Application of the NCHPAD F.I.T.T. principles for adults with disabilities (Box 17.3) in the aquatic PA environment can be a successful means of engaging adults with disabilities in moderate- to high-intensity aerobic exercise.

- ▪ School is an opportune environment for children with disabilities to spend time being physically active. Physical educators and recess monitors can support the PA of children with disabilities by establishing play partnerships (i.e., child/adolescent with disability and a child/adolescent without disability) to aid in the successful application of reciprocal peer tutoring.

▓ Resources

While research provides best-practice strategies for constructing and implementing exercise interventions for people with disabilities, further guidelines can be found using the following evidence-based resources:

- ▪ U.S. Office of Disease Prevention and Health Promotion: health.gov
  - ● Healthy People 2020: www.healthypeople.gov
  - ● Physical Activity Guidelines for Americans: https://health.gov/paguidelines/guidelines
- ▪ National Center on Physical Activity and Disability
  - ● For healthcare providers: https://www.nchpad.org/Health~Care~Providers
  - ● For fitness professionals: https://www.nchpad.org/Fitness~Professionals
- ▪ Step It Up! The Surgeon General's Call to Action to Promote Walking and Walkable Communities: https://www.surgeongeneral.gov/library/calls/walking-and-walkable-communities/exec-summary.html
- ▪ Centers for Disease Control and Prevention: www.cdc.gov
  - ● Division of Nutrition, Physical Activity, and Obesity: https://www.cdc.gov/nccdphp/dnpao/state-local-programs/health-equity/index.html
  - ● Health Equity Toolkit: https://www.cdc.gov/nccdphp/dnpao/state-local-programs/health-equity/pdf/toolkit.pdf

References

1. Rimmer JH, Chen MD, Hsieh K. A conceptual model for identifying, preventing, and managing secondary conditions in people with disabilities. *Phys Ther.* December 2011;91(12):1728–1739. doi:10.2522/ptj.20100410

2. World Health Organization. *How to Use the ICF: A Practical Manual for Using the International Classification of Functioning, Disability and Health (ICF). Exposure Draft for Comment.* Geneva: World Health Organization; 2013.

3. Schalock RL, Borthwick-Duffy SA, Buntinx WHE, et al. *Intellectual Disability: Definition, Classification, and Systems of Supports.* 11th ed. Washington, DC: American Association on Intellectual and Developmental Disabilities; 2010.

4. Buchner D. Health benefits of physical activity. In: Centers for Disease Control. *Promoting Physical Activity.* 2nd ed. Champaign, IL: Human Kinetics; 2010:3–20.

5. Gretebeck RJ, Ferraro KF, Black DR, et al. Longitudinal change in physical activity disability in adults. *Am J Health Behav.* March 2012;36(3):385–394. doi:10.5993/AJHB.36.3.9

6. Levinson LJ, Reid G. The effects of exercise intensity on the stereotypic behaviors of individuals with autism. *Adapt Phys Activ Q.* July 1993;10(3):255–268. doi:10.1123/apaq.10.3.255

7. Prupas A, Reid G. Effects of exercise frequency on stereotypic behaviors of children with developmental disabilities. *Educ Training Ment Retard Dev Disabil.* June 2001;36(2):196–206. Available at: http://www.jstor.org/stable/23879735

8. Todd T, Reid G, Butler-Kisber L. Cycling for students with ASD: self-regulation promotes sustained physical activity. *Adapt Phys Activ Q.* July 2010;27(3):226–241. doi:10.1123/apaq.27.3.226

9. Lytle R, Todd T. Stress and the student with autism spectrum disorders: strategies for stress reduction and enhanced learning. *Teach Except Child.* March 2009;41(4):36–42. doi:10.1177/004005990904100404

10. Johnson CC. The benefits of physical activity for youth with developmental disabilities: a systematic review. *Am J Health Promot.* January-February 2009;23(3):157–167. doi:10.4278/ajhp.070930103

11. Ortega F, Ruiz JR, Castillo MJ, et al. Physical fitness in childhood and adolescence: a powerful marker in health. *Int J Obes (Lond).* January 2008;32(1):1–11. doi:10.1038/sj.ijo.0803774

12. Heller T, Ying GS, Rimmer JH, et al. Determinants of exercise in adults with cerebral palsy. *Public Health Nurs.* May-June 2002;19(3):223–231. doi:10.1046/j.0737-1209.2002.19311.x

13. Hsieh K, Heller T, Bershadsky J, et al. Impact of adulthood stage and social-environmental context on body mass index and physical activity of individuals with intellectual disability. *Intellect Dev Disabil.* April 2015;53(2):100–113. doi:10.1352/1934-9556-53.2.100

14. Stanish HI, Temple VA, Frey GC. Health-promoting physical activity of adults with mental retardation. *Ment Retard Dev Disabil Res Rev.* 2006;12(1):13–21. doi:10.1002/mrdd.20090

15. Bodde AE, Seo DC, Frey GC, et al. Correlates of moderate-to-vigorous physical activity participation in adults with intellectual disabilities. *Health Promot Pract.* September 2013;14(5):663–670. doi:10.1177/1524839912462395

16. Van Schijndel-Speet M, Evenhuis HM, van Wijck R, et al. Facilitators and barriers to physical activity as perceived by older adults with intellectual disability. *Intellect Dev Disabil.* June 2014;52(3):175–186. doi:10.1352/1934-9556-52.3.175

17. Stanish HI, Curtin C, Must A, et al. Physical activity enjoyment, perceived barriers, and beliefs among adolescents with and without intellectual disabilities. *J Phys Act Health.* January 2016;13(1):102–110. doi:10.1123/jpah.2014-0548

18. Stanish H, Curtin C, Must A, et al. Enjoyment, barriers, and beliefs about physical activity in adolescents with and without autism spectrum disorder. *Adapt Phys Activ Q.* October 2015;32(4):302–317. doi:10.1123/APAQ.2015-0038

19. Pan CY, Frey GC. Identifying physical activity determinants in youth with autistic spectrum disorders. *J Phys Act Health.* October 2005;2(4):412–422. doi:10.1123/jpah.2.4.412

20. Jones RA, Downing K, Rinehart NJ, et al. Physical activity, sedentary behavior and their correlates in children with autism spectrum disorder: a systematic review. *PLOS ONE.* February 28, 2017;12(2):e0172482. doi:10.1371/journal.pone.0172482

21. Ayvazoglu NR, Kozub FM, Butera G, et al. Determinants and challenges in physical activity participation in families with children with high functioning autism spectrum disorders from a family systems perspective. *Res Dev Disabil.* December 2015;47:93–105. doi:10.1016/j.ridd.2015.08.015
22. Downs SJ, Boddy LM, Knowles ZR, et al. Exploring opportunities available and perceived barriers to physical activity engagement in children and young people with Down syndrome. *Eur J Spec Needs Educ.* 2013;28(3):270–287. doi:10.1080/08856257.2013.768453
23. Hutzler Y, Korsensky O. Motivational correlates of physical activity in persons with an intellectual disability: a systematic literature review. *J Intellect Disabil Res.* September 2010;54(9):767–786. doi:10.1111/j.1365-2788.2010.01313.x
24. Yazdani S, Yee CT, Chung PJ. Factors predicting physical activity among children with special needs. *Prev Chronic Dis.* July 18, 2013;10:E119. doi:10.5888/pcd10.120283
25. Carroll DD, Courtney-Long EA, Stevens AC, et al. Vital signs: disability and physical activity—United States, 2009–2012. Centers for Disease Control and Prevention. *MMWR Morb Mortal Wkly Rep.* May 9, 2014;63(18):407–413.
26. Martin Ginis KA, Ma JK, Latimer-Cheung AE, et al. A systematic review of review articles addressing factors related to physical activity participation among children and adults with physical disabilities. *Health Psychol Rev.* December 2016;10(4):478–494. doi:10.1080/17437199.2016.1198240
27. Richardson EV, Smith B, Papathomas A. Disability and the gym: experiences, barriers and facilitators of gym use for individuals with physical disabilities. *Disabil Rehabil.* September 2017;39(19):1950–1957. doi:10.1080/09638288.2016.1213893
28. Williams TL, Ma JK, Martin Ginis KA. Participant experiences and perceptions of physical activity-enhancing interventions for people with physical impairments and mobility limitations: a meta-synthesis of qualitative research evidence. *Health Psychol Rev.* June 2017;11(2):179–196. doi:10.1080/17437199.2017.1299027
29. Bult MK, Verschuren O, Jongmans MJ, et al. What influences participation in leisure activities of children and youth with physical disabilities? A systematic review. *Res Dev Disabil.* September-October 2011;32(5):1521–1529. doi:10.1016/j.ridd.2011.01.045
30. King G, Law M, Petrenchik T, et al. Psychosocial determinants of out of school activity participation for children with and without physical disabilities. *Phys Occup Ther Pediatr.* November 2013;33(4):384–404. doi:10.3109/01942638.2013.791915
31. Bloemen MA, Backx FJ, Takken T, et al. Factors associated with physical activity in children and adolescents with a physical disability: a systematic review. *Dev Med Child Neurol.* February 2015;57(2):137–148. doi:10.1111/dmcn.12624
32. Shields N, Synnot AJ, Barr M. Perceived barriers and facilitators to physical activity for children with disability: a systematic review. *Br J Sports Med.* November 2012;46(14):989–997. doi:10.1136/bjsports-2011-090236
33. Li R, Sit CHP, Yu JJ, et al. Correlates of physical activity in children and adolescents with physical disabilities: a systematic review. *Prev Med.* August 2016;89:184–193. doi:10.1016/j.ypmed.2016.05.029
34. Hinckson EA, Curtis A. Measuring physical activity in children and youth living with intellectual disabilities: a systematic review. *Res Dev Disabil.* January 2013;34(1):72–86. doi:10.1016/j.ridd.2012.07.022
35. Lai B, Young HJ, Bickel CS, et al. Current trends in exercise intervention research, technology, and behavioral change strategies for people with disabilities: a scoping review. *Am J Phys Med Rehabil.* October 2017;96(10):748–761. doi:10.1097/PHM.0000000000000743
36. Pan CY, Hsu PJ, Chung IC, et al. Physical activity during the segmented school day in adolescents with and without autism spectrum disorders. *Res Autism Spectrum Disord.* July 2015;15:21–28. doi:10.1016/j.rasd.2015.04.003
37. Rimmer JH, Chen MD, McCubbin JA, et al. Exercise intervention research on persons with disabilities: what we know and where we need to go. *Am J Phys Med Rehabil.* March 2010;89(3):249–263. doi:10.1097/PHM.0b013e3181c9fa9d
38. Tyler K, MacDonald M, Menear K. Physical activity and physical fitness of school-aged children and youth with autism spectrum disorders. *Autism Res Treat.* 2014;2014:312163.

39. Physical Activity Guidelines Advisory Committee. *Physical Activity Guidelines Advisory Committee Report, 2008*. Washington, DC: US Department of Health and Human Services; 2008. Available at: https://health.gov/paguidelines/report/pdf/committeereport.pdf. Accessed May 16, 2018.

40. Tyler K, Cook NM, MacDonald M. Physical activity and children with disabilities. *Palaestra*. 2014;28(4):17–22.

41. Caspersen CJ, Powell KE, Christenson GM. Physical activity, exercise, and physical fitness: definitions and distinctions for health-related research. *Public Health Rep*. March-April 1985;100(2):126–131.

42. Mendonca GV, Pereira FD, Fernhall B. Effects of combined aerobic and resistance exercise training in adults with and without Down syndrome. *Arch Phys Med Rehabil*. January 2011;92(1):37–45. doi:10.1016/j.apmr.2010.09.015

43. Stanish HI, Temple VA. Efficacy of a peer-guided exercise programme for adolescents with intellectual disability. *J Appl Res Intellect Disabil*. July 2012;25(4):319–328. doi:10.1111/j.1468-3148.2011.00668.x

44. McGarty AM, Downs SJ, Melville CA, et al. A systematic review and meta-analysis of interventions to increase physical activity in children and adolescents with intellectual disabilities. *J Intellect Disabil Res*. April 2018;62(4):312–329. doi:10.1111/jir.12467

45. Castro O, Ng K, Novoradovskaya E, et al. A scoping review on interventions to promote physical activity among adults with disabilities. *Disabil Health*. April 2018;11(2):174–183. doi:10.10.1016/j.dhjo.2017.10.013

46. McGarty AM, Penpraze V, Melville CA. Accelerometer use during field-based physical activity research in children and adolescents with intellectual disabilities: a systematic review. *Res Dev Disabil*. May 2014;35(5):973–981. doi:10.1016/j.ridd.2014.02.009

47. McGarty AM, Penpraze V, Melville CA. Calibration and cross-validation of the ActiGraph wGT3X+ accelerometer for the estimation of physical activity intensity in children with intellectual disabilities. *PLOS ONE*. October 2016;11(10):e0164928. doi:10.1371/journal.pone.0164928

PHYSICAL ACTIVITY IN URBAN POPULATIONS

AMY A. EYLER | WILLIAM J. DAVIS

LEARNING OBJECTIVES

By the end of this chapter, the student should be able to

1. Differentiate between the classification levels of urban populations.
2. Examine the socio-ecological factors related to physical activity (PA) in urban environments.
3. Compare and contrast aspects of the urban infrastructure that influence PA.
4. Distinguish factors of a health impact assessment that would help inform an urban PA intervention.
5. Assess examples of PA interventions in urban settings.

Introduction

What is urban? The definition of the word *urban* is "relating to or characteristic of a city or town," but the concept is more complex than that, especially when it comes to physical activity (PA) interventions. Other terms used to describe urban areas are developed, dense, industrialized, and more populated than rural areas. The U.S. Census Bureau definition of urban has evolved since first developed in 1910 because the environments themselves have changed immensely in the past century. Since 2010, urban is defined by the U.S. Census Bureau as densely developed geographic delineation that encompasses residential, commercial, and other nonresidential urban land uses, differentiated in two ways. A place is designated an **Urban Area** if it consists of 50,000 or more people. **Urban Clusters** are places with a population between 2,500 and 50,000 (1). To be considered urban, there must be a minimum population of at least 2,500 people. Nearly 81% of the American population lives in either of these urban classifications. The U.S. Department

© Springer Publishing Company DOI: 10.1891/9780826134592.0018

of Agriculture uses a different categorization to differentiate geographic patterns based on measures of population density, urbanization, and daily commuting. The codes range from 1 to 10, with 1 being a metropolitan area and 10 being rural. These codes help identify urban cores and adjacent territories that are economically integrated with those cores (2). These ways of classifying urban are important to researching PA and implementing PA interventions, particularly given the importance of mobility within and/or around urban settings.

Traffic is an important consideration for urban-setting PA interventions. Peak-period congestion, especially when traveling by automobile, is an issue in urban areas. In 2014, drivers in the largest 79 urban areas in the United States spent the equivalent of 42 hours annually per rush-hour commuter in extra travel time due to traffic congestion (3). Persistent urban sprawl, separated land uses, and lower residential densities have all contributed to negative trends in urban mobility, resulting in adverse effects on public health through reduced PA, prolonged sitting, injuries, air pollution, social isolation, noise, stress, compromised personal safety, unhealthy diets, urban heat island effects, and greenhouse gas emissions driving climate change (4). Furthermore, travel time reliability, measuring the extent of unexpected delay, continues to worsen due to urban mobility congestion (5). Negative trends in urban mobility are resulting in adverse impacts on movement of goods and people, sustainability, and public health.

There is evidence to suggest that adults tend to be more physically active when they live in higher density, mixed-use neighborhoods with destinations such as parks and shops within walking distance (6). There is also evidence that in general, adults who live in urban areas walk more and are less sedentary than those residing in rural areas (7). Figuring out what factors in urban environments contribute to greater activity is important for intervention planning, particularly as it relates to the built environment. The socio-ecological model has been applied to urban PA to help frame these factors and theorize potential interactions among the levels. See Figure 18.1.

Environmental characteristics are particularly significant to PA in urban areas. Supportive environments can make PA an easy choice or serve as a barrier to this important behavior. An urban environment can also support individual and interpersonal factors. For example, if you are motivated to walk to gain health benefits and have a friend who has committed to walk with you, a safe, walkable neighborhood can support these efforts. Conversely, a high-traffic neighborhood without sidewalks or trails might be the factor that keeps you from walking despite your motivation and social support. Living in the most supportive environment could help the average person achieve at least half of the recommended amount of 150 minutes of PA per week (6–8). Environmental characteristics that enhance this support are integral parts of community design, street design, transportation planning, and city development. Because many of the terms used to describe these characteristics come from fields outside of public health such as urban planning and transportation, it is important to define and clarify them with relevant examples to foster an understanding of the relationship between the urban environment and PA.

Walkability. This term is used to describe pedestrian friendliness of specified geographic areas. One common measure of walkability is WalkScore (www.walkscore.com), an aggregate score from 1 to 100 based on factors such as population, pedestrian design, complete streets, and public spaces. The more supportive the environment is for walking, the more likely it is that people will choose to do so for recreation or travel. Walkability is related to health benefits and is also associated with a healthier environment due to lower pollution.

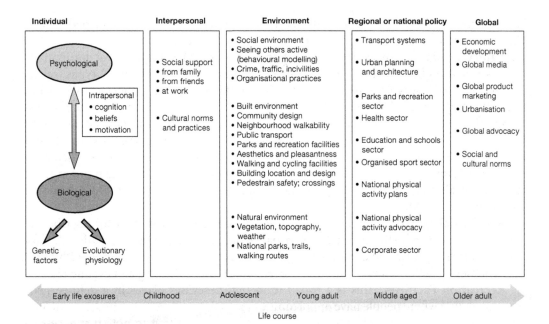

FIGURE 18.1 Socio-ecological factors related to PA in urban environments. PA, physical activity.

Source: Bauman A, Reis R, Sallis J, et al. Correlates of physical activity: why are some people physically active and others not? *Lancet.* 2012;380(9838):258-271. doi:10.1016/S0140-6736(12)60735-1

Bikeability. This term is used to describe bicycle friendliness of the physical and operational conditions for on-street (lanes, bike lanes) and off-street (multiuse paths) travel. For on-street facilities, traffic volume, traffic speed, and width are critical inputs to bikeability, formally evaluated under multimodal mobility using 2016 Highway Capacity Manual procedures (9). For off-street multiuse paths, bicycle and pedestrian use, path width, alignment, and intersection characteristics are important components for bikeability of these types of facilities. How paths and routes are connected with one another is an essential element for both types of bicycling facilities, as well as other amenities such as lighting, security, shade, water fountains, benches, bike parking, and interface with other modes of travel. Cycling as a day-to-day means of travel in urban areas provides measurable health benefits including a 52% lower risk of dying from heart disease and a 40% lower risk of dying from cancer, as shown in a recent 5-year study from the United Kingdom (10). The need for a well-connected network of bicycle-specific infrastructure in urban areas including multiuse paths and on-street facilities is critical to encourage more bicycling among adults and therefore the potential to positively influence health outcomes (11).

Traffic Speed and Volume. The posted (and actual) speed of vehicles as well as the number of vehicles on a road can impact safety for pedestrians and cyclists. Engineering and design about alignment, width, shoulder, and median all play a crucial role in determining the speed motor vehicles travel along U.S. roadways. For every incremental reduction in speed from 35 to 25 miles per hour, considerable operational benefits result in improving the safety of cyclists traveling within mixed traffic flows (12). Traffic calming measures such as speed bumps or chicanes (a series of narrowing or curb extensions that alternate from one side of the street to the other forming S-shaped curves) have been used to slow traffic and increase pedestrian safety (13).

Land Use Mix. This measures the average neighborhood-level diversity of destinations across a metropolitan area based on the mix of eight different employment types (office, retail, industrial, service, entertainment, education, health, and public sector) within each block group of that area. The scores are from 0 to 1 where 1 offers the widest range of convenient access to a wide range of jobs and services (14). Handy et al., found that the number of different businesses within 800 m of home was associated with walking to these destinations. Trends in mixed-use development (sometimes called New Urbanism) support better and healthier mobility patterns by encouraging more walking (17.2%) of all trips and trip purposes as compared with 7.3% in more conventional neighborhoods (15).

Residential Density. This urban planning and design term is used to describe the number of people who live in a specified urban area in contrast to the population density of that area. People who live in high residential density areas in combination with other environmental factors such as land use mix engage in more walking and cycling (8).

Recreation Facilities. This is a broad term that describes places in a defined geographic region where people have opportunities to be physically active. These can include recreation centers, parks, playgrounds, and trails. It is important to note that access to these facilities is an important aspect, too. If a community has recreation centers, but they charge high use fees or have inconvenient hours, they may not influence PA.

Urban Green Space. This is defined as publicly owned and publicly accessible open space with a high degree of vegetative cover and connection to other green space within city boundaries. They provide safe and equitable places for PA and are important to social interaction and mental health (16).

Multiuse Paths and Greenways. Multiuse paths are developed for multiple modes of active transportation such as walking, running, and bicycling. Urban greenways often extend along water fronts, water courses, and transportation, utility, and/or converted rails-to-trails corridors. Walkers and bicyclists are drawn to these types of highly desirable, off-street facilities, and provision of urban greenways leads to longer active transportation trips (17).

Connectivity. Urban environments typically have a more compact development pattern and more intersections that offer direct and alternate routes to destinations that support walking (18). This, in combination with mixed land use, can facilitate PA. It makes intuitive sense that the more connected destinations are, the easier they are to access.

Complete Streets. An emerging movement in urban transportation is being advanced through adoption of complete street policies by numerous jurisdictions and transportation agencies. Policies are focused on providing facility designs within the road right of way that more equitably accommodate diverse and often competing travel modes, including motor vehicles, public transit, bicycles, and pedestrians. In 2014, 25.2% of all U.S. municipalities with a population of 1,000 or larger reported adopting complete street policies (19).

Multimodal Urban Trips, Green Travel Modes. Walking and bicycling combined with public transit system use are considered green travel modes and are found to support sustainability principles and increase PA outcomes (20). These modes of travel also decrease urban congestion, decrease energy consumption, improve air quality, and increase PA. Walking and bicycling to transit stations for everyday trip making generally occur within a 0.5-mile radii and 1.0-mile radii, respectively, and some research suggests these distances are even larger (21). The combined effect of green mode travel results in a measurable increase in PA for urban travelers (22).

Health Impact Assessment (HIA). This is a process that is used to evaluate potential health effects of a plan, project, or policy prior to adoption or implementation. HIAs are used to identify positive and negative impacts for consideration in guiding the decision-making process to influence projects involving transportation and land use to support more desirable health outcomes (23). For walking and bicycling, HIAs commonly weigh benefits of active transportation against detrimental effects of traffic incidents and air pollution exposure on health.

It is important to note that these factors (as well as others) often work together to create the most supportive urban environments for PA. For example, a community with high walkability and an integrated public transportation system seems likely to have more physically active residents than a low-walkability, car-dependent city. Also, safety features such as well-maintained sidewalks, lower speed limits, and crosswalks can work together to enable people to feel safer when out on the streets walking for transportation or for leisure. Seeing the added value of multiple strategies, the Community Preventive Services Task Force recommends a combination of interventions to improve pedestrian and bicycle transportation systems with land use and environmental design interventions to positively influence PA (24).

Community Preventive Services Task Force Built Environment Recommendations

Transportation system interventions:

- Street connectivity, complete streets, bike boulevards
- Sidewalk, multiuse path, and trail infrastructure
- Bicycle infrastructure, bike share programs
- Public transit infrastructure and multimodal connectivity

Land use and environmental design interventions:

- Mixed land use environments to increase the diversity and proximity of local destinations
- Access to parks and other public or private recreational facilities
- Transit-oriented development
- Neotraditional neighborhood development
- Blue Zones Project Communities

There has been an increase in the research evidence related to built environments and PA within the past decade. As indicated by the Community Guide recommendations, several reviews have reported that adults tend to be more physically active when they live in a higher density, mixed-use neighborhood with parks and shops within walking distance (7). In a 2012 review, Bauman et al., found several factors that were correlates of PA in urban environments. See Table 18.1. Evidence shows that the way urban areas are planned and developed (and maintained) can influence PA for children, adolescents, and adults, and the features most relevant to this influence may vary among these age groups. Separating correlates by age is especially important for tailoring interventions. If high traffic speed and volume influence the perception of safety by parents, modifications to these factors may result in them feeling more confident in letting children walk and bicycle in these environments.

There is also a global interest in urban correlates of PA. In a multicountry study, Sallis et al., found several urban environmental attributes that accounted for variability in adult PA (6). Residential density, public transportation density, and park density were related to PA. These findings can help inform design of urban environments to have the most positive impact on PA, particularly because of the health burden related to the global PA pandemic.

TABLE 18.1. Correlates of PA in urban areas by age group

GROUP	MOST ROBUST CORRELATES
Children	■ Walkability ■ Traffic speed and volume (inverse) ■ Land use mix ■ Residential density ■ Access or proximity to recreation facilities
Adolescents	■ Land use mix ■ Residential density
Adults	■ Recreation facilities and location ■ Transportation environment ■ Aesthetics

NOTE: PA, physical activity.

■ Urban PA Interventions

There are many examples in the United States and internationally of strategies, programs, and policies to increase PA among urban residents (see Box 18.1). One of the first to be implemented (and evaluated) was the Ciclovia project in Bogota, Colombia. Ciclovias (translates to "bicycle path" or "cycle way") are initiatives where the streets in a certain area are temporarily closed to automobile traffic and open to pedestrians and cyclists in an effort to promote PA, social connectedness, social capital, economic growth, and sustainability (25). Bogota's Ciclovia Recreativa project began in 1976 and, over time, has evolved into a weekly event. For 7 hours every Sunday, over 100 km of roads are closed to motor vehicles to allow for people to safely walk or bike along the route. It is estimated that over one million people participate each Sunday. Evaluation of this initiative shows that participants in Ciclovias are likely to meet the recommended amounts of weekly PA (26) and that hosting these events is cost beneficial (27). The success of Ciclovias has caused an increase in these types of events all over the world. As of 2017, 122 U.S. cities have hosted similar events (28). While they vary in frequency, length, and duration, these events are an excellent example of an urban initiative that has benefits beyond just providing an opportunity for PA.

Another example of an urban initiative to increase PA is bike sharing. Bike sharing is a transportation program that provides users with the ability to pick up a bicycle at any self-serve bike station and return it to any bike station located within the system's service area. These programs are usually designed for short distance trips (0.5–3 miles) and fit well with the density of an urban area. In 2008, Washington, DC became the first major city in the United States to implement a bike share program; due to its success, many other cities followed. As of 2017, 119 U.S. cities had bike share programs (29). Most bike share programs rely on self-serve technology with automated kiosks for checkout and return. However, dockless bike share programs are becoming more common. Bike share programs may facilitate planned and spontaneous trips and can complement the use of public transportation systems. Some literature exists on the benefits of bike share programs, but more rigorous evaluations are needed to identify the impact on PA for leisure and transport among urban bike share users (30).

Technology is making systems such as bike share more user-friendly, and it also has the potential to influence urban PA in other ways. Global Positioning Software (GPS) has been integrated into programs that help people track their walking, running, and cycling trips. These programs sync to wearable PA tracking devices and to websites where routes, mileage, and time can be compared with other users. This aggregate data can also be helpful to urban planners to identify the most used routes for walking, running, and cycling. This data can inform development of new streets or detect areas that might be safety concerns.

Another way technology can influence urban PA is the increasing popularity of interactive mobile phone apps. For example, apps have been developed for self-guided walking tours of many major United States and international cities (31). These apps provide maps and specific details about walking destinations, and can even provide audio instructions and destination information. This technology is relatively new and quickly evolving, making evaluation challenging. However, technology will no doubt be an increasingly common aspect of urban PA interventions in the future.

BOX 18.1

New York City's High Line

Urban centers are known for being densely populated, and while this can be a correlate for PA, it can also take a toll on mental health and increase the need for peaceful respite. Parks and urban greenspaces can be places for residents to get away from the negative aspects of city life, but also to be physically active in ways that city streets or indoor recreation centers might not accommodate. Gaining space for parks can be challenging in urban areas where undeveloped real estate may be scarce.

In 2016, New York City was the most populated and population-dense city in the United States (32). Even though it is home to Central Park, which encompasses 843 acres within city limits, developers found an opportunity to create another park through innovative public space transformation. The High Line has history dating back to 1934, where it was originally built as a rail line. After decades of success in facilitating the transport of freight, the increasing use of highways for trucking resulted in closure of the rail line in 1980. Seen as an opportunity for a new kind of park, developers began planning this recreational space in 2002. Community input was solicited, and in 2009 the first section was open to the public. Currently, the elevated park is 2.4 km and is home to walkways, plants, and gardens. The High Line promotes walking tours that attract millions of visitors as well as residents (www.thehighline.org).

(continued)

(*continued*)

The development of the High Line falls in line with the *Active Design Guidelines*: *Promoting Physical Activity and Health in Design,* which was developed by a partnership of the New York City Departments of Design and Construction, Health and Mental Hygiene, Transportation, City Planning, and Office of Management and Budget, as well as many other stakeholders (33). It is worth noting the diversity of organizations represented in this project. As was discussed in Chapter 6, building PA coalitions with diverse members who can benefit strategically from participating in the coalition often leads to successful outcomes. The purpose of these guidelines is to be a resource for strategies for creating healthier buildings, streets, and urban spaces, based on the latest evidence and practice. The guidelines include

- Urban design strategies for creating neighborhoods, streets, and outdoor spaces that encourage walking, bicycling, and active transportation, and recreation
- Building design strategies for promoting active living where we work and live and play, through the placement and design of stairs, elevators, and indoor and outdoor spaces
- Discussion of synergies between active design with sustainable and universal design initiatives

Source: https://centerforactivedesign.org/guidelines

PA, physical activity.

Transit-Oriented Development, Denver, Colorado

A widely used anecdote to urban sprawl and traffic congestion is adoption of land use policies that encourage transit-oriented development (TOD). Denver, Colorado, is a city that has expanded its public transit system to include eight light rail lines and two commuter rail lines with 63 stations and 87.5 miles of track, with extensive plans to further extend coverage into additional urbanized areas (34). TOD largely focuses on the area within a half-mile radius, or what is taken to be a walkable distance, to a transit station. Increased land use densities, from moderate to high, are frequently allowed and encouraged through special zoning regulations by offering developers incentives for constructing desirable projects that efficiently connect with nearby transit stations. Wide-scale implementation of TOD in Denver was achieved through supportive partnerships between the Denver Regional Transit District, City of Denver, County of Denver, and Regional Council of Governments. This collaboration led to the adoption of "Blueprint Denver" in 2002 that changed zoning near transit stations and led to creation of a TOD strategic plan, which right-sized explicit zoning and overlay approaches for each specific transit station location (35).

Neotraditional Residential Developments

The residential and commercial development industry is responding to the overwhelming desire of the public to live and work in walkable communities. Amounts of PA related to walking and bicycling increase when the scale and balance of important elements are addressed through planning and design (8). Table 18.2 provides a comparison of three nationally recognized walkable community developments in Colorado, South Carolina, and North Carolina. Common design elements of these neotraditional developments include (a) ample amounts of open space, (b) balanced and blended single-family homes and rental residences, (c) comparatively equal employment and residential populations,

(d) inclusion of some institutional facilities that serve as destination trip generators, and (e) presence of widespread multiuse path systems. There is a growing demand for these mixed-use walkable developments to provide quality healthy, active, and connected urban lifestyles.

TABLE 18.2. Common design elements for nationally recognized walkable communities

	STAPLETON	DANIEL ISLAND	MEADMOUNT
Location	Denver, CO	Charleston, SC	Chapel Hill, NC
Total area (acres)	4,700	4,000	435
Open space (acres)	1,700	400	70
SF	13,000,000	250,000	200,000
Single-family homes	8,000	1,800	700
Rental homes	4,000	1,700	700
Resident population	30,000	10,000	1,800
Employment	35,000	11,000	1,200
Institutional elements	Multiple K-12 schools	K-8 neighborhood school	UNC satellite campus building
Other key elements	Average of 12 residential units per acre	Two major sports venues	UNC Wellness Center facility

NOTE: SF, commercial space.

SOURCE: https://trid.trb.org/view/1320811.

Walking and Bicycling Audits, Bellevue, Washington

This approach involves field collection of data to assess walking and bicycling conditions to conduct an unbiased objective examination/evaluation of block by block conditions, with an emphasis on identifying barriers or challenges to these modes of active transportation. These types of area assessment audits are often focused around schools as part of a Safe Routes to School program. Audits can be used to conduct before and after comparisons, assess corridor and network mobility, and identify potential alternatives or optimal solutions. Audits should be conducted by multidisciplinary teams of trained professionals including engineers, planners, and pedestrian/bicycle specialists. A wide number of audit tools, checklists, survey forms, prompt lists, and guidelines are available to conduct data-driven assessments of walking and bicycling conditions (36). Results from these data-intensive audits can be used to empower community leaders, engage decision makers, identify pedestrian–bike savvy solutions to network connectivity issues, influence transportation design, inform long-range planning, and enlist stakeholder advocacy. Feet First spearheaded an effective and comprehensive walking audit of downtown Bellevue, Washington, the results of which served as a catalyst for helping maintain a walkable and livable core including pedestrian paths and complete streets linking residential, commercial, and recreational destinations (37).

Bicycle Boulevards, Portland, Oregon

Bicycle boulevards are low-speed streets that discourage cut-through motor vehicle traffic and optimize mobility for bicycle travel by accommodating through movements for bicycles, and pedestrians, only along extended corridor lengths. Motor vehicle traffic is required to turn onto side streets at strategic intersection locations through use of physical traffic diverters, which include pass-throughs for bicyclists and pedestrians. This corridor approach has been used as a low-cost means to create a connected network of streets supporting comfortable, safe, and efficient active transportation. Implementing bicycle boulevards commonly results in lower speeds, less motor vehicle traffic, comfortable free-flowing bicycle travel, and enhanced livability for surrounding land uses, which are typically residential. The City of Portland, Oregon, adopted the "Portland Bicycle Master Plan" in 1996, leading to expansion of bicycle infrastructure from an initial 190 miles to 630 miles in 20 years. This plan includes 70 miles of completed bicycle boulevards, also referred to as neighborhood greenways. These active transportation policies and programs have resulted in an 8% bicycle mode share for all trips in the Portland area. Future program goals include increasing bicycle mode share from 8% to 25% and expanding residents living within a half mile of a bicycle facility from 25% to 80%. Key bicycle boulevard elements include traffic calming elements, network guide signing, four-way intersection bike sharrow (shared lanes) paving markings, park-like feeling of corridor, complementary stormwater improvements, and enhanced feeling of community. Adoption of uniform planning and design standards played a crucial role in the wide-scale success of bicycle boulevard implementation (38).

Pedestrian-Oriented Development, Greenville, South Carolina

Greenville, South Carolina, is part of an 885,975 population metropolitan statistical area (MSA), with a city limits population of 67,453 in 2016 (39). The city went through a 30-year revitalization of their downtown central business district, which included transforming public rights of way and parks to be more pedestrian friendly. Public–private partnerships were a critically important component of the success of the reinvigoration of this lively downtown area which includes a public park with a signature pedestrian bridge, reconfigured main street (with frequent auto free periods), pedestrian-oriented businesses, public gathering places, signage/wayfinding, public art, new civic attractions, new sports venues, and residential-oriented developments. In addition to the transformation of the downtown area, numerous spin-off active transportation-oriented projects followed, the most significant of which, from a mobility perspective, is the 20.6-mile long Swamp Rabbit multiuse trail extending north to outlying communities, primarily along an abandoned railroad right of way. In year one of opening the trail to the public, trail use greatly exceeded expectations. Furthermore, desirable business and land use transformation occurred along the trail to support trail users and respond to the overwhelming popularity of the facility (Box 18.2).

BOX 18.2

Built environment elements of walkable communities

1. Mixed-use development using human-scale design principles
2. Interconnected transportation multimodal options

(continued)

(continued)

> 3. Unique and identifiable public spaces, with sense of place
> 4. Lower speed complete streets, with context-sensitive design
> 5. Interconnected street grid patterns, with short block size
> 6. Relative close proximity of desirable destinations

Regional Trail System, Raleigh–Durham, North Carolina

A regional trail system can be aligned to serve as the collective spine for a dispersed network of community pedestrian and bicycle facilities. Having local networks that connect to a regional trail system provides a well-configured and interconnected mobility hierarchy of facility classification types, which parallels common mobility infrastructure configuration principles used for many other modes of transportation. In the Raleigh–Durham area of central North Carolina, a regional trail system has been developed and implemented as part of the East Coast Greenway. The local trail extends for a length of 70 miles, connects with numerous other trail systems, and provides an enjoyable way for residents to access parks, downtowns, college campuses, museums, shopping areas, entertainment districts, sporting venues, historic sites, and countless other everyday destinations. This regional trail system includes sections extending along rails-to-trails, natural water course right-of-way buffers, public parks, complete streets, and forested preserve areas. Continuity, along the 70-mile extended length of this extremely popular multiuse path facility, is preserved through numerous grade-separated bridge crossings of busy roadway thoroughfares, including five major interstate highway multiuse path bridges constructed as a result of considerable investment from public transportation funding sources. As a result of the high-order design standards used for this unique facility, the regional trail experiences considerable use with an estimated 22,000,000 miles of biking and walking occurring annually, equating to an estimated total of 3,592,000 hours of PA per year (40). Regional active transportation projects such as this can serve as a catalyst in transforming community mobility values and substantially enhancing desirable health and sustainability outcomes (41).

▨ Limitations of Information on Effectiveness of Urban Physical Activity Interventions

While there is a growing interest in investigating and evaluating aspects of urban PA, it is important to note the evidence base is neither solid nor conclusive. Research in this area is challenging for several reasons. First, much of the research is limited to a cross-sectional study design. While informative, the findings from these studies cannot indicate causality. There is a need for well-designed and rigorous studies or randomized controlled trials, but many of the aspects of interest cannot be experimentally manipulated. One option is to study the urban built environment through "natural experiments." Natural experiments capitalize on events or issues that are planned to occur, allowing researchers to collect baseline data needed to examine the causal connections between the urban environment and PA (42). For example, using the development of a new bus network that included a traffic-free path for pedestrians as the natural experiment, Ogilvie and colleagues were able to determine an increase in the proportion of commuting trips involving active travel from the time before the new network was built (43). The value of these natural experiments is increasing, but complex logistics and funding for such studies remain challenging.

Another issue related to urban PA interventions is the use of different measures and inconsistent definitions. It is difficult to build a body of evidence and compare results across intervention studies when study factors are different. For example, there are differing views of the acceptable distance for measurement of the space between an intervention and residential location. When a new park is built in a city, what is the entire field of the intervention area? Should it be 0.5 mile from the park or 1 mile from the park? Consistent measurement and reporting is needed.

The scalability of urban PA interventions should be considered, too. Developing strategies to increase PA among urban residents with the intention to implement them broadly across similar environments is key to scalability. A good example of this is the Ciclovia initiatives described earlier in this chapter. It started locally in Bogota and now is implemented in many cities around the world. Rigorous process and outcome evaluation information can help facilitate support for enhancing scalability.

Equity is another issue related to strategies to improve PA in urban environments. Improvements and renovations made to urban communities that result in making them more walkable and attractive to new residents also make them less affordable for segments of the population. This concept is called gentrification and can create unequal opportunities for living in better environments. Researchers and practitioners seeking to improve PA in urban environments should consider equity when planning and implementing interventions. Underserved population groups are likely the most at risk for physical inactivity and subsequent poor health outcomes (see Box 18.3). Involving community members and stakeholders can help ensure equitable interventions and outcomes.

■ Summary

People who live in urban environments are generally found to be more physically active than rural residents. Research findings indicate that factors inherent to urban areas such as high population density and characteristics of the built environment such as mixed land use contribute to increased PA. There are several examples of interventions within urban environments, but determining a causal effect is challenging due to measurement issues and moderating factors. Increased application of technology and the use of natural experiments can help build the evidence base for creating urban environments that are supportive of population PA.

BOX 18.3

Cultural Considerations

PA interventions in urban settings need to carefully consider equity throughout planning, implementation, and evaluation. Many urban areas have wide income disparities, and oftentimes, the lowest resource areas and populations within a city are also the ones that would benefit the most from interventions. However, without policies on prioritizing these areas and populations, they get overlooked to the detriment of their health-promoting PA behaviors and result in lasting

(continued)

(continued)

> negative health impact. Having representation from all facets of the community will help ensure broad input and, ultimately, a more equitable intervention.
>
> PA, physical activity.

■ Things to Consider

- ■ Even though there are government definitions of what qualifies as "urban," urban settings can be very unique in population, culture, and infrastructure. Assessing the environment and tailoring interventions is essential to success.

- ■ PA interventions in urban settings need the input from a broad group of stakeholders. Representatives from government, business, urban design, city planning, and transportation are all needed within stakeholder groups.

- ■ There are many examples of successful PA interventions in urban settings. Level of support, local priority, and feasibility are important factors to consider for replicability.

■ References

1. United States Census Bureau. 2010 Census urban and rural classification and urban area criteria. 2010. Available at: https://www.census.gov/geo/reference/ua/urban-rural-2010.html. Accessed January 18, 2018.
2. Ecomonic Research Service. 2010 Rural-Urban Commuting Area (RUCA) codes. 2010. https://www.ers.usda.gov/data-products/rural-urban-commuting-area-codes/documentation/. Accessed January 18, 2018.
3. Texas A & M Transportation Institute Summary tables—congestion levels and trends. 2018. Available at: https://mobility.tamu.edu/ums/national-congestion-tables/. Accessed April 9, 2018.
4. Sallis J, Bull F, Burdett R, et al. Use of science to guide city planning policy and practice: how to achieve healthy and sustainable future cities. *The Lancet*. 2016;388(10062):2936–2947. doi:10.1016/S0140-6736(16)30068-X
5. Federal Highway Administration. *2016 Urban Congestion Trends*. Washington, DC: 2016. Available at: https://ops.fhwa.dot.gov/publications/fhwahop17010/fhwahop17010.pdf
6. Sallis JF, Cerin E, Conway TL, et al. Physical activity in relation to urban environments in 14 cities worldwide: a cross-sectional study. *Lancet*. 2016;387(10034):2207–2217. doi:10.1016/S0140-6736(15)01284-2
7. Bauman A, Reis R, Sallis J, et al. Correlates of physical activity: why are some people physically active and others not? *Lancet*. 2012;380(9838):258–271. doi:10.1016/S0140-6736(12)60735-1
8. Saelens B, Sallis J, Black J, et al. Neighborhood-based differences in physical activity: an environment scale evaluation. *Am J Public Health*. 2003;93(9):1552–1558. doi:10.2105/AJPH.93.9.1552
9. Transportation Research Board Modal Characteristics. *Highway Capacity Manual*. Washington, DC: The National Academies of Science, Engineering, Medicine; 2016:1–38.
10. Celis-Morales C, Lyall D, Welsh P, et al. Association between active commuting and incident cardiovascular disease, cancer, and mortality: prospective cohort study. *BMJ*. 2017;357:j1456. doi:10.1136/bmj.j1456
11. Dill J. Bicycling for transportation and health: the role of infrastructure. *J Public Health Policy*. 2009;30(1):S95–S110. doi:10.1057/jphp.2008.56
12. McCabe K, Schoneman K, Arcaya M. *Community Speed Reducation and Public Health: A Technical Report*. Boston, MA; 2013. Health Resources in Action and Metroploitan Area Planning Council;.

13. Institute of Transportation Engineers. Traffic Calming Fact Sheets: Chicane. 2018. Available at: https://www.ite.org/pub/?id=29df6928%2D0059%2D96b7%2Dcfb7%2Dc79b3585a17d. Accessed April 25, 2018.
14. United States Department of Transportation. Land use mix. 2016. Available at: https://www.transportation.gov/mission/health/land-use-mix. Accessed Febuary 8, 2018.
15. Khattak A, Rodriguez D. Travel behavior in neo-traditional neighborhood developments: a case study in USA. *Transp Res Part A*. 2005;39(6):481–500. doi:10.1016/j.tra.2005.02.009
16. World Health Organization. Health and sustainable development: urban green spaces. 2012. Available at: http://www.who.int/sustainable-development/cities/health-risks/urban-green-space/en/. Accessed Febuary 9, 2018.
17. Krizek K, El-Geneidy A, Thompson K. A detailed analysis of how an urban trail system affects cyclists' travel. *Transportation*. 2007;34(5):611–624. doi:10.1007/s11116-007-9130-z
18. McCormack G, Shiell A. search of causality: a systematic review of the relationship between the built environment and physical activity among adults. *Intl J Behav Nutr Phys Act*. 2011;8:125. doi:10.1186/1479-5868-8-125
19. Carlson S, Paul P, Kumar G, et al. Prevalence of complete streets policies in U.S. municipalities. *J Transp Health*. 2017;5:142–150. doi:10.1016/j.jth.2016.11.003
20. Li H. Study on green transportation system of international metropolises. *Procedia Eng*. 2016;137:762–771. doi:10.1016/j.proeng.2016.01.314
21. Durand C, Tang X, Gabriel K, et al. The association of trip distance with walking to reach public transit: data from the California household travel survey. *J Transp Health*. 2016;3(2):154–160. doi:10.1016/j.jth.2015.08.007
22. Morency C, Trépanier M, Demers M. Walking to transit: an unexpected source of physical activity. *Transp Policy*. 2011;18(6):800–806. doi:10.1016/j.tranpol.2011.03.010
23. Centers for Disease Control and Prevention Healthy places: health impact assessment. 2016. Available at: https://www.cdc.gov/healthyplaces/hia.htm. Accessed April 27, 2018.
24. Community Preventive Services Taskforce. Physical activity: built environment approaches combining transportation system interventions with land use and environmental design. 2016. Available at: https://www.thecommunityguide.org/findings/physical-activity-built-environment-approaches. Accessed May 1, 2018.
25. Sarmiento O, Torres A, Jacoby E, et al. The ciclovia-recreativa: a mass-recreational program with public health potential. *J Phys Act Health*. 2010;7(suppl 2):S163–180.
26. Torres A, Sarmiento OL, Stauber C, et al. The Ciclovia and Cicloruta programs: promising interventions to promote physical activity and social capital in Bogota, Colombia. *Am J Public Health*. 2013;103(2):e23–30. doi:10.2105/AJPH.2012.301142
27. Montes F, Sarmiento OL, Zarama R, et al. Do health benefits outweigh the costs of mass recreational programs? An economic analysis of four Ciclovia programs. *J Urban Health*. 2012;89(1):153–170. doi:10.1007/s11524-011-9628-8
28. Open Streets Project. About open streets. 2018. Available at: Available at: http://openstreetsproject.org/about-open-streets/. Accessed Febuary 18, 2018.
29. Greater Greater Washington. All 119 U.S. bikeshare systems, ranked by size. 2017. https://ggwash.org/view/62137/all-119-us-bikeshare-systems-ranked-by-size. Accessed Nov 11, 2018.
30. Fishman E, Washington S, Haworth N. Bike share: a synthesis of the literature. *Trans Rev*. 2013;33(2):148–165. doi:10.1080/01441647.2013.775612
31. Cushing A, Cowan B. Walk1916: exploring how a mobile walking tour app can provide value for LAMs. *Proc Assoc Inf Sci Technol*. 2016;53(1):1–5. doi:10.1002/pra2.2016.14505301147
32. United States Census Bureau. Quick facts: New York City, New York. 2016. Available at: https://www.census.gov/quickfacts/fact/table/newyorkcitynewyork/PST045216. Accessed April 27, 2018.
33. Lee K. Developing and implementing the active design guidelines in New York City. *Health Place*. 2012;18(1):5–7. doi:10.1016/j.healthplace.2011.09.009
34. Regional Transportation District. Fastracks facts and figures. 2017. Available at: http://www.rtd-denver.com/factsAndFigures.shtml. Accessed April 27, 2018.

35. Ratner K, Goetz A. The reshaping of land use and urban form in Denver through transit-oriented development. *Cities*. 2013;30:31–46. doi:10.1016/j.cities.2012.08.007
36. Center PaBI. Audits. 2016. Available at: http://www.pedbikeinfo.org/planning/tools_audits.cfm. Accessed April 27, 2018.
37. Feet First. *Downtown Bellevue Walking Audit Report*. Seattle, WA: Feet First. Available at: http://feetfirst.org/wp-content/uploads/2013/02/Bellevue_2012.pdf. January, 2012. Accessed February 20, 2018.
38. Walker L, Tresidder M, Birk M. Fundamentals of Bicycle Boulevard Planning and Design. 2009. Available at: https://www.pdx.edu/sites/www.pdx.edu.syndication/files/BicycleBoulevardGuidebook.pdf. Accessed November 16, 2018.
39. Greenville Area Development Corporation. Demographics. 2017. Available at: http://www.greenvilleeconomicdevelopment.com/demographics.php. Accessed Febuary 20, 2018.
40. Alta Planning and Design. *The Impact of Greenways in the Triangle*. Kirkwood, MO; 2017.
41. Rails to Trails Conservancy. Benefits of trails. 2018. Available at: https://www.railstotrails.org/experience-trails/benefits-of-trails/. Accessed April 27, 2018.
42. Craig P, Katikireddi SV, Leyland A, et al. Natural experiments: an overview of methods, approaches, and contributions to public health intervention research. *Annu Rev Public Health*. 2017;38:39–56. doi:10.1146/annurev-publhealth-031816-044327
43. Ogilvie D, Griffin S, Jones A, et al. Commuting and health in Cambridge: a study of a 'natural experiment' in the provision of new transport infrastructure. *BMC Public Health*. 2010;10(1):703. doi:10.1186/1471-2458-10-703

PHYSICAL ACTIVITY IN RURAL POPULATIONS

M. RENÉE UMSTATTD MEYER | MICHAEL B. EDWARDS |
LINDSAY ELLIOTT JORGENSON | JUSTIN B. MOORE

LEARNING OBJECTIVES

By the end of this chapter, the student should be able to

1. Define the term *rural* as it relates to opportunities for physical activity (PA).
2. Describe social and physical environmental characteristics of rural communities that are supportive or prohibitive of PA interventions.
3. Describe challenges to the design of policies to promote PA in rural communities.
4. Explain the role of schools and school facilities in promotion of PA in rural communities.
5. Describe the role and importance of multisectoral partnerships to the design and implementation of PA interventions in rural communities.

■ Introduction

The country, remote, countryside, land, space outside of town, away from a city, not urban, not metro, not a big city, small towns, villages, one stop light, agricultural areas, farms, hills, mountains, hollers, nature, natural settings, ranches, woods, backwoods, fields, prairies, deserts, plains, villages, fewer people, no people, quiet, isolated, frontier, a lot of space, the boonies, boondocks, the bush, backwaters, the sticks, dirt road country, middle of nowhere, "If you blink, you'll miss it" . . .

All of these words have been used to describe what a rural area is, and we are certain that if you grew up in "the country" or have visited a rural place that you can add a few of your own words to this list. Given the variety of terms listed earlier as examples for how people in everyday conversations convey what rural is, it should be of no surprise that there are also vast differences in how rural is officially defined and described as is

© Springer Publishing Company DOI: 10.1891/9780826134592.0019

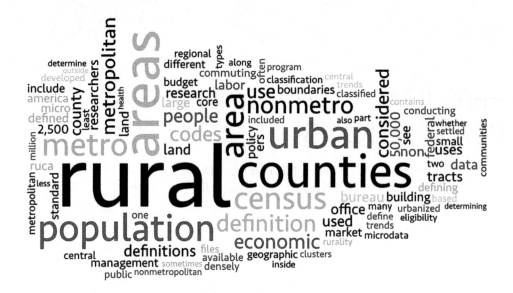

FIGURE 19.1 Word cloud using federal language to describe rural.

demonstrated visually in the word cloud shown in Figure 19.1 displaying current federal language used to describe or define rural (1–3), highlighting that rural is often identified or described "as what is not urban—that is, after defining individual urban areas, rural is what is left" (3).

Similar to race, some contend that "rural" is a socially constructed concept; however, also like race, having a definition of "rural" is useful in fields associated with public health and physical activity (PA) (4). In literature incorporating or focused on rural America, authors will describe a study setting as "rural," but will often provide no or limited information regarding the rural designation. Other definitions of rural range from "not being urban," low population, or low population density (5). Researchers also often use various governmental agency designations as a proxy for rural. These designations range from the U.S. Office of Management and Budget (non-metropolitan < 10,000 county population) or the U.S. Census Bureau (non-metropolitan areas < 50,000 county population) approach of county classifications to more continuum-based definitions out of the U.S. Department of Agriculture (e.g., Rural-Urban Commuting Area [RUCA] codes, Rural-Urban Continuum Codes [RUCC]) or the U.S. Department of Education's Common Core Data (1, 2). These continuum-based definitions consider both population size and density, in addition to adjacency to urban areas (5). Please see the map shown in Figure 19.2 detailing rurality in the United States based on one of these continuum-based code sets, the RUCC (1).

Discussions where rural is described as contrasted to urban or metro areas (e.g., nonmetro/nonurban) can leave us with an image of rural as a small town or small city—for example, rural is like a big city, but smaller in scale. While there are small towns within many rural areas in the United States, which can function both similarly to and differently than large cities, these "towns" only make up a small portion of the geographical space identified as rural. This is important to note as the majority of rural areas have even greater dispersion and sprawl than town centers or main streets located within rural areas or counties, as is evidenced in agricultural communities built around farming or ranching with miles between residences. This example highlights

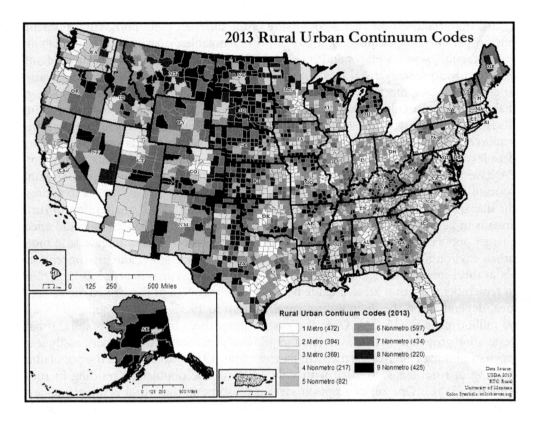

FIGURE 19.2 A U.S. map of RUCC.
RUCC, Rural-Urban Continuum Codes.

how heterogeneous rural communities are, which can be lost when rural is framed as the opposite of urban, suggesting that rural is more homogenous than it is. It is also important to note that most designations of rurality are made at a county level, even though there is often great variability in rurality even within a county, as is demonstrated when considering that the Grand Canyon is located in an "urban" or metropolitan designated county (2, 6). We present the complexity in describing and defining rural as it is relevant when it comes to various federal funding lines, and also to help you better understand how much variation there is not only in defining rural, but also how much variation there is between and among various rural areas in the United States (e.g., rural Maine as compared to rural North Carolina or rural Arizona).

BOX 19.1

Defining Rural

Defining rural is complex, with no clearly agreed upon definition. Rural can be a small town with a main street core or a dispersed expanse of farmland. Organizations use multiple different definitions to designate rural areas of the country and each of these has limitations.

It is important to note that across many of the different definitions, rural residents often experience intense poverty and demonstrate notable disparities in the availability and accessibility to PA places and resources when compared to more urban residents. Perhaps unsurprisingly, rural residents also face great health disparities when it comes to chronic disease mortality and morbidity rates related with physical inactivity (e.g., diabetes, cardiovascular disease, obesity, cancer) (7–13), in addition to experiencing disparities in access to preventative care and treatment, as there are simply fewer resources in rural communities (5, 13, 14). Yet, most of the efforts over the past few decades researching ways to improve physical and social environments to promote PA have focused in urban areas. Considering these disparities, you might be asking yourself the question, "Why haven't we focused more efforts and resources to address the disparities seen in rural communities here in the U.S.?" Lack of attention to rural areas is in part due to perception of impact, given changes in urban areas would affect a larger population; convenience, since it is easier to research and/or intervene in more urban environments given proximity to most research universities; and misconceptions about rural environments, many of which are highlighted in this chapter. It is important to remember that rural areas include between 72% and 97% of the United States' land area, depending on the definition of rural, and up to 19.3% of the population (about 60 million people) (15, 16). Over the past century, there has been substantial urban population growth as well as associated migration from rural to urban areas, easily seen when examining American settlement patterns from 1910 with 54.4% of the population residing in rural areas, to 2010 with only 19.3% of the population residing in rural America (3, 16). One misconception viewed by some is that rural residents achieve sufficient PA through their occupations under the perception that all rural occupations require physical labor (e.g., agriculture, forestry, mining . . .). While it is true that the majority of the agricultural and many other labor-intensive industries occur in rural areas, there are two characteristics that need to be considered: the increase in machine labor in these industries (vs. human physical labor), and recent trends demonstrating that the largest rural industry growth for decades is in retail and service (17).

As you have seen in this text, Sallis and colleagues' ecological model of PA can be used to examine various environments or settings that influence and/or are related with PA in all types of areas, including rural communities (18). Sallis suggests that there are crosscutting environments—information, social-cultural, natural, and policy—that each simultaneously influences someone's PA, which occurs in and is influenced by four domains: active transport, active recreation, household activities, and occupational activities. PA within each of these domains is influenced by interactions between the individual, intrapersonal factors, perceived and physical environments, and PA behavior itself. While this framework provides a useful tool in understanding PA from multiple points of influence, we should remain mindful when applying these concepts in rural communities, since it also was designed and fashioned from an urban perspective. This is apparent when observing how open/natural spaces are viewed within the active living ecological framework. While open and natural spaces are amenities and strengths within many rural communities (e.g., there are woods, fields, or other open spaces to play in), these characteristics are often viewed as barriers within the ecological framework, since there are fewer "built structures" or "planned" walking areas. Given its utility and universality, we focus this chapter on identifying unique characteristics, strengths, and challenges of PA within rural areas using the crosscutting environments and settings identified within the active living ecological model; however, the focus is only on the portions of this model that need special consideration in rural areas. While we acknowledge that all of the components of the active living ecological framework are important, not all require special consideration in a rural context (18).

■ Current Issues in Rural PA From an Active Living Ecological Lens

Characteristics of rural areas call for special consideration in multiple areas of the active living ecological model, including the social-cultural, natural, and policy environments and active transport, recreation, and school settings and domains. While the information environment and household and workplace environments remain critically important for PA of rural residents, specifically considering the lack of infrastructure and opportunities in many rural areas, evidence does not suggest rurality as a moderator of these relationships. Evidence-based approaches in workplaces, home environments, and the information environment should be more heavily considered in intervention design since these spaces are available for most rural residents.

Social-Cultural Environment

Rural communities have experienced a drastic shift in the past 100 years, with employment changes from agriculture to industry, and from small-scale family farming to large-scale corporate agriculture (19). Additionally, globalization has led to a reduced dependence on rural America as much of the world's primary source of agricultural products and many manufactured goods (19). With this economic change, most of the U.S. population has shifted to urban areas in search of sustainable employment, leaving those in rural areas behind with a very different social fabric from previous generations. For many rural residents, the transformation of rural life over the past two decades, and the accompanying shifts in social and cultural institutions, has been perceived in almost traumatic terms (20). In addition, the movement to labor-intensive crops has brought an influx of immigrant and migrant workers to rural areas (21). Thus, individuals working in rural areas to promote PA often encounter a much different and complex social and cultural environment than expected. This environment, particularly in the context of social and cultural changes, presents a unique set of challenges and opportunities.

Race, Ethnicity, and Culture

As in urban and suburban areas, the demographics of rural areas should be considered when selecting strategies for PA promotion. It has been previously shown that racial composition is associated with resource allocation in the rural South. Rural areas in this region that are predominantly White often have greater natural and built supports for PA (22, 23). Additionally, historical segregation of rural communities continues to influence residential patterns and perceptions of access to recreational spaces within communities (24). Previous research also suggests that American Indian, Black, Hispanic, and White park users have different preferences and uses for shared recreational resources (e.g., in comparison to other groups, Hispanic users are more likely to visit parks in large family groups and use picnic shelters) (25, 26). In light of these considerations, interventionists working in diverse rural areas should be especially aware and mindful when locating or allocating limited resources to promote PA areas across the community and not overlook preferences of micro-populations potentially residing in the community.

Crime and Safety

As in urban areas, crime and safety are concerns of rural residents, although they may manifest in different ways around different threats. For example, traffic is often reported as a concern in urban areas due to the density of traffic networks or speed at which traffic travels (27, 28). Conversely, rural residents often cite traffic as a concern, but it may be related to the presence of trucks or other large vehicles, which is compounded by the lack of bike lanes, sidewalks, or even shoulders along roads (29). Similarly, crime can be a concern in both urban and rural areas. However, rural residents may be more worried about isolation and loose animals such as dogs as risk factors than urban residents, which should be considered when designing interventions.

Social Support

Social support is also a concept that should be carefully considered in rural areas. While many rural residents report strong social connections, their lack of proximity to their friends and neighbors can present a challenge when trying to mobilize their social networks to promote PA. As such, it is important to assess the type and function of social support among rural residents. For example, social support can come from peers, family, partners/spouses, or church family, among other sources (30). This support can take many forms such as informational, logistic, companionship, and/or emotional (31). For rural residents, it has been shown that logistic support can be especially important in youth who may lack transportation or other resources to be physically active (32). Similarly, companionship support might be important in overcoming concerns about crime or isolation for adults who would like to start a walking program.

Natural Environments

Traditionally, natural environments are less often considered than built environments in the design of PA interventions. For urban-focused interventions, this approach makes sense as access to natural spaces and settings are typically lower in cities. The efficacy of developing supportive built environments would expectedly be more appropriate in urban settings. In fact, when natural environments are considered in urban contexts, they are often presented as elements that create a barrier to PA (e.g., hilly terrain or extreme weather) (22, 33). Examining natural environments solely from this perspective, natural barriers to PA, especially extreme climate and weather, may be more significant in rural areas, where indoor spaces for PA are less available than in urban areas (34). However, what should also be examined is how proximate natural environments in rural areas may also be an asset in designing interventions to promote PA in these communities.

BOX 19.2

Many rural areas have natural environments nearby, which may be important starting places when designing interventions to promote PA for rural residents. Natural environments can lend themselves to low-cost strategies for PA (e.g., mowing out a pathway underneath an electric line). Researchers need to explore how this unique asset can be better utilized in rural communities.

While less explored than built environments, research suggests that the proximity of natural environments may be associated with higher levels of PA in rural settings (33, 35). An Australian study suggested that local natural environments (e.g., forests, meadows, or farmland) provided opportunities to develop walking paths and mountain bike trails that facilitated active transportation and recreation in a rural community (36). Similarly, in the United States, utilitarian walking in rural communities has been shown to be positively associated with the availability of natural areas in which to walk, as well as the presence of suitable destinations, such as a post office (37).

Despite their promise in potentially promoting PA, there are some unique barriers associated with natural environments in rural areas that must be considered. A lack of structured interventions (e.g., walking groups or similar social activities) may be more likely to inhibit use of natural environments for PA than similar resources in urban areas (36). Additionally, rural residents have identified issues with loose dogs, use of all-terrain vehicles, potential for criminal behavior, and general fear of vacant land and undeveloped natural areas as barriers to feeling secure in using natural environments for PA (34, 38).

Thus, important to maximizing the potential of natural environments to facilitate PA is to develop conditions that are attractive to visitors, reduce fears of the outdoors, and promote social activities (39). For example, regularly thinning forests, providing marked trails and visible directional signage, can help people maintain their bearings and feel safer in natural areas. Additionally, rather than solely promoting traditional PA interventions, developing interventions that utilize the natural environments (e.g., obstacle races, geocaching clubs, or environmental education interventions) may have potential to further promote PA in rural areas (40).

Policy Environment

Very little is known about rural-specific policies to support PA, and much of the policy research has been conducted in urban areas or considered urban and rural areas concurrently. As such, most of what is known about policy adoption and effectiveness has limited applicability in rural areas (41). Policy approaches can also face financial barriers in rural areas, due to lack of capital for large-scale interventions or lack of capacity to leverage the political system or compete for external funding.

Additionally, some evidence exists to suggest that rural organizations such as health departments are less likely to take policy approaches (42), or that unique barriers exist when trying to adopt or implement them (43). For example, rural residents are often perceived as resistant to government mandates, taxes, or incentives (44). Despite these challenges, evidence exists that these might be overcome through nontraditional partnerships (45) or regional partnerships that allow for the pooling of resources (46). For example, the Appalachian Diabetes Control and Translation Project has experienced success in pooling resources and seeking funding in a collaborative manner (see the following Box).

BOX 19.3

The Appalachian Diabetes Control and Translation Project

The Appalachian Diabetes Control and Translation Project is working in 78 distressed Appalachian counties to reduce the impact of diabetes through promotion of PA and healthy eating. In one initiative launched in 2014, the Appalachian Diabetes Control and Translation Project began to offer minigrants to support dissemination and implementation efforts for the National Diabetes Prevention Program. By awarding $2,000 minigrants to coalitions marketing and recruiting to the program, more than 132 participants have enrolled in evidence-based, diabetes prevention programs (as of December 2015). For more information, see www.cdc.gov/diabetes/programs/appalachian.html.

In addition to barriers to policy development, adoption, and implementation, an additional challenge faced is the incongruence with urban-developed policies and rural realities. For example, Complete Streets legislation may not be applicable in rural areas due to the lack of incorporated areas for their application. Similarly, while interventions such as Safe Routes to School have been effective in rural areas, they have been less effective in rural areas where drop zones need to be created to have places to safely walk to school. As such, policy efforts in rural areas have limited reach and tend to be restrained to strategies shown effective in urban areas, such as Comprehensive School PA Programs implemented in schools. While these types of strategies can be effective, they do not address unique challenges for rural residents.

Transportation Settings

Active transport is usually described as someone getting from point A to point B in a physically active way (e.g., walking to school or a store, riding a bike to work) (47). Many rural areas lack some or all of the environmental characteristics and/or features that have been identified in the literature as supportive for active transport. For instance, people live further apart from one another in rural areas and further from most destinations within rural communities, requiring people to travel greater distances and making active transport a more significant time commitment for rural residents. In addition, there are often fewer developed open spaces (trails, parks); intersection density and segment density (how close intersections and street segments are to other intersections and street segments) are less developed; public transit is often limited if present at all; rural roads are designed to support higher speed traffic and seldom provide bike lanes, shoulders, footpaths, or sidewalks; and parking is plentiful in most rural areas (48). Some evidence also suggests that "active transportation" means something different in rural communities that have greater geographic dispersion, where active transportation often means availability of transportation to get to and from a PA place (5). This is seen both in terms of transportation to and/or from schools, which can be used for their physical space and for out-of-school PA interventions, and also to other destinations for PA, including natural resources.

Despite the challenges to how active transport is traditionally framed using an urban lens, residents in some rural areas do achieve higher active transportation rates than suburban areas and current evidence examining these characteristics as they relate to active transport are mixed. For example, recent work in rural Georgia suggests that sidewalks and utilitarian destinations might not be as important for walkability and active transport in rural areas, proposing the importance of safe streets to walk in or next to with less formal infrastructure required (49, 50). This work has also highlighted a different potential facilitator to walking in rural areas, where walking for travel or transport purposes is not as important, or possibly feasible. In rural areas, walking to support social interactions should be considered, which can be fostered through walkable communities and neighborhoods (50) and potentially interventions that build upon social interactions (e.g., walking groups). Creating more walkable rural communities must be combined with, or folded into, small town planning; involve local decision makers and town administrators; and often requires creative solutions. For example, in some rural communities walking groups meet and walk inside big box stores (e.g., Walmart, in parking lots, or at other available indoor or outdoor spaces.

BOX 19.4

Creative Solutions: Creating a Pop-up Bike Lane

The town of Whitefish, Montana, used traffic cones to create a "pop-up" style bicycle lane in conjunction with a "bike to school" day to support active transportation during this event, and while this was not a permanent solution it provided a creative solution and the infrastructure necessary for children to participate in this event (51).

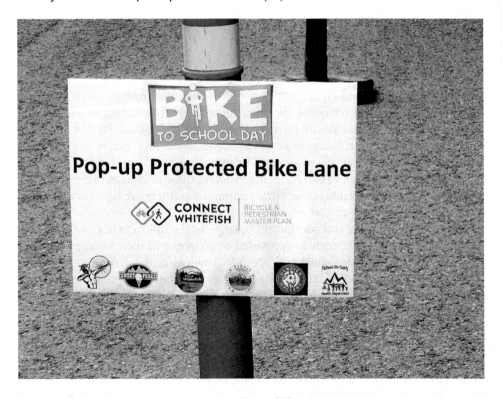

(*continued*)

(continued)

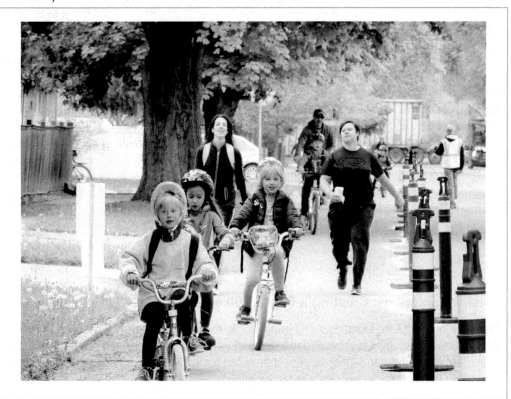

Recreation Settings

Recreation settings in rural communities are often different from those in more urban areas. For example, rural residents are often more likely than urban residents to have access to larger yards that could provide settings for individual PA (34). Generally, residents of rural communities have access to adequate outdoor spaces (e.g., parks) and even informal open natural spaces where PA can occur (29, 48), and are often willing to drive greater distances than urban residents to access these resources (52, 53). However, despite these potential advantages for rural communities, there are significant challenges to providing suitable recreational opportunities.

Interestingly, for many rural communities, large local employers (e.g., manufacturing or extraction companies) historically provided employees and their families with spaces and sponsored programs for sport and PA (54). The loss of these companies has often left a void in the provision of recreational settings and the rural public sector is often more likely to have constrained budgets and a lack of political will to fully replace these opportunities (55). While parks might be available, rural residents often perceive them as neglected and uninviting—providing outdated and poorly maintained equipment and amenities (38, 55). Rural residents also perceive a lack of safe places to walk (38). Additionally, rural communities often have few indoor spaces for PA (34) and structured PA interventions (55). Indoor recreational spaces and structured interventions that are available are often inaccessible to many residents. On one hand, the small number of private settings (e.g., dance studios or health clubs) may be cost prohibitive to low-income residents. On the other hand, public indoor settings (e.g., school gymnasiums) may be closed to nonstudent access without personal connections with facility managers (55). Additionally, public interventions (e.g., recreational sport programs) may have limited availability or sustainability due to a lack of volunteers or create transportation barriers for families who are unable to drive to practices or classes (56).

Despite the challenges to providing supportive recreational settings in rural communities, there are some opportunities that may help inform more successful interventions. There is potential for interventions focused on enhancing existing facilities and equipment in rural areas, rather than developing new parks and facilities, to be successful (41, 55). The development of trails may also provide a cost-effective means to promote walking in rural communities and can incorporate existing environments typical to these areas (52, 57). For example, Rails-to-Trails Conservancy has successfully developed many trails from abandoned rail beds that are abundant in rural areas (58). Additionally, Kids in Parks (part of the Blue Ridge Parkway Foundation) has created 160 trails in small towns and rural areas in 10 states designed to make natural environments more accessible to children and families (59). Multisectorial partnerships may also be important for building community capacity and leveraging limited resources to provide access to PA resources, including indoor spaces and PA interventions (56). Developing networks that include both governmental (e.g., parks and recreation agencies, schools, or housing authorities) and nongovernmental (e.g., faith communities, nonprofits, and health centers) have demonstrated unique successes in supporting PA interventions in rural communities. For example, many rural churches have gymnasiums that are open to the public and provide fitness classes for church members. The development of shared-use agreements for the use of recreational spaces and promotion of recreational programs and classes, especially with faith communities, may be a unique opportunity for rural communities (60).

BOX 19.5

Case Study: Creative Solutions Through Multisectorial Partnerships: How the Community of Princeville, North Carolina, Is Coming Together to Advocate for a Greenway

Princeville, North Carolina, was the first U.S. municipality incorporated by freed African American slaves. The 2,000 people that call Princeville "home" share a common identity that is steeped in American history, racism, adversity, and resilience. In addition to this, Princeville was settled on low-lying land in the Tar River floodplain, meaning the town has faced significant trauma from natural disasters.

In 1999, Hurricane Floyd left Princeville 23 feet underneath water that had risen to the town's stop lights. The devastation of the flooding displaced many residents for years, and some indefinitely. The town slowly rebuilt over the following 17 years until 2016, when significant flooding from Hurricane Matthew once again left the town underwater. Today, in 2018, most of the 450 homes that were damaged are still marked with red "X's" on their front doors (61). Many Princeville residents reside in nearby hotels and few have been provided with clear guidelines for how to rebuild their homes. The town's school is still closed, and the town's only community center just reopened. The historic markers of hope and freedom—historic churches and homes—are stained with remnants of water damage.

(continued)

(continued)

What most people would see as a grim landscape, the people of Princeville have seen as opportunity. In 2017, groups of residents known as the Freedom Hill Fighters began working with the town's elected officials, community members, and North Carolina State University's College of Design to hold a community charrette to discuss topics of recovery and regeneration. Many of the redevelopment ideas focused on rebuilding the town around social interaction with ultimate goals of promoting community health and well-being, history and heritage, and overall quality of life (61).

While efforts are still underway, NC State Architecture and Design faculty have worked with residents to develop plans around a well-designed greenway along a 500-year floodplain that can prevent flooding while following the tracks of slavery walked by Princeville's founders. This walking path would highlight the town's history while providing a much-needed amenity for community residents.

While PA would certainly be an outcome for this project, should it move forward, efforts for a greenway have not come from the simple need for recreation or PA. Rather, the greenway efforts represent a long and windy process of bright and passionate people. It shows the importance of collaboration, not only within a community, but across the urban–rural divides. Whether or not you are working in a rural area, you can affect change within rural spaces.

Princeville residents are turning oppressive human-led systems and natural disasters to tell stories of resilience and hope, and their vision represents the apex of creative problem solving that can occur in rural places when groups work together for common good.

School Settings

Schools act as anchor institutions within their communities. This is especially true in rural settings, where schools serve a multitude of functions that extend beyond the education of children and youth. In rural America, schools are often the center of their community's social, cultural, and civic life (62). They link community members to performing arts, adult learning, sports events, and other community activities, and in doing so, they help facilitate and maintain a community's sense of place and identity (63). Rural schools are therefore uniquely trusted by the community members they serve.

Use of School Facilities

Rural schools are positioned to meet a wide array of community needs because of their facilities. Schools have libraries, cafeterias, theaters, playgrounds, athletic fields, and gyms—assets that are otherwise unavailable or unmaintained under the stressed economic climate of many rural municipalities. School playgrounds, athletic fields, and gyms are particularly important facilities that can be leveraged for PA through formal or informal shared-use "agreements" between two or more organizations. While shared use is a promising avenue for rural health promotion, it is underutilized. A 2014 survey of 1,182 North Carolina school principals showed that only 67% of principals reported opening their school's gym for public use, 33% opened their school's baseball/softball field, 18% opened their school's playground, and 16% opened their school's track for public use (64). The most commonly reported reason why a school without shared use did not open their facilities to the public was "no one has asked" (64). In the field, liability is often voiced as the main concern that prevents schools from opening their facilities to the public. Given the ubiquity of schools across rural America, public health advocates entering the rural landscape should partner with schools to establish and implement shared-use agreements that meet the community's PA needs.

Rural Schools and PA

In addition to promoting community PA, schools also play the well-known role of promoting, or hindering, child and youth PA. Rural schools are crucial in this role because their youth are more likely to be obese than their urban and suburban counterparts (65).

There are two primary avenues for youth to engage in school-sponsored PA: physical education and extracurricular activities (66). Physical education curriculum is legislated at the state level and implemented with slight (or sizable) variance based on a school's interpretation. While there is not currently a clear understanding of whether these standards are implemented differently across the urban–rural continuum, it is important to note that rural youth are less likely to walk or ride their bicycle to school, increasing their need for PA within the school day (67).

Even more than physical education, extracurricular PA—primarily school-sponsored sports—differs unmethodically across rural communities. Some rural schools offer an array of competitive sports while some have just two. Others, typically in more underserved areas, are forced to end certain sports programs because not enough youth have basic knowledge of the sport, equipment, or transportation to practices/games. Regardless of the disparities, the main point is this: in rural communities, school sports may be the only youth sports program in the area—club sports simply may not exist. If a school does not have soccer, then there is no soccer in that community. If they do have soccer, the program will likely accommodate a wide range of skill levels.

Public health practitioners should take special consideration of equity within the context of school sports. Ethnic/racial minority children, or those from resource-limited families, have fewer opportunities to engage in school-sponsored sports (68–70). Rural America is ethnographically changing. There were 55% more minority youth enrolled in rural schools in 2004 than there were 10 years prior, and minority youth now represent 23% of all rural students (71). This shift in diversity offers an exciting opportunity for schools, public health practitioners, and other health advocates to find creative ways to accommodate the sports needs of their youth.

School Siting

School siting refers to a school's location within its community. The term is often used in the planning of a new school or the consolidation of existing schools. Because of rural depopulation, the consolidation of two existing schools is a common approach used by local county governments to preserve resources. While the approach may save resources (though this is quite debatable), consolidation puts schools further from the students they serve, making it more difficult for students to walk or bike to school (72–74). It also compromises participation in after-school PA, as youth spend significantly more time on busses to travel cross county for school. An example is Northampton County, North Carolina. In 2012, a 6-1 decision was made to consolidate two high schools that served a 551-square feet county where some students now sit on the bus up to 4 hours each day (75). Efforts to keep schools close to students, especially in rural areas, are needed. School siting debates can allow public health advocates to work across sectors with local county governments, planners, and school administrators to advocate for PA in school siting decision making.

The education sector, while traditionally overlooked as a key public health partner, is trusted in the community and positioned to affect change within a variety of settings that influence childhood and adult health. Public health practitioners are equipped with the skills, knowledge, and resources needed to support rural schools' role in promoting healthier communities.

BOX 19.6

Case Study: Drop-In Soccer and Small-Town Kansas: How an English Teacher Grew a Multiethnic Program

Goodland, Kansas, is a frontier town located 15 miles east of the Colorado border. The town is home to 4,480 residents, 83% of whom identify as "White alone" and 13% as "Hispanic/Latino" (76). One-fifth of Goodland residents live at or below the federal poverty level (76).

Goodland has one business corridor, Main Street, with historic brick buildings that sit along both sides of its eight-block stretch. Main Street itself is brick, adding an element of small-town charm. Goodland has a library, a Walmart, a technical college, a regional medical center, and a small selection of Mexican, Chinese, and American-style restaurants. All of this is surrounded by a vast expanse of farmland. Goodland has three schools—an elementary, middle, and high school. Goodland High School is classified as a Title 1 school; 15% of students identify as Hispanic/Latino and 32% qualify for free or reduced lunch (77).

While Goodland High School offered a wide range of athletics in 2015—golf, track and field, baseball, basketball, wrestling, and football—it did not offer soccer, the sport of interest to most Hispanic/Latino students. That was partially because few schools in Western Kansas offered soccer, so Goodland High School would have been required to travel long distances for games. Noticing this gap in access, in 2015 one of the high school's English teachers, himself a soccer player, started a drop-in soccer program through an informal shared-use agreement.

The program was granted permission by the principal and started within the first month of school at a nearby community park. The program was well-supported by the school and its Board of Directors, one of whom brought water to the games. By November, the weekly drop-in games were attended by an average of 15 to 20 players, including students as well as community members of various racial/ethnic and socioeconomic backgrounds. But with November came cold weather, and the town's $5 per visit indoor community gym was inaccessible for many players. Thus, the teacher approached the Superintendent for permission to move the drop-in games to the school's gymnasium after school hours. The Superintendent agreed, despite fears that the soccer ball would damage the scoreboards. The teacher was given permission to use the school's gym under the condition that a foam ball would be used. Games ensued, and then a normal soccer ball started being used (after some convincing). No written shared-use agreement was in place for this program, making it an informal "handshake" agreement.

The program ran for 1.5 years until it was ended by the school's administration after an altercation broke out between community members during a basketball open-use gym practice (after the soccer program started, a different teacher started open-use basketball for the community). None of the soccer players were present during the altercation.

Even while it was short lived, the program was successful in several regards. It provided youth who were not otherwise reached by the school's athletic program an opportunity to participate in a structured and supervised sport. This was important given that Hispanic/Latino youth, who

(continued)

(continued)

were the majority of the student soccer players, experience greater health risk factors and are less likely to participate in school-sponsored sports (78–80). According to the teacher, students were also more engaged in their English education and some expressed their first interest in pursuing college through collegiate soccer. Paradoxically, transportation was not a barrier to participation. Most White youth were driven by parents, while Hispanic/Latino youth carpooled with one another or community members. The program also accommodated a wide range of skill levels and it did not require a financial commitment or weekly attendance from students or their parents. The program integrated students and community members, allowing students who lived on the outskirts of town an opportunity to engage in interactive ways with others in their community. And lastly, the program positioned the school to engage community members' recreational interests.

Operating the program was challenging. Because there was not a formal agreement established with terms of use, soccer was second to other school-sponsored sports. As such, scheduling for gym time was challenging and inconsistent—several weeks might pass when no evenings were available for soccer. And, because there was no written agreement, the league eventually ended when liability concerns rose.

What Are the Lessons Learned?

Shared use should be more widely disseminated. It is for the rural school of 200 youth as much as the urban school of 2,000. Informal "handshake" agreements, while they have a purpose and place, can make valuable programs more vulnerable. Had the teacher been equipped with shared-use tools and knowledge, he may have had the resources needed to formalize the program and delay or prevent its eventual end.

Liability will always be a concern. Public health practitioners should know the ins and outs of liability when working in the realm of shared use. For private landowners, states have recreational land use statutes that protect landowners from liability when their land is open for recreational purposes. Schools are also protected under Sovereign Immunity or Governmental Immunity. While formal shared-use agreements can be written with terms of use, they can also offer a contractual transfer of liability between two entities. These distinctions are important for public health practitioners.

Lastly and most importantly, anyone can shape a rural community. The English teacher certainly did not have a public health understanding of shared use, he simply wanted his students to have an avenue to be more involved with their school and community through a shared enjoyment of soccer. He was not trying to curb the obesity epidemic or address issues of health equity; however, he did. Community champions, such as this teacher, are key partners for public health practitioners, and equipping such champions should be a priority in the field of public health.

■ Summary

Although there are numerous other details and examples that could be provided to highlight the unique challenges and assets related with promoting PA in rural areas, our aim is for you to walk away from this chapter realizing how complex working with rural communities is. At the heart of this, complexity is the diversity within and across rural communities; rural communities are each unique, they are not just small cities, and the people within each community are also not all the same, demanding cultural considerations. Diversity in terms of race, ethnicity, socioeconomic status, and occupations needs to be considered to ensure that all voices in a community are heard and included.

The changing context of rural America will continue to isolate rural communities and contribute to health and PA disparities evident for these residents. PA promotion in rural areas needs to consider and address the unique characteristics identified within this chapter. Additional research and evaluation is also needed to identify evidence-based approaches for rural communities, specifically to better understand how to address the unique challenges and incorporate unique assets seen in many rural areas. Addressing health needs and PA promotion in rural areas demands creative, multisector solutions that draw from the strengths of a community, acknowledging and addressing barriers along the way. Given this complexity, diversity, and these demands, there are a number of things to consider when working to promote PA in rural areas.

Things to Consider

- It is essential to identify and build relationships with key stakeholders and "gatekeepers" within a rural community, which takes time; take the time.
- It is also important to listen to multiple voices and viewpoints within the community, not just the loudest voice.
- Cross-sector partnerships are extremely important in rural communities where often public health interventions are being implemented by nontraditional community members (e.g., mayors, teachers). Plan to identify and engage traditional and nontraditional partners in PA promotion planning and implementation. Time needs to be spent cultivating local leaders to support these efforts, in capacity building, and to identify avenues to provide technical assistance. Partnerships with academic institutions should be fostered as one such avenue.
- Rural communities are not always what you think they are. It takes intentionality, relationships with multiple people, and time to identify these nuances, which can include characteristics such as race/ethnicity, migrant populations, culture, and environmental challenges/facilitators. These nuances must be understood and considered when thinking about PA interventions in rural communities, as was emphasized in the case study about the community soccer program.
- Environmental characteristics unique to rural communities must be considered and addressed in PA promotion, including distance between places and transportation needs, fewer built areas within communities, and the availability of more space, often including natural environments.
- And, finally, working with rural communities demands creative solutions given limited resources and competing demands, which requires PA promotion efforts to incorporate the earlier key points in planning, implementation, and evaluation phases. This not only requires knowledge of evidence-based approaches, but also of broader community needs, goals, and assets. The case study provided describing efforts in the North Carolina town of Princeville highlights one example of this.

References

1. Economic Research Service. Rural classifications. Available at: https://www.ers.usda.gov/topics/rural-economy-population/rural-classifications/. Accessed December 4, 2017.
2. Federal Office of Rural Health Policy. Defining rural population. Available at: https://www.hrsa.gov/rural-health/about-us/definition/index.html. Accessed December 4, 2017.
3. Ratcliffe M, Burd C, Holder K, et al. Defining Rural at the U.S. Census Bureau. *American Community Survey and Geography Brief*. Washington, DC: U.S. Census Bureau; 2016.
4. Trussell DE, Shaw SM. Changing family life in the rural context: women's perspectives of family leisure on the farm. *Leis Sci*. 2009;31(5):434–449. doi:10.1080/01490400903199468
5. Umstattd Meyer MR, Moore JB, Abildso C, et al. Rural active living: a call to action. *J Public Health Manag Pract*. 2016;22(5):E11–E20.
6. Isserman AM. In the national interest: defining rural and urban correctly in research and public policy. *Int Regional Sci Rev*. 2005;28(4):465–499. doi:10.1177/0160017605279000
7. Befort CA, Nazir N, Perri MG. Prevalence of obesity among adults from rural and urban areas of the United States: findings from NHANES (2005-2008). *J Rural Health*. 2012;28(4):392–397. doi:10.1111/j.1748-0361.2012.00411.x
8. Trivedi T, Liu J, Probst J, et al. Obesity and obesity-related behaviors among rural and urban adults in the USA. *Rural Remote Health*. 2015;15(3267):1999–2006.
9. Go AS, Mozaffarian D, Roger VL, et al. Heart disease and stroke statistics 2014 update: a report from the American Heart Association. *Circulation*. 2014;129(3):e28–e292. doi:10.1161/01.cir.0000441139.02102.80
10. Singh GK, Siahpush M. Widening rural–urban disparities in life expectancy, U.S., 1969–2009. *Am J Prev Med*. 2014;46(2):e19–e29. doi:10.1016/j.amepre.2013.10.017
11. O'Connor A, Wellenius G. Rural–urban disparities in the prevalence of diabetes and coronary heart disease. *Public Health*. 2012;126(10):813–820. doi:10.1016/j.puhe.2012.05.029
12. Henley SJ, Anderson RN, Thomas CC, et al. Invasive cancer incidence, 2004-2013, and deaths, 2006-2015, in nonmetropolitan and metropolitan counties—United States. *Morb Mortal Wkly Rep*. 2017;66(14):1–13. doi:10.15585/mmwr.ss6614a1
13. National Rural Health Association. About rural health care. Available at: https://www.ruralhealthweb.org/about-nrha/about-rural-health-care. Accessed December 18, 2017.
14. Yousefian Hansen A, Umstattd Meyer MR, Lenardson JD, et al. Built environments and active living in rural and remote areas: a review of the literature. *Curr Obes Rep*. 2015;4(4):484–493. doi:10.1007/s13679-015-0180-9
15. Economic Research Service. *Rural America at a Glance: 2017 Edition*. Washington, DC: USDA; November 2017.
16. United States Census Bureau. *Measuring American: Our Changing Landscape*. 2016.
17. Economic Research Service. Rural economy & population. Available at: https://www.ers.usda.gov/topics/rural-economy-population/. Accessed November 20, 2017.
18. Sallis JF, Cervero RB, Ascher W, et al. An ecological approach to creating active living communities. *Annu Rev Public Health*. 2006;27:297–322. doi:10.1146/annurev.publhealth.27.021405.102100
19. Satterthwaite D, McGranahan G, Tacoli C. Urbanization and its implications for food and farming. *Philos Trans R Soc Lond B Biol Sci*. 2010;365(1554):2809–2820. doi:10.1098/rstb.2010.0136
20. McCormick BP. "People aren't together too much anymore": social interaction among rural elderly. *J Park Recreat Admi*. 1994;12(4):47–63.
21. Martin P, Taylor JE. *Ripe With Change: Evolving Farm Labor Markets in the United States, Mexico, and Central America*. Washington, DC: Migration Policy Institute; 2013.
22. Edwards MB, Jilcott SB, Floyd MF, et al. County-level disparities in access to recreational resources and associations with obesity. *J Park Recreat Admi*. 2011;29(2):39–54.
23. Abercrombie LC, Sallis JF, Conway TL, et al. Income and racial disparities in access to public parks and private recreation facilities. *Am J Prev Med*. 2008;34(1):9–15. doi:10.1016/j.amepre.2007.09.030

24. Edwards MB, Cunningham G. Examining the associations of perceived community racism with self-reported physical activity levels and health among older racial minority adults. *J Phys Act Health.* 2013;10(7):932–939. doi:10.1123/jpah.10.7.932

25. Tinsley HEA, Tinsley DJ, Croskeys CE. Park usage, social milieu, and psychosocial benefits of park use reported by older urban park users from four ethnic groups. *Leis Sci.* 2002;24(2):199–218. doi:10.1080/01490400252900158

26. Payne LL, Mowen AJ, Orsega-Smith E. An examination of park preferences and behaviors among urban residents: the role of residential location, race, and age. *Leis Sci.* 2002;24(2):181–198. doi:10.1080/01490400252900149

27. Frost SS, Goins RT, Hunter RH, et al. Effects of the built environment on physical activity of adults living in rural settings. *Am J Health Promot.* 2010;24(4):267–283. doi:10.4278/ajhp.08040532

28. Moore JB, Jilcott SB, Shores KA, et al. A qualitative examination of perceived barriers and facilitators of physical activity for urban and rural youth. *Health Educ Res.* 2010;25(2):355–367. doi:10.1093/her/cyq004

29. Yousefian A, Ziller E, Swartz J, et al. Active living for rural youth: addressing physical inactivity in rural communities. *J Public Health Manag Pract.* 2009;15(3):223–231. doi:10.1097/PHH.0b013e3181a11822

30. Kegler MC, Swan DW, Alcantara I, et al. Environmental influences on physical activity in rural adults: the relative contributions of home, church and work settings. *J Phys Act Health.* 2012;9(7):996–1003. doi:10.1123/jpah.9.7.996

31. Scarapicchia TMF, Amireault S, Faulkner G, et al. Social support and physical activity participation among healthy adults: a systematic review of prospective studies. *Int Rev Sport Exerc Psychol.* 2017;10(1):50–83. doi:10.1080/1750984X.2016.1183222

32. Moore JB, Davis CL, Baxter SD, et al. Physical activity, metabolic syndrome, and overweight in rural youth. *J Rural Health.* 2008;24(2):136–142. doi:10.1111/j.1748-0361.2008.00144.x

33. Jilcott Pitts SB, Edwards MB, Moore JB, et al. Obesity is inversely associated with natural amenities and recreation facilities per capita. *J Phys Act Health.* 2013;10(7):1032–1038. doi:10.1123/jpah.10.7.1032

34. Hennessy E, Kraak VI, Hyatt RR, et al. Active living for rural children: community perspectives using PhotoVOICE. *Am J Prev Med.* 2010;39(6):537–545. doi:10.1016/j.amepre.2010.09.013

35. Michimi A, Wimberly MC. Natural environments, obesity, and physical activity in nonmetropolitan areas of the United States. *J Rural Health.* 2012;28(4):398–407. doi:10.1111/j.1748-0361.2012.00413.x

36. Cleland V, Hughes C, Thornton L, et al. Environmental barriers and enablers to PA participation among rural adults: a qualitative study. *Health Promot J Austr.* 2015;26(2):99–104. doi:10.1071/HE14115

37. Doescher MP, Lee C, Berke EM, et al. The built environment and utilitarian walking in small US towns. *Prev Med.* 2014;69:80–86. doi:10.1016/j.ypmed.2014.08.027

38. Maley M, Warren BS, Devine CM. Perceptions of the environment for eating and exercise in a rural community. *J Nutr Educ Behav.* 2010;42(3):185–191. doi:10.1016/j.jneb.2009.04.002

39. Rajnoch M. Forestry—recreation and education objects. In: *Public Recreation and Landscape Protection—With Man Hand in Hand.* Brno, Czech Republic; 2013.

40. Karašniece K. Motivation for students to participate in non-traditional outdoor activities. Paper presented at: 9th International Scientific Conference "Rural Environment. Education. Personality (REEP)"; May 13-14, 2016; Jelgava, Latvia.

41. Umstattd Meyer MR, Perry CK, Sumrall JC, et al. Physical activity–related policy and environmental strategies to prevent obesity in rural communities: a systematic review of the literature, 2002–2013. *Prev Chronic Dis.* 2016;13:E03. doi:10.5888/pcd13.150406

42. Harris JK, Mueller NL. Policy activity and policy adoption in rural, suburban, and urban local health departments. *J Public Health Manag Pract.* 2013;19(2):E1–8. doi:10.1097/PHH.0b013e318252ee8c

43. Calancie L, Leeman J, Jilcott Pitts SB, et al. Nutrition-related policy and environmental strategies to prevent obesity in rural communities: a systematic review of the literature, 2002–2013. *Prev Chronic Dis.* 2015;12:140540. doi:10.5888/pcd12.140540

44. Jilcott Pitts SB, Smith TW, Thayer LM, et al. Addressing rural health disparities through policy change in the stroke belt. *J Public Health Manag Pract*. 2013;19(6):503–510. doi:10.1097/PHH.0b013e3182893bbb

45. Barnidge EK, Radvanyi C, Duggan K, et al. Understanding and addressing barriers to implementation of environmental and policy interventions to support physical activity and healthy eating in rural communities. *J Rural Health*. 2013;29(1):97–105. doi:10.1111/j.1748-0361.2012.00431.x

46. Barnidge EK, Baker EA, Estlund A, et al. A participatory regional partnership approach to promote nutrition and physical activity through environmental and policy change in rural Missouri. *Prev Chronic Dis*. 2015;12:E92. doi:10.5888/pcd12.140593

47. Sallis JF, Frank LD, Saelens BE, et al. Active transportation and physical activity: opportunities for collaboration on transportation and public health research. *Transp Res Part A Policy Pract*. 2004;38(4):249–268. doi:10.1016/j.tra.2003.11.003

48. King KE, Clarke PJ. A disadvantaged advantage in walkability: findings from socioeconomic and geographical analysis of national built environment data in the United States. *Am J Epidemiol*. 2015;181(1):17–25. doi:10.1093/aje/kwu310

49. Kegler MC, Swan DW, Alcantara I, et al. The influence of rural home and neighborhood environments on healthy eating, physical activity, and weight. *Prev Sci*. 2014;15(1):1–11. doi:10.1007/s11121-012-0349-3

50. Kegler MC, Alcantara I, Haardörfer R, et al. Rural neighborhood walkability: implications for assessment. *J Phys Act Health*. 2015;12(6 suppl):S40–S45. doi:10.1123/jpah.2013-0431

51. Downing J. Bike to School Day. [twitter photo]. 2016. Available at: https://twitter.com/jessdowning. Accessed December 4, 2017.

52. Abildso CG, Zizzi S, Abildso LC, et al. Built environment and psychosocial factors associated with trail proximity and use. *Am J Health Behav*. 2007;31(4):374–383. doi:10.5993/AJHB.31.4.4

53. Brownson RC, Housemann RA, Brown DR, et al. Promoting physical activity in rural communities: walking trail access, use, and effects. *Am J Prev Med*. 2000;18(3):235–241. doi:10.1016/S0749-3797(99)00165-8

54. Oncescu J. Rural restructuring and its impact on community recreation opportunities. *Ann Leis Res*. 2015;18(1):83–104. doi:10.1080/11745398.2014.980834

55. Lo B, Morgan E, Folta S, et al. Environmental influences on physical activity among rural adults in Montana, United States: views from built environment audits, resident focus groups, and key informant interviews. *Int J Environ Res Public Health*. 2017;14(10):1173. doi:10.3390/ijerph14101173

56. Edwards MB, Theriault DS, Shores KA, et al. Promoting youth physical activity in rural southern communities: practitioner perceptions of environmental opportunities and barriers. *J Rural Health*. 2014;30(4):379–387. doi:10.1111/jrh.12072

57. Troped PJ, Saunders RP, Pate RR, et al. Associations between self-reported and objective physical environmental factors and use of a community rail-trail. *Prev Med*. 2001;32(2):191–200. doi:10.1006/pmed.2000.0788

58. Rails-to-Trails Conservancy. n.d. About us. Available at: https://www.railstotrails.org/about/. Accessed November 27, 2017.

59. Kids in Parks. About Kids in Parks. n.d. Available at: http://www.kidsinparks.com/about. Accessed November 27, 2017.

60. Hardison-Moody A, Edwards MB, Bocarro JN, et al. Shared use of physical activity facilities among North Carolina faith communities, 2013. *Prev Chronic Dis*. 2017;14:E11. doi:10.5888/pcd14.160393

61. Allen T, Boone K, Flink CA, II, et al. *Home Place: A Conversation Guide for the Princeville Community, Rebuilding After Hurricane Matthew*. North Carolina State University; 2017.

62. Lyson TA. What does a school mean to a community? Assessing the social and economic benefits of schools to rural villages in New York. *J Res Rural Educ*. 2002;17(3):131–137.

63. Schafft KA, Jackson AY. *Rural Education for the Twenty-First Century: Identity, Place, and Community in a Globalizing World*. University Park, PA: The Pennsylvania State University Press; 2010.

64. Kanters MA, Bocarro JN, Moore R, et al. Afterschool shared use of public school facilities for physical activity in North Carolina. *Prev Med.* 2014;69(suppl 1):S44–S48. doi:10.1016/j.ypmed.2014.10.003

65. Johnson JA III, Johnson AM. Urban-rural differences in childhood and adolescent obesity in the United States: a systematic review and meta-analysis. *Child Obes.* 2015;11(3):233–241. doi:10.1089/chi.2014.0085

66. Edwards MB. *Place Disparities in Access to Supportive Environments for Extracurricular Sport and Physical Activity in North Carolina Middle Schools.* Raleigh, NC: University of North Carolina; 2009.

67. Turner L, Chriqui JF, Chaloupka FJ. Walking school bus programs in U.S. public elementary schools. *J Phys Act Health.* 2013;10(5):641–645. doi:10.1123/jpah.10.5.641

68. Beaulieu L, Butterfield SA, Pratt PJR. Physical activity opportunities in United States Public Elementary Schools. *J Res.* 2009;5(2):6–9.

69. Powell LM, Slater S, Chaloupka FJ. The relationship between community physical activity settings and race, ethnicity and socioeconomic status. *Evid-Based Prev Med.* 2004;1(2):135–144.

70. Simons-Morton BG, McKenzie TJ, Stone E, et al. Physical activity in a multiethnic population of third graders in four states. *Am J Public Health.* 1997;87(1):45–50. doi:10.2105/AJPH.87.1.45

71. Johnson J, Strange M. *Why Rural Matters 2007: The Realities of Rural Education Growth.* Washington, DC: Rural School and Community Trust; 2007.

72. McDonald NC. Children's mode choice for the school trip: the role of distance and school location in walking to school. *Transportation.* 2008;35(1):23–35. doi:10.1007/s11116-007-9135-7

73. The Rural School and Community Trust. Consolidation fight-back toolkit. 2016. Available at: http://www.ruraledu.org/articles.php?id=2425. Accessed December 11, 2017.

74. Laboratory RE. Rural school district consolidation. 2009. Available at: http://cesu.schoolfusion.us/modules/groups/homepagefiles/cms/1556877/File/School_Boards/MERGER%202/REL%20Reports/RD162-2009-05-15_Rural_Consolida_Final-2.pdf. Accessed December 11, 2017.

75. VanDerBroek A. High school merger ratified. *Roanoke-Chowan News-Herald.* March 8, 2012. Available at: https://www.roanoke-chowannewsherald.com/2012/03/08/high-school-merger-ratified

76. United States Census Bureau. *2012-2016 American Community Survey 5-Year Estimates.* Available at https://factfinder.census.gov/faces/tableservices/jsf/pages/productview.xhtml?src=bkmk

77. United States Census Bureau. *2015: 2015 American Community Survey 5-Year Estimates.*

78. Zambrana RE, Logie LA. Latino child health: need for inclusion in the US national discourse. *Am J Public Health.* 2000;90(12):1827–1833. doi:10.2105/AJPH.90.12.1827

79. Johnston LD, Delva J, O'Malley PM. Sports participation and physical education in American secondary schools: current levels and racial/ethnic and socioeconomic disparities. *Am J Prev Med.* 2007;33(4 suppl):S195–S208. doi:10.1016/j.amepre.2007.07.015

80. Yu SM, Newport-Berra M, Liu J. Out-of-school time activity participation among US-immigrant youth. *J Sch Health.* 2015;85(5):281–288. doi:10.1111/josh.12255

IV

EVALUATING YOUR INTERVENTION AND DISSEMINATING THE RESULTS

EVALUATION OF PHYSICAL ACTIVITY INTERVENTIONS: IMPACT, OUTCOME, AND COST EVALUATION

JUSTIN B. MOORE | JAY E. MADDOCK | CAMELIA R. SINGLETARY | THERESA M. ONIFFREY

LEARNING OBJECTIVES

By the end of this chapter, the student should be able to

1. List and define the types of evaluation that can be conducted on **physical activity (PA) interventions**.
2. Describe the evaluation planning process and identification of relevant questions for the evaluation.
3. Create SMART objectives.
4. Describe characteristics of reliable and valid measurement instruments.
5. List and describe threats to internal validity.
6. List and define the aspects of impact evaluation that are relevant to PA interventions.

■ Introduction to Evaluation

What Is Evaluation?

Evaluation is a systematic method for collecting, analyzing, and using data to examine the effectiveness of programs. This includes aspects such as determining if your program is reaching the intended population, if the program is carried out as true to your original plans, the impact on policy or behavior in the target settings and populations, and effectiveness relative to the cost of delivering the program (called *cost-effectiveness*). Evaluation is often overlooked or considered an afterthought to the delivery of the intervention, but it should be treated as an important component of the overall intervention strategy, including the planning phase. Just as *Implementation Monitoring* (see Chapter 21) is crucial to understanding if you are implementing your intervention with full fidelity, comprehensive impact, outcome, and cost evaluation is of critical importance to show stakeholders the significance, benefit, and return on investment of the intervention. As such, thorough and continuous evaluation is integral to the success of your program and the potential of your receiving support for future interventions.

Types of Evaluation

Evaluation should be considered from the onset of program planning and well before implementation. It should be in the forefront from the development of program materials; in short-term goals; identification of policy, environmental, and behavioral impacts; and, ultimately, outcomes. There are three primary evaluation types to be considered. Process evaluation is a combination of formative evaluation and implementation monitoring. *Formative evaluation* typically occurs before the start of the intervention, and the data generated are used to improve the design of the intervention and evaluation. Conversely, *implementation monitoring* is conducted during the delivery of the intervention to determine if the intervention is being delivered as designed, and to identify areas for improvement so that feedback can be given for improvement of processes and activities that directly affect a program's impacts and outcomes. Implementation monitoring can be affected by intervention and evaluation plans/activities, which is why it should be thoroughly considered (and why it is addressed in a separate chapter). Impact and outcome evaluations allow researchers to identify markers of success for interventions (e.g., behavior change, improvement in markers of health).

- *Process evaluation* focuses on program components and activities that are directly related to the delivery of a program or intervention to its intended audience. Process evaluation encompasses formative evaluation and implementation monitoring. Formative evaluation is concerned with collecting data to assess aspects of the intervention target (e.g., school setting, workplace, participant characteristics) to determine the suitability and feasibility of the intervention, and considers factors such as readability of materials, training of staff, and cultural appropriateness of the materials. Implementation monitoring refers to activities to evaluate the active delivery of the intervention, including the completeness of delivery, dose delivered, and fidelity to planned activities (1).

- *Impact evaluation* measures any short-term changes in the target population or delivery setting related to the intervention. This can be changes in knowledge, skills, attitudes, policies, systems, environments, and behaviors. Impact evaluation is important, since it assesses more short-term changes that can lead to changes in healthy behaviors (e.g., physical activity [PA]), which should in turn impact health outcomes. Impact evaluation also includes cost evaluation, which often involves assessing the cost of the intervention relative to standard practice. Once cost is evaluated, it can be used to determine the cost-effectiveness, cost-benefit, or return on investment for the intervention.

- *Outcome evaluation* determines if the program or intervention has been successful in effectively addressing the health issue that was identified at the beginning of the planning process. Many times, desired outcome evaluation targets (e.g., heart disease) can be beyond the scope or resources of the intervention team; however, more proximal health-related measures may be appropriate (e.g., blood pressure) to use as indicators/markers of long-term outcomes. Ultimately, the focus of outcome evaluation is improvement of health status or quality of life.

Planning an Evaluation

Conducting PA interventions can be exciting. It is a time when you get to actually make a difference in people's lives by helping them be active. Often, we rush to get programs and projects started, forgetting about one of the most important elements . . . evaluation! This could be based on our own enthusiasm, from political or leadership pressure, or based on funding timelines, but one thing is certain; to demonstrate an intervention's success, you will need to evaluate. In this section, we are going to examine a few things that need to be done with evaluation before you start your program.

Initial Thoughts for Planning the Evaluation

One essential phrase to remember when conducting an effective evaluation is, "Prior planning prevents poor performance." The development of the evaluation and implementation plans should occur well before any interventions or activities are conducted. One of the biggest reasons evaluations fail to produce useful information is a lack of careful consideration about the evaluation early enough in the process. To state it simply, when you are planning your intervention, also make sure to plan your evaluation.

Once you have made the commitment to start planning the evaluation, determining who will lead the evaluation is the next step. Evaluations may be done by the program implementer, a newly hired internal person, or by an external evaluator. These decisions depend a lot on the size and scope of the intervention, existing skills and abilities, and experience in evaluations. Roughly, you should consider devoting a minimum of 10% of your total intervention budget to the evaluation. The complexity of the evaluation should match the complexity of the intervention. A large community-wide intervention will need a much more sophisticated evaluation than evaluating a series of training workshops. Whatever methods you choose to evaluate the program, the program developer needs to be centrally involved. Even if an external evaluator is used, the people conducting the intervention need to be centrally involved to make sure the right questions are asked, the right data are collected, and the findings are used. However, it is important for the evaluator (if he/she is not the implementer) to have independence from the persons conducting the intervention. If it is necessary that the implementer is also the evaluator, it is important to incorporate opportunities for external feedback (e.g., an advisory board) to ensure objectivity of the evaluation.

Identifying Evaluation Questions of Interest

Once it has been decided who will be leading the evaluation, it is time to figure out what questions to ask. The Centers for Disease Control and Prevention (CDC) framework for program evaluation (2), a six-step evaluation model, provides a step-by-step framework. Step one of this model is to engage stakeholders. Who are your stakeholders? They are anyone who will be interested/concerned about the results of your intervention. Step one is to make a list of everyone who might be a stakeholder. This might include your core team, school boards, elected officials, department of health staff, coalitions, community members, religious organizations, parent organizations, and so forth. This is also a good time to listen to those who might oppose your efforts. The biggest critics of the project should be engaged up front. What type of data will they believe? What do they think is the biggest stumbling block that you will encounter? Why do they think your program will not work? By engaging these people early in the process, you can use their input to plan a better evaluation. Please also refer to Chapter 6, which provides an in-depth discussion of how best to engage stakeholders. Also, engaging the right people in your project before it starts may help them to become advocates rather than critics. People like to be involved, so bring them into your group and learn what they have to tell you.

BOX 20.1

Who are your stakeholders?

Imagine that you are planning to implement a Complete Streets policy in a downtown business district, which will include traffic calming, bike lanes, and sidewalks. Make a list of everyone that you need to talk to about your program before it happens. Make sure to think of people who may be critical of the project, too.

Once you have this list, it is time to go on a *listening tour*. The concept of a listening tour dates back to at least George Washington and can be a useful tool in planning for evaluation. The goal of the tour is to find out what questions your stakeholders want answered. Town hall meetings can be an excellent mechanism for collecting this feedback. For a PA intervention, questions that stakeholders want answered might include:

Process

- How many people were served by the program?
- Did people enjoy the program?
- How much did it cost?
- Can the program continue after the grant is done?

Impact

- Are people more physically active than before the intervention?
- Did the program work with different types of people (i.e., ethnic minority, low income, low education, handicap)?

Outcome

- Are people healthier than before the intervention?

There are lots of questions that can be asked, so you want to make sure that you are hearing the most important ones from the most relevant stakeholders. For instance, an elected official who is funding the program may be very concerned about how the program is being received in the community and the long-term funding of this program may rely on this person's support. An example of an evaluation question here would be, "What is the perception of the program among the target population?" The other question you will want to ask your stakeholders is what type of data they are most interested in considering. Quantitative data from surveys is certainly important but there are many types of data that speak to different people. Policy makers may not care about statistical significance but would prefer stories or quotes to highlight findings. Nontraditional types of data are also helpful in evaluation. For example, before and after photographs of a trail that was renovated to improve PA access within a community or testimonials or success stories from people affected by your intervention can be powerful pieces of data. Information and data of interest might also be nonhealth data like reduced traffic in a neighborhood or increased sales in businesses in more walkable communities. Measures of increased productivity in the workplace are good examples of a nonhealth outcome that is important to measure in PA intervention evaluations. In one recent study assessing the impact of standing desks in a call center, results showed that workers with standing desks completed 45% more calls than those with traditional desks (3). In this case, a business owner would benefit from information not only on health outcomes, but on productivity and improved sales.

BOX 20.2

Stakeholder Exercise

Using the Complete Streets example from earlier in the chapter, make your list of questions for stakeholders. Take a few minutes to write down the questions that you want to ask stakeholders about your project. Do not forget to include which type of data they will believe and what they want to see happen with the project.

Describing the Intervention

Once you have completed your listening tour with your stakeholders, it is time to really start examining your intervention. What exactly are you planning to do? How will the program be delivered and who will deliver it? How will you recruit people? When will it occur? It is essential to think through everything step by step. Write down everything you are planning on doing in the program. (This is where the CDC guide is helpful!) Most individual and group-based programs follow a step-by-step progression from recruitment to intervention delivery. Intervention delivery often gets the most attention but it is essential to focus on recruitment and retention as well.

Recruitment is essential. You can have the best intervention in the world, but if no one participates, it is worthless. Here are a few questions to think about in the recruitment phase:

1. Who is your target audience? What type of person do you want to enroll in your program (e.g., sedentary, overweight, employees, women, older adults)?
2. Are there people who cannot participate in your program (e.g., too young, no insurance, too active)?
3. Which members of your target audience (e.g., older adults) are at most need for your program but might be the most difficult to recruit (e.g., those >75 years of age)?
4. What might keep your target audience from participating? For example, if you are targeting women, you might want to find out if lack of child care would be a barrier.

Other questions about participation also need to be considered.

1. How many people can you include in the program at one time?
2. What are you going to do if more people sign up than expected? Fewer?
3. What is the time commitment expected of participants?
4. Where will the intervention be delivered?
5. Where/how will you recruit people?
6. Will incentives be used? Are they appropriate for the audience?

Retention of participants is also key to a successful intervention:

As anyone who goes to the gym at the first of the year knows, early January is a lot busier than it is a few months later. A lot of people make resolutions to get active, but only a few of these actually stick. What are the things that might cause people to drop out of your program? You will need to get input on things like time, location, transportation, child care, cost, or other factors that might be barriers to participation. One way to do this is to conduct a simple benefit/barrier analysis of why people may or may not participate. For example, benefits may include getting in shape, losing weight, and having stronger social connections, as well as others. Barriers could include inconvenient time/day, lack of transportation or child care, dislike the activities presented, and so forth.

BOX 20.3

Exercise: Potential Benefits

Using the Complete Streets example from earlier in the chapter, make a list of the potential benefits of and barriers to your planned intervention from a participant perspective. How would you maximize each of the benefits, while reducing each of the barriers?

After you have refined your recruitment strategy and considered retention efforts, it is time to describe your intervention. As it relates to your evaluation, you will want to document all the activities that you will engage in during the course of the intervention. At the simplest level, whether those activities were actually delivered the way you intended them to be delivered constitutes implementation monitoring, whether they actually changed anything relates to your impact evaluation, and whether they improved the health of the target population is the foundational question of your outcome evaluation.

Once you have fully developed your intervention plan, documented the activities that constitute your intervention, and identified simple overarching goals to inform the specific questions that will form the core of your evaluation, you can create your evaluation plan. A typical mistake when making an evaluation plan is to focus exclusively on behavioral impacts of the intervention. While behavioral impacts are important, they are most important for research-oriented projects that are focusing on the efficacy (i.e., does the intervention work in ideal situations) or effectiveness (i.e., does the intervention work in the "real world") of the intervention in question. For example, Coordinated Approach to Child Health (CATCH) is an evidence-based tested program for physical education in schools (4). In numerous research studies, it has been shown to increase PA in children (5, 6). If you are planning to implement it at your school district, you do not need to show that it works. That has already been established. However, you do need to know information about who was trained to deliver the program and the level to which they were proficient in the curriculum at the end of training. You will also have to track the children who participated in the program (e.g., number, gender, ethnicity). Equally important is evaluating implementation fidelity, or the extent that your intervention is delivered as designed. This could form the basis for your implementation monitoring plan. Whether proposed policy or environmental changes occurred, systems within the intervention setting worked better, or participants' skills increased could be more important than short-term gains in PA behaviors and should therefore be carefully measured.

Developing SMART Objectives

Once you decide what is important and what you want to measure in your evaluation, it is time to develop objectives. People often get confused between goals and objectives. It is easiest to think of it this way: Goals are big picture ideas and objectives are specific accomplishments. Here is an example:

> *Goal:* Children who attend Windwood Elementary are physically fit, healthy, and ready to learn.
>
> *Objective:* By the end of the semester, 80% of children in the third grade at Windwood Elementary will pass the state physical fitness assessment.

This example shows the broad scope of the goal and the more detailed aspects of the objective that will help achieve the goal. It might take several objectives to address your overall goal. In this example, the objective addresses the goal idea of "physically fit" but you would need other objectives to measure healthy and ready to learn. As you begin your project, you should develop one to two goal statements. These are the big picture and what you want to achieve with the project. They tend to be easy to remember and to discuss with people in the community but will not be easily measurable. That is why the next step is to develop *SMART objectives* (7). A SMART objective is one that is

> *Specific:* What are you going to do and how will you know when it is done?
>
> *Measurable*: How can you assess if it is done? From the previous example, "fit" is not measurable but passing a state PA assessment is a way to measure fitness.
>
> *Achievable:* If everything goes well, can you reasonably expect that this is going to happen? By the end of the year, all students will achieve the fitness standard vs. by the end of the year, 5% more students will achieve the fitness standard.
>
> *Relevant:* Does this actually address the goals that you are trying to achieve?
>
> *Time-specific*: What is the time frame in which this objective will be completed?

Good objectives are essential to developing a strong evaluation. As you develop your objectives, think about ways in which you could measure what is stated in the objective. Objectives can be measured in different ways. For example, you might use an online survey, observation measures, photos, interviews, or devices (i.e., pedometers, accelerometers, etc.). It is always best to choose tools and measurement strategies that have been previously tested and known to be reliable and valid. While surveys can be useful tools to measure your objectives, it is important to consider other options. For example, let us say your program objective is 12 months after the installation of protected bike lanes on Maddock Road, automobile–bicycle crashes will be reduced by 80%.

One of the best ways to measure the achievement of this objective would be to use accident data from the Department of Transportation.

Selecting Instruments to Measure Objectives

Reliability and *validity* are important facets of any measurement tool. Reliability means measuring the same thing over and over again and you get the same result. Validity assesses if the tool is actually measuring what it is designed to measure. Something can be reliable but not valid, but it cannot be valid and not reliable. For example, a scale that gives you the same weight all the time but reads 10 pounds less than you really are is reliable but not valid. If you are planning a PA intervention, it is best to use a tool where reliability and validity have already been measured. The Active Living Research website (see the section "Resources") has a great list of tools. There are also several articles like Sylvia and colleagues (8) and Ainsworth and colleagues (9) that can help you in selecting strong tools to measure PA; Chapter 2 in this book covers measurement in detail. If you do need to develop your own surveys, keep the questions very simple. Questions like, "Did you attend our exercise session today?" will give you more valid and reliable results than questions like, "All things considered, do you feel that our program has increased the likelihood of how much you will exercise in the next 3 years, on a scale from 1-100?"

No evaluation is perfect, as it is difficult to balance *internal validity* versus *external validity*. External validity is a fairly simple concept: Are the results of the intervention representative of those you would expect in a real-world setting? For evaluations of programs delivered by practitioners in community settings, external validity is usually high because your program takes place in the real world. For research studies, it can be considerably lower. Often in randomized trials, there are strict protocols about who can be involved, how often, and when. In real-world programs, the goal is to make a difference in as many people as possible. If you hire 10 people in your company in the middle of a worksite wellness program and they want to join in, you will usually let them. This would be much less likely to be true in a randomized trial. However, this high level of external validity makes getting acceptable internal validity more difficult. Internal validity is the extent that your intervention actually affected the variable that you are interested in. The way you design your evaluation can greatly affect this (Table 20.1).

There are eight main threats to internal validity that one should consider: *ambiguous timing, selection, history, maturation, regression to the mean, attrition, testing exposure,* and *instrumentation* (10). *Ambiguous timing* can affect your conclusions when it is unclear the temporal order (i.e., sequence in time) of things believed to be cause or effect. For example, it would be unclear whether exercise class attendance increased enjoyment of exercise if you measured both attendance and enjoyment at the same time (i.e., the enjoyment of being active might have caused the attendance, rather than the other way around). *Selection* looks at the people willing to be part of an intervention or an evaluation. For example, are healthier or more active individuals more likely to enroll in an exercise program? If so, it might affect your evaluation results. *History* relates to the extraneous events that happen during the course of your intervention that could cause the observed effects. An example: If you are running a walking program and the sedentary, overweight mayor of the town dies from a heart attack in the middle of the program, this historical event could affect the results of the walking program. *Maturation* is an acknowledgment that people, especially children, change over time and that these natural changes can explain change (or lack of change) that your evaluation detects. Considering

TABLE 20.1. Potential threats to internal validity of an evaluation

POTENTIAL THREAT	EXPLANATION
Ambiguous timing	When the timing of variables is unclear and makes it difficult to discern which variable affected the other. You are unable to establish the direction of cause and effect between variables.
Selection	The manner in which the participants are selected for the study differs across conditions. For example, children in school-based interventions are selected to participate if they are on a sports team, while children in the comparison condition are chosen from the general student population.
History	External situations/events that happen simultaneously (or in close proximity) with your intervention, which may be the cause of any observed shifts in data collected during that time. For example, if you are distributing a survey on pedestrian safety, and a pedestrian/car accident occurs at a local high school during your last wave of surveys.
Maturation	Natural processes that introduce change over time concurrently with the intervention and could cause effects similar to expected effects of the intervention. Ex: Gathering adiposity data from adolescents during a PA study could be biased by effects of puberty.
Regression to the mean	If participants are chosen because of their extreme nature (e.g., high levels of time spent sedentary), they are likely to have less extreme values if measured again. This can appear to be in response to your intervention.
Attrition	A loss of participants from an intervention or data collection that is not random can give the appearance of an intervention effect when none has occurred. For example, the least active participants from your baseline assessment do not complete the follow-up measures.
Testing exposure	An individual given the same test more than once might improve his or her score due to familiarity with the measure rather than a true improvement in knowledge.
Instrumentation	Changes in tools or measures that occur over time during data collection could have an influence that is mistaken as a treatment effect.
Additive and interactive effects of threats to internal validity	Combinations of bias may result in a summative effect, or possibly the effect of the combination depends on the type of biases introduced and how much.

SOURCE: Adapted from Shadish WR, Cook TD, Campbell DT. *Experimental and Quasi-Experimental Designs for Generalized Causal Inference*. Belmont, CA: Wadsworth/Cengage; 2002.

that children tend to become less active as they get older, is an intervention that shows that sixth-grade girls engage in the same amount of PA at the beginning and end of the school year a failure or a success? *Regression to the mean* refers to the concept that extreme values tend to move toward the average over time. For example, imagine a city where pedestrian fatalities increase from an average of 10 per year to 25 over the most recent year, and the mayor creates a traffic safety advisory board in response. The board then organizes and conducts several pedestrian safety events, after which pedestrian deaths fall back to 10 in the following year. The results could very well be a result of regression to the mean. *Attrition* is a similar issue related to recruitment and retention, which is also referred to as differential dropout (i.e., are those who leave the study different than those who stay). Much like selection bias, people who stop participating in an evaluation may be more likely to be the less successful people in the program. *Testing exposure* is the concept that simply being familiar with a measurement tool can affect your scores on that tool in subsequent assessments. This is particularly relevant for tools that assess knowledge or skills. Finally, *Instrumentation* refers to the effect that changing measurement tools can have on your results. For example, a one item measure of PA might be replaced with a more comprehensive assessment in a longitudinal surveillance study as it becomes available, but this change in instrumentation will mean that estimates of PA from earlier in the study will not be comparable to those after the measurement instrument changes.

◼ Process Evaluation

Process evaluation is a crucial component to any intervention and can be the difference between successful implementation and producing suboptimal results. Process evaluation is comprised of two separate types of evaluation: *formative evaluation* and *implementation monitoring* (11).

Formative Evaluation

Formative evaluation, as the name would suggest, refers to evaluation that provides data to inform the development of the evaluation and implementation of the intervention. Formative evaluation might be conducted to assess the knowledge, skills, and attitudes of the target population or the policies, systems, and environments in which they function where the intervention will be implemented. Formative evaluation can be important for developing or tailoring intervention materials to ensure that they are consistent with the language, culture, and literacy level of the target population and the change agents who will implement the intervention. Formative evaluation can take many forms and levels of complexity. For example, the program planning model *PRECEDE–PROCEED* (see Table 20.2) specifies four steps that are important to formative evaluation (12), and may prove helpful in planning a formative evaluation. Regardless of the specific application of formative evaluation, it should be a well thought-out and purposeful process because it is foundational to planning and conducting subsequent evaluations. Thorough investigation of the aspects of the target setting, target population, and key stakeholder input will inform elements of program planning and development, as well as future implementation and evaluation strategies.

TABLE 20.2. Planning phases from the PRECEDE–PROCEED model

Phase 1: Social assessment	Identify societal needs and desires affecting quality of life of a community.
Phase 2: Epidemiological, behavioral, and environmental assessment	Identify health problems, and the reciprocal relationship between behavioral and environmental factors.
Phase 3: Educational and ecological assessment	Identify the predisposing, enabling, and reinforcing factors that can affect the behaviors, attitudes, and environmental factors.
Phase 4: Administrative and policy assessment and intervention alignment	Identify current and needed policies to determine the best method for creating and sustaining changes in health policies.

SOURCE: Green LW, Kreuter MW. *Health Program Planning: An Educational and Ecological Approach.* New York, NY: McGraw-Hill; 2005 (13).

Implementation Monitoring

Implementation monitoring is covered in greater detail in Chapter 21, but briefly, it is comprised of two major components: (a) the identification and quantification of the components of complete and acceptable delivery and (b) strategies to measure and monitor those components. Specifically, components of the intervention should be defined in terms of the fidelity, dose, and reach so that benchmarks can be set and a monitoring strategy can be developed (11). For example, if a worksite exercise program is being evaluated, one might want to know who is attending exercise classes (reach), how many classes are being delivered (dose), how well the classes are being attended (dose), and how well the instructors are delivering the classes as designed (fidelity). While some of these components are relatively easy to assess (e.g., number of people attending a class), others (e.g., fidelity of instructors to the lesson plan) will take careful planning to measure accurately and consistently. A greatly expanded description of implementation monitoring and how it can be conducted is found in Chapter 21.

■ Impact Evaluation

Impact evaluation measures the types of variables and constructs most people associate with the word *evaluation* in the context of PA interventions; most notably, changes in PA behaviors. However, impact evaluation is much more than simply identifying behavioral change. Impact evaluation should encompass all aspects of the intervention setting and target population that can be expected to change in response to intervention activities. These include knowledge, skills, attitudes, policies, systems, environments, and behaviors. Recently, costs associated with the intervention activities relative to the health or behavior changes of the target population have garnered more attention and should also be considered under the impact evaluation umbrella. While there are certainly several ways impact can be conceptualized (see Table 20.3), the framework we propose can accommodate the vast majority of interventions. Additionally, it is possible that your intervention is being designed and delivered through a collaborative effort, such as a coalition. If this is the case, there may be members of the coalition (e.g., transportation

TABLE 20.3. Domains of impact evaluation with examples and potential measures

CONSTRUCT	EXAMPLE	MEASURE
Knowledge	Compared to preintervention, participants are able to explain the difference between light and vigorous activity	Three-item questionnaire matching terminology with light, moderate, and vigorous PA
Skills	Participants are able to measure their own heart rate	Observational skills checklist
Attitudes/beliefs	Changes in outcome expectancies related to PA in youth	PA outcome expectancies questionnaire (14)
Policies	Increase in intervention schools that require documentation of the schools' physical education programs to follow specific physical education standards or guidelines	S-PAPA (15)
Systems	Coordination of statewide surveillance procedures for PA programs	Number of local health departments using a core set of PA measures
Environments	Changes in the number and quality of environmental features supportive of PA	PARA (16)
Behaviors	Minutes of MVPA	Accelerometers (see Chapter 2)
Costs	Cost of offering three weekly exercise classes in a local church gymnasium relative to the observed increase in PA	Direct, indirect, and capital costs to perform a cost-effective analysis

NOTE: MVPA, moderate-to-vigorous physical activity; PARA, physical activity resource assessment; S-PAPA, school physical activity policy assessment.

planners) who could help broaden the scope of the impact of your evaluation (e.g., reduction in traffic congestion) while also providing valid and reliable instruments for measuring this broader impact.

Knowledge

Knowledge is pretty straightforward from a conceptual basis, as it represents what is known about a specific topic by the individual in question. However, operationalizing knowledge can be challenging depending on the domain you intend to measure. For example, measuring knowledge about PA resources in a community might be a variable of interest, but it is unlikely that a community-specific measure exists. This might require you to catalog all the available resources in the community and come up with a checklist that a participant can complete to indicate his or her knowledge or awareness of those resources. This would require some degree of preliminary (i.e., pilot) work to establish evidence for validity and reliability before one could be confident in the results. Related, one must be careful not to conflate knowledge with other constructs such as skills or attitudes. For example, knowledge of using a gym facility might entail properly describing the process of setting up exercise machines, the number of set and repetitions of exercises, the uses for the various pieces of equipment, and so forth. However, skill would be demonstrated through the actual use of the equipment with proper form, resistance settings, and so forth. As such, it is important to clearly define each construct before choosing or developing measures.

Skills

As previously noted, skills are to be differentiated from knowledge in that they are the application of knowledge in a practical sense. For example, knowing how to (theoretically) ride a bike is not the same as riding a bike, and bike riding skill can vary within regular riders considerably due to years of experience and frequency of riding. Skill is often going to be assessed with hands-on demonstrations of skill or observation of individuals in the proper setting. Any assessment is going to require a valid and reliable process for systematic observation to ensure that skill assessment is independent of the individual conducting the assessment. These types of assessments are common in clinical settings, but the principles are the same in community settings. For example, the evaluation of a cycling program for youth might assess whether participants can properly fit a helmet for themselves following a safety demonstration. This would require determining criteria for success (e.g., no movement of the helmet, helmet level to head) that would be assessed on a standard form.

Attitudes

Attitudes can normally be thought of as the perceptions, feelings, thoughts, and beliefs individuals hold for persons and things. In this context, "attitudes" is an umbrella term for anything that does not fall under the knowledge and skills category. Attitudes might include characteristics, emotions, or affective states that might change due to a PA intervention (e.g., enjoyment of PA, self-efficacy, self-confidence), but health-related clinical conditions such as anxiety, depression, and disordered eating would be considered outcomes. Attitudes are often measured with questionnaires but could also be assessed via interview or open-ended questions.

Policies

Many PA interventions target organizational policies to promote PA (see Chapter 5) in those working, learning, playing, or praying in the affected organizations. For example, a school district might change the policy related to the number of minutes allocated for physical education in a school day or might implement a joint use agreement so that a walking track can be used by community members outside of school hours. As such, a complete evaluation plan should consider the direct and indirect policy implications of the proposed intervention and develop ways to monitor and measure changes. This can be as simple as surveying decision makers within an organization at the beginning and end of an intervention period, or reviewing content of policy documents (e.g., school wellness plans, operating manuals) to document changes over time. Evaluation of policies can become more complicated when assessing changes in enforcement or quality of a policy, as this can involve layers of policy elements overlapping with systems, environmental, and behavioral changes in order to examine the qualitative changes of the policy.

Systems

Many individuals work in formal systems such as those in healthcare, education, and transportation. Monitoring the form and function of those systems can be challenging and complex but can reveal very interesting information relevant to PA promotion. For example, a city public bus system has many facets such as the number, timing, and coverage of routes. An intervention to promote public transportation utilization and active transport might seek to increase the number of stops, percentage of population within one-quarter mile of a bus stop, and frequency of pickups. These would be important characteristics to monitor since they might lead to increased utilization and result in more individuals walking as part of their commute. Informal systems, or networks, might also be important to measure. For example, a peer-led intervention might be expected to increase the number and density of connections between individuals, and these connections might facilitate the spread of informational and logistic peer support. Assessing whether the connections increase as a mediator of the effectiveness of the peer-led intervention might give useful information regarding the impact of the intervention itself.

Environments

Environmental changes are often an integral part of PA interventions (see Chapter 14). These changes might be simple, reversible changes such as signage to take the stairs, or reminders to walk at lunch, or more permanent changes, such as the installation of a walking trail or an onsite gym at a corporate facility. Environmental changes can be expansive, such as complete streets during road renovations, or relatively minor, such as playground markings at an elementary school. These changes might even be temporary, such as park landscaping, event setup for race routes, or litter pickup at a greenway. Evaluation of these changes might be as simple as documenting their presence (e.g., a new walking trail at a high school), or might take a more systematic format, such as the PA resource assessment (PARA) instrument (16). The PARA documents the presence and qualities of various community resources such as parks, gyms, or community centers, and can be used to document large-scale changes to communities over time. Similarly, tools exist to measure park features, attributes of roads, and school settings. Regardless of the method used, measurement of environmental features and evaluation of changes in them can be valuable in determining intervention effectiveness.

Behaviors

PA behavior change is probably the one impact that an intervention can have that most implementers do not need to be reminded to evaluate. As laid out in Chapter 2, there are many methods that can be used to measure PA or a specific modality. While PA is a relatively straightforward construct, it is a multidimensional one that can take many forms and combinations of its application regarding type/mode, intent/reason, and intensity (light to moderate-to-vigorous PA [MVPA]) of the activity. For example, an individual might be active for transportation (e.g., active commuting), leisure (e.g., walking in the park), or occupation (e.g., picking vegetables). Within a domain, that activity might take different modalities. For example, within the leisure domain, one might engage in walking, basketball, swimming, or any number of other pursuits. However, as suggested in Chapter 2, not all measures can capture all domains or modalities. *Therefore, it is paramount to tie the measurement strategy to the intervention objectives or goals.* For example, if one were interested in the effectiveness of a walking program, measuring total PA might not be as meaningful as measuring the number of steps participants engaged in. Similarly, one would not want to use a measure of occupational PA in an evaluation of an intervention to increase leisure-time PA.

Costs

Since public health resources are finite, it is imperative that monies allocated to PA interventions are spent in a manner to maximize the benefit received in terms of the impacts and outcomes of the intervention. This is an important and growing area of evaluation (17). Costs can take on many forms, from the more conspicuous dollars spent directly on the intervention in the form of supplies, equipment, and staff time, to those that are easier to overlook, such as mileage to attend trainings, volunteer time, or time spent during technical assistance. When assessing costs, procedures can get complicated rather quickly, as equipment should be considered against its "useful economic life" since something like exercise equipment is expected to last and provide value for many years. Once costs are assessed, they can be used to calculate three values that might prove useful for decision makers when determining whether to sustain investment in a particular intervention or when choosing one strategy over another. The **cost-effectiveness** analyses measure the cost of the intervention per unit of change in an impact or outcome variable (e.g., minutes per day of PA) over a comparison period. **Cost-benefit analyses** are similar but require all consequences to be measured in monetary terms. For example, if an exercise program in diabetics produces a cost savings related to reductions in necessary medications, a cost-benefit analysis gives the gain of the intervention after subtracting the costs of the intervention. Related, **return on investment** is the ratio of the cost-benefit divided by the cost of the intervention, which shows how many dollars are saved by the program for every dollar invested.

◼ Outcome Evaluation

Outcome evaluation is traditionally and primarily concerned with changes in physical or mental health as a result of the program or intervention. As such, true outcome evaluation is rarely conducted with PA interventions due to their short-term nature and cost associated with collecting markers of health. However, if the intervention time frame is long enough to expect clinically meaningful changes in markers of health (i.e., biomarkers), the evaluation budget is robust enough, and resources are sustainable for the duration of the evaluation, then there are a number of biomarkers that can be considered. For example, PA in adults and youth has been shown to have beneficial effects on body composition, cardiorespiratory fitness, resting heart rate, metabolic risk score, blood pressure, lipids, insulin, glucose, sleep quality, and triglycerides (18, 19). Similarly, PA has been shown to have beneficial effects on markers of depression, anxiety, and self-esteem in adults and youth (20). Any of these markers of health benefits could be the target of an outcome evaluation. Unfortunately, the relationship between PA and health is complex, and not all domains and modalities of PA would be expected to affect all potential health outcomes. For example, some modalities of PA are more likely to result in body composition changes than others (21), so you would want to choose a biomarker that has been empirically supported to change in response to the type of intervention you are conducting. Similarly, an intervention targeting a higher level policy (e.g., school physical education policy) would be unlikely to impact a biomarker such as blood pressure, and therefore it would be unwise to dedicate resources to that type of measurement.

■ Data Management, Cleaning, Analyses, and Reporting

Before data are collected, it is very important to put thought into data management. This includes designing a database and a data entry strategy (if a paper survey is used) or data import procedures (if an online survey is used). Managing data is crucial, since failure at this step can lead to data that are potentially less useful, harmful to participants, or, in extreme cases, unusable. Data management should be discussed early in the project when deciding how to capture, store, and protect the data. For example, a simple variable such as the age of a participant can prove to be complicated. Should you capture date of birth, age, or age range (i.e., 25–30 years) as a categorical variable? If you choose date of birth, some participants might refuse to respond due to privacy concerns. If you choose age, you run the risk of losing specificity, which might be important in studies of rapidly growing children. Age range is especially nonspecific but might be sufficient if you just wish to describe your sample. As can be seen in this example, data questions can get relatively complex quickly, thus necessitating thought for any data that are to be captured. In the end, it is important to think about how each variable will be used, and capture/store them accordingly. Ideally, someone evaluating a project would have a dedicated database administrator who could build and manage a relational database to store data that are collected; in reality, relatively few health departments or universities have the capacity, even if the expertise exists within the organization. It often falls upon the evaluator(s) to develop a way to enter and store the data. If the evaluator has experience and training in database administration, designing the database for most interventions is relatively easy, but in many situations, this is not the case. Therefore, it is important to carefully consider a number of questions when designing the database and the data dictionary in preparation for cleaning and analyses.

BOX 20.4

Types of Variables

- Nominal variable—It has two or more categories, but with no specific ordering (i.e., hair color, gender).
- Ordinal variable—It has two or more categories, but there is a clear ordering (i.e., economic status, education).
- Interval variable—It has equally spaced intervals in between values (i.e., the gap between $10 and $20 is the same as the gap between $20 and $30).
- Ratio variable—It has the properties of the interval variable, except that it includes an absolute zero, with zero being the absence of the variable (i.e., number of children, years of experience).

Database Design

A database is where the data are stored, and the form it takes will determine how they may be retrieved or exported for reporting and analyses. Ideally, a database should be constructed in a database program since it allows for relational storage of data. For example, a participant can be given a unique identification code that would link all data sheets together so that all data for a participant could be connected. Participant data could also be linked by setting (e.g., school, worksite) or other grouping variables (e.g., teacher, job code). Unfortunately, database administration is a complex skill, and most evaluators lack the expensive software or training to create a relational database. As such, many people use a series of spreadsheets to capture data and create the data dictionary. While not ideal, a spreadsheet program (e.g., Microsoft Excel) or statistical software (e.g., Stata, SAS, SPSS) can be used, but may require extra training to be used properly.

Regardless of the program or method used to create a database, a number of questions should be considered during the development process. Specifically:

- Who will be responsible for creating and maintaining the database?
- Who needs access to the data and should they be password protected?
- Where will the data be stored, and what is the plan for creating regular backups?
- Who will enter the data and what steps will be taken to assure accuracy of the data?
- Who will the data be shared with, and what is the process for requesting data access?
- Will the data be identifiable?

Related to these questions are a series of best practices that should be considered when designing the database:

- When creating variable names, use lowercase words with numbers. Avoid spaces in the variable names or long names. A few popular analyses programs are case sensitive and require that spaces be omitted from variable names.
- Use consistent formats for repeating waves of data (e.g., age1, age2) or use a wave variable to differentiate the different waves.
- For categorical data, create codes in the data dictionary instead of using the categories themselves. For example, use 1 = red, 2 = green, rather than writing the words red or green and use consecutive numbers. If zero is meaningful, use zero as a code (e.g., 0 = no servings of fruit). If the variable is dichotomous, use zero to represent the absences of that quality (e.g., 1 = yes, 0 = no).
- Store the data as the appropriate data type (e.g., date, numerical) rather than a general format or as text unless the data are text (e.g., names).
- If multiple responses are possible, create additional codes to represent combinations of responses.
- Store data in the most granular format possible. For example, do not collapse age into categories during data collection if you have individual ages.
- Create codes to represent missing data rather than leaving missing data blank, especially if participants are able to skip or refuse to answer certain questions. Use different codes to represent the different reasons for missingness, which should also be documented and defined in the data dictionary you have created.

Data Dictionary

A data dictionary that defines your variables and their interpretation is a necessary step and will allow you to understand your data in absence of a data entry key, an original data collection form, or the survey instrument. A data dictionary should always accompany the data, except in rare circumstances (e.g., sensitive data). In the data dictionary, all variables should be listed with additional columns providing information about the variables. Examples of descriptive columns might include a descriptive label, the units of measurement, the text of the question, a description of the response categories, and any notes on the variable. In short, the data dictionary should replace all other documentation you have about the data and allow anyone with the data and the data dictionary to understand your variables and run any necessary analyses. A few best practices should be considered when creating your data dictionary:

- A data dictionary should be self-contained. As such, avoid nonstandard abbreviations, slang, or technical terms that the person analyzing the data might not understand.
- If entering questionnaire data, give the entire question and response in the description. The data dictionary should replace the questionnaire.
- Always have a column for units for biological data.
- If transferring to an analytical program, use the data dictionary to label the data in the new program. Many programs like Stata and SPSS allow the data dictionary to be incorporated into the dataset.
- Include coding and definitions for every type of *missingness* identified in the data.

Data Cleaning

Data cleaning refers to the process of ensuring that data are accurately entered and accurately reflect the data were collected. In addition, data should be screened to ensure that all values are plausible. For example, a variable such as age will have upper and lower limits that are possible within the population. Deviations from this range represent either a failure to screen participants properly or a data entry error. It is very important to screen all variables in the dataset to ensure accuracy, and a number of strategies are available to assist in these efforts. Specifically:

- Examine the range of the variable and pay special attention to missing values. Are the number and type of missing values reasonable, and is the range practically and biologically plausible? For example, does an item with four response categories have a range of 1 to 5? If so, something is amiss.
- For outliers, check with the original data collection form if possible before deleting the variable. It is always possible that a wayward keystroke during data entry caused your outlying variable.
- Consider multivariate outliers, which are combinations of two variables that are unlikely. You can identify these with histograms and box-plots where you plot one variable against the other. Identification of outliers can be challenging, but some will be easier to spot (e.g., a 6-foot-tall 5-year-old girl).

■ Check for the normality of your variables, especially if you intend to use inferential statistics. You can examine this graphically with a frequency distribution plot or with statistics such as skewness and kurtosis.

■ Consider what is considered a complete case (e.g., if someone only answered 75% of the questions, should they be counted?).

Reporting Evaluation Results

When reporting evaluation results, it is important to consider the audience. Very few reporting documents work for all audiences, so you will want to consider having a large report with multiple sections or multiple documents tailored for specific stakeholders. For example, a comprehensive report should start with an executive summary. If a stakeholder only reads the executive summary, at least he or she will be familiar with the most important results of the intervention. Similarly, you might consider different formats for different stakeholders. An infographic that summarizes the highlights of the evaluation might work best for the public, while a two-page policy brief might be useful for relaying results to elected officials, policy makers, or those responsible for funding the program. A more comprehensive exploration of dissemination of results can be found in Chapter 22.

BOX 20.5

Cultural Considerations for Evaluating PA Interventions

■ In implementation and evaluation, consider any language barriers that may be encountered. Make sure that you have a staff member available who is able to act as a gatekeeper that can effectively communicate with your target population, and vice versa.

■ Remember that language is not culture. Just because an instrument has been translated into the target population's native language does not mean that the terminology or tone is culturally appropriate. Be sure to have members of the target population review and translate instruments to ensure cultural sensitivity.

■ Explore attitudes, beliefs, and behaviors that are central to the target population's ideas surrounding health. Try to understand what they know about certain conditions and causes of conditions and choose your impact measures accordingly. You do not want to miss a potential benefit or harm of an intervention because you did not know to measure it.

■ Different cultures define family and community differently. Determine what constitutes family/community or forms of social support if you seek to assess it as part of your evaluation.

■ A self-assessment of how your culture affects your behavior and values can be valuable when working with a new culture or community. Look within yourself to assess your background and the things that formed your preferences, attitudes, and motivations. Also, try to think about any preconceived notions that you may have formed about a particular group before you attempt to work with them and explore the origins of these preconceptions.

▓ Things to Consider

- Start with evaluation in mind during the program planning process.
- Aside from garnering the support of stakeholders, it is also important to provide consistent updates and to effectively disseminate information to keep them engaged. This includes the actual population that you are targeting as well.
- Record all results of the intervention. During the evaluation process, it is important to both understand what works and what does not work. Use mishaps, barriers, and successes as a learning tool to refine implementation, the intervention, and evaluation.

▓ Resources

CDC Evaluation Template:
https://www.cdc.gov/eval/framework/index.htm
Active Living Research. Tools and Measures: http://activelivingresearch.org/toolsand resources/toolsandmeasures
Developing SMART Objectives:
https://www.cdc.gov/phcommunities/resourcekit/evaluate/smart_objectives.html
National Collaborative on Childhood Obesity Research. Measures Registry: https://tools.nccor.org/measures

▓ References

1. Saunders RP. *Implementation Monitoring and Process Evaluation*. Thousand Oaks, CA: Sage Publications; 2015.
2. Centers for Disease Control and Prevention A framework for program evaluation; 2017. Available at: https://www.cdc.gov/eval/framework/index.htm. Accessed January 15, 2018.
3. Garrett G, Benden M, Mehta R, et al. Call center productivity over 6 months following a standing desk intervention. *IIE Trans Occup*. 2016;4(2-3):188–195.
4. Perry CL, Stone EJ, Parcel GS, et al. School-based cardiovascular health promotion: the child and adolescent trial for cardiovascular health (CATCH). *J Sch Health*. 1990;60(8):406–413. doi:10.1111/j.1746-1561.1990.tb05960.x
5. Luepker RV, Perry CL, McKinlay SM, et al. Outcomes of a field trial to improve children's dietary patterns and physical activity. The Child and Adolescent Trial for Cardiovascular Health. CATCH collaborative group. *JAMA*. 1996;275(10):768–776. doi:10.1001/jama.1996.03530340032026
6. Nader PR, Stone EJ, Lytle LA, et al. Three-year maintenance of improved diet and physical activity: the CATCH cohort Child and Adolescent Trial for Cardiovascular Health. *Arch Pediatr Adolesc Med*. 1999;153(7):695–704. doi:10.1001/archpedi.153.7.695
7. Centers for Disease Control and Prevention. Develop SMART objectives. 2011. Available at: https://www.cdc.gov/phcommunities/resourcekit/evaluate/smart_objectives.html. Accessed January 15, 2018
8. Sylvia LG, Bernstein EE, Hubbard JL, et al. Practical guide to measuring physical activity. *J Acad Nutr Diet*. 2014;114(2):199–208. doi:10.1016/j.jand.2013.09.018
9. Ainsworth B, Cahalin L, Buman M, et al. The current state of physical activity assessment tools. *Prog Cardiovasc Dis*. 2015;57(4):387–395. doi:10.1016/j.pcad.2014.10.005
10. Shadish WR, Cook TD, Campbell DT. *Experimental and Quasi-Experimental Designs for Generalized Causal Inference*. Belmont, CA: Wadsworth Cengage Learning; 2002.

11. Saunders RP, Evans MH, Joshi P. Developing a process-evaluation plan for assessing health promotion program implementation: a how-to guide. *Health Promot Pract*. 2005;6(2): 134–147. doi:10.1177/1524839904273387

12. Carson Gielen A, McDonald EM, Gary TL, et al. Using the PRECEDE-PROCEED model to apply health behavior theories. In: Glanz K, Rimer BK, Vishwanath K., eds. *Health Behavior and Health Education: Theory, Research, and Practice*. San Francisco, CA: Jossey-Bass; 2008.

13. Green LW, Kreuter MW. *Health Program Planning: An Educational and Ecological Approach*. New York, NY: McGraw-Hill; 2005.

14. Lee RE, Booth KM, Reese-Smith JY, et al. The Physical Activity Resource Assessment (PARA) instrument: evaluating features, amenities and incivilities of physical activity resources in urban neighborhoods. *Int J Behav Nutr Phys Act*. 2005;2(1):13. doi:10.1186/1479-5868-2-13

15. Moore JB, Heboyan V, Oniffrey TM, et al. Cost-effectiveness of community-based minigrants to increase physical activity in youth. *J Public Health Manag Pract*. 2017;23(4): 364–369. doi:10.1097/PHH.0000000000000486

16. Story M, Sherwood NE, Himes JH, et al. An after-school obesity prevention program for African-American girls: the Minnesota GEMS pilot study. *Ethn Dis*. 2003;13(1 suppl 1): S54–S64.

17. Lounsbery MA, McKenzie TL, Morrow JR, Jr. School physical activity policy assessment. *J Phys Act Health*. 2013;10(4):496–503. doi:10.1123/jpah.10.4.496

18. Gralla MH, McDonald SM, Breneman C, et al. Associations of objectively measured vigorous physical activity with body composition, cardiorespiratory fitness, and cardiometabolic health in youth. *Am J Lifestyle Med*. 2016. doi:10.1177/1559827615624417

19. Warburton DE, Nicol CW, Bredin SS. Health benefits of physical activity: the evidence. *Can Med Assoc J*. 2006;174(6):801–809. doi:10.1503/cmaj.051351

20. Fox KR. The influence of physical activity on mental well-being. *Public Health Nutr*. 1999;2(3A):411–418. doi:10.1017/S1368980099000567

21. Cox KL, Burke V, Beilin LJ, et al. A comparison of the effects of swimming and walking on body weight, fat distribution, lipids, glucose, and insulin in older women—the Sedentary Women Exercise Adherence Trial 2. *Metabolism*. 2010;59(11):1562–1573. doi:10.1016/j.metabol.2010.02.001

IMPLEMENTATION MONITORING FOR PHYSICAL ACTIVITY INTERVENTIONS

JUSTIN B. MOORE | THERESA M. ONIFFREY

LEARNING OBJECTIVES

By the end of this chapter, the student should be able to

1. Define implementation monitoring and why it is important for physical activity (PA) interventions.
2. Describe the steps in planning for implementation monitoring.
3. Compare and contrast the benefits and limitations of using qualitative and quantitative data in implementation monitoring.
4. Create an implementation monitoring plan for a PA intervention.
5. Describe how the results of implementation monitoring can be used to improve the effectiveness of a PA intervention.

▦ Introduction

Implementation monitoring can be thought of as the measurement of what is actually happening during an intervention compared to what is supposed to be happening in an intervention (1). Implementation monitoring is one of the most important components of a comprehensive evaluation plan, since summative evaluation results are often less encouraging than one initially hopes. For example, if a walking program enrolls 100 women, and the results of the impact evaluation show that the average participant walked an additional 5 minutes more per week than he or she did at baseline, then most people would conclude that the program was not a success, since they would hope for a bigger increase. However, if a systematic implementation monitoring plan was in place, you might learn that a number of factors impacted the program's success, such as a lack of attendance at workshop sessions, a failure to actually deliver the sessions, or poor

© Springer Publishing Company DOI: 10.1891/9780826134592.0021

instruction during the sessions. Therefore, you might come to a very different conclusion related to the feasibility, acceptability, or effectiveness of the walking intervention.

Why Monitor Implementation?

There are a number of reasons that a comprehensive implementation monitoring plan should accompany all interventions.

1.   Implementation monitoring can provide feedback to the interventionists regarding the quality of the implementation of the intervention so that necessary adjustments can be made during the delivery of the intervention. To use our previous example, an implementation monitoring plan might have included observations of the walking intervention sessions. These observations would catch deviations from the lesson plans, which could be relayed to the interventionists who would then address them with the instructor of the sessions. This would allow correction before the intervention was finished, while there is still time to salvage the intervention.

2.   Implementation monitoring data can answer a crucial question for programs that are ineffective or less effective than expected. Specifically, was the failure attributable to a failure of the intervention (i.e., the program does not work), or a failure of the implementation (i.e., the program was not delivered correctly) (2)? Determining this distinction can be very valuable in making a decision to continue or discontinue an intervention, since even interventions with proven efficacy in controlled settings can fail in more natural settings even if implemented correctly. If a failure is due to lack of fidelity to the intervention, this can be potentially addressed and corrected, resulting in a more effective intervention without starting over from the beginning.

3.   Implementation monitoring can be useful even when the intervention is a success, as it can highlight aspects of the intervention that were necessarily modified to implement the program (3). As discussed later in this chapter, not all settings are alike, and modifications will need to be made at the local level to implement any intervention. For example, after-school programs might be delivered in a number of different settings (e.g., schools, community organizations, churches) that have great variability in the type of space and equipment available (4). As such, there might be considerable adaptation of curricula or specific games during the implementation of an evidence-based intervention. These changes might not be a bad thing. For example, Weaver and colleagues found considerable variability in the implementation of a physical activity (PA) intervention, even among the sites that were implementing successfully (3).

Unfortunately, the importance of collecting evaluation data is often minimized or overlooked amid the equally complex orchestration of implementing an intervention. Recent reviews of the literature suggest that process evaluation results, especially those related to implementation monitoring, are infrequently or incompletely reported (5). This lack of implementation data can make it difficult to select and implement an evidence-based strategy when a complete picture of the challenges associated with implementation are not available.

Planning for Implementation Monitoring

As with any other aspect of evaluation, planning is imperative to conduct implementation monitoring. Purposeful preparation is needed to collect useful information that can aid the implementation team in determining the success and opportunities for improvement of the intervention (6). Much like implementation planning and impact evaluation, implementation monitoring can seem unnecessarily complex when one is first beginning the process. Ultimately, implementation monitoring can be reduced to one thing: what was supposed to be done versus what was actually done. Implementation monitoring should start with a clear, documented understanding of what the intervention should be under ideal circumstances. Since interventions are rarely delivered under ideal circumstances, a clear set of criteria should be developed for each step of the intervention with strategies developed to assess the intervention activities against the criteria. This all begins with establishing the *gold standard* against which activities will be compared.

Steps in Planning for Implementation Monitoring

The Gold Standard

In popular use, the term "gold standard" has become synonymous with the prototypical or exemplar version of something to which other variations are compared. For the purposes of implementation monitoring, it is the "complete and acceptable" implementation of a specific program (6). For example, a church-based walking program might be designed to include a finite number of activities that should be performed in a particular manner. These might include 10 peer-led walking classes, weekly messages for the church bulletin, weekly reminders to be delivered by the pastor, signage for the church, and markers around the gym to help walkers chart their progress. Ideally, each of these components would be monitored or audited to ensure that they were implemented correctly; for example, were the walking classes the proper duration, did the instructor deliver the curriculum correctly, were all the activities successfully completed, and did everything occur how and where it was designed to occur? In this example, we could have an instructor arrive late, cut some of the material out for timing reasons, and skip some prescribed activities because the gym was being used by another group. As such, the reality of this particular class could be considerably deviant from the "gold standard," which would likely impact the effectiveness of the walking program in the short and long term.

As suggested by Saunders et al. (1, 6) and Glasgow and colleagues (7), defining the gold standard (also called "complete and acceptable delivery") requires consideration of several elements. We propose collecting a blend of those most commonly used. Specifically:

- *Reach:* This can be thought of as the target audience (all possible participants) of the intervention in the broadest sense. It should be considered from a participant, site, and "intervention agent" (i.e., those who deliver the intervention) level. For example, if you are offering a walking program to a company with multiple worksites, reach would be the proportion of workers, sites, and local wellness managers that were invited to join the program.

- *Adoption:* Very similar to reach, adoption is the proportion of the target audience (those reach-ed) who agree to participate. Again, it should be considered from participant, site, and intervention agent perspectives. In our worksite wellness program, this would show the representativeness of the participants, the sites who chose to deliver the program, and those who actually delivered the program.

- *Fidelity:* The most complex component of establishing the gold standard that you will use to measure and compare your intervention, fidelity results from the comparison of the activities that were conducted versus those that were planned. To make this comparison, one must have a complete checklist of measurable activities that constitute complete delivery. These will likely have a mixture of quantitative and qualitative components. For example, in our worksite walking program, we might establish that five, 30-minute classes be delivered. The number and duration of these classes could then be documented. However, if a standard curriculum is to be utilized, it would be necessary to do some type of assessment (e.g., observation of teaching, lesson plan review) to examine if the classes were being taught as intended by the standard curriculum. Measurement of fidelity can have many components, which may vary in value or utility to the overall evaluation. It will be crucial to list and prioritize those that are believed to be most important to the success of the intervention so that measurement strategies and tools can be identified or developed.

- *Dose delivered/received*: Closely related to fidelity are the dose delivered and the dose received. These should be thought about from both the perspective of the participant and the intervention agent. For example, the number of walking classes delivered (as mentioned in fidelity) and the average number of classes attended would be good participant-level data to collect. Similarly, the number of training sessions delivered and attended for the teachers of the walking classes would be a useful measure from the intervention agent perspective.

- *Context:* Often overlooked, context (i.e., the physical, social, and policy environments) can be very important to understanding the other data collected during implementation monitoring. For example, you may find that the number of participants attending walking classes varies based on environmental factors such as the quality of the walking surface (e.g., nice track vs. parking lot) available at the worksite, indoor/outdoor (i.e., weather controlled), or location (i.e., conveniently accessible, safe, ample parking). Similarly, you might find that utilization of walking tracks around worksites are used more frequently where employers have flexible scheduling policies that allow the workday to start early or late for those enrolled in the walking program. Without assessing context, these important moderators of the program's effectiveness would be misattributed or overlooked completely.

The Role of Theory

Ideally, theory should inform the intervention that you are implementing (1), and should be observable in the activities of the intervention. For example, *Self-Determination Theory* could form the basis for a youth summer day camp intervention, with one of the objectives of the program being to increase the intrinsic motivation for PA of the children in attendance. If this is the case, an evaluator would expect to see the staff interacting with the children in a manner consistent with the theory; for example, not using PA (like sprints) as punishment. Therefore, to properly monitor the delivery of an intervention, it is important to have an appreciation for *how* an intervention is supposed to work from a theoretical perspective when designing the implementation monitoring plan. In this example, we would expect the camp activities to increase intrinsic motivation (operationalized as enjoyment of PA), and that increase would lead to more PA during free play and/or outside of the camp setting. While measuring the impact of the intervention is important (i.e., measuring enjoyment and PA), you would also want to employ an observation tool such as the System for Observing Staff Promotion of Activity and Nutrition (8) that could capture staff behaviors that are supportive or discouraging of intrinsic motivation, such as letting the children have input into the games played, being verbally supportive, and modeling of PA. The theoretical underpinnings of the intervention should be evident in the tools that are used during implementation monitoring, especially those related to the delivery of components by staff or other agents of change (e.g., see Yin et al.) (9).

BOX 21.1

Self-Determination Theory

Self-Determination Theory was initially developed by Drs. Edward L. Deci and Richard M. Ryan to explain behavioral tendencies based on different sources and types of motivation. To learn more about Self-Determination Theory, visit selfdeterminationtheory.org.

Stakeholders

When possible, stakeholders should be involved in the development of an implementation monitoring plan. Since implementation monitoring often seeks to assess the quantity and quality of programmatic activities and participant engagement in these activities, designing an effective implementation monitoring plan requires an intimate knowledge of the activities being delivered. For example, if you were implementing a classroom-based PA intervention for third-grade youth, you would need to understand early child education to assess whether lessons were being delivered appropriately. Therefore, it would be important to have one or more elementary-level teachers involved in planning to inform the strategies and measurement instruments to ensure that they were appropriate for the setting and population. One of the biggest mistakes one can make when working in communities is to underestimate the complexity of the setting you are seeking to evaluate (10). Engaging stakeholders in the planning process can bring these complexities to light and often produce solutions to accommodate them in a manner that will bring validity to the evaluation results (11).

Objectives

While objectives should drive the impact evaluation for an intervention, they can also be very useful for implementation monitoring, as they can help quantify the components of interest for ideal and complete implementation. These might include aspects such as the number and type of environmental changes, the number of sessions to be delivered, provision of equipment, or any number of other necessary ingredients for success of an intervention. As with any other type of evaluation, these objectives should be SMART (Specific, Measurable, Achievable, Realistic, and Time-bound), to ensure that they are appropriate for the monitoring plan (see Chapter 20). For example, a park-based intervention that includes dance classes might include an implementation monitoring objective of delivering five, 1-hour Zumba classes within the first 2 months of the intervention taught by a certified instructor.

Data Sources—Qualitative Versus Quantitative

As with any type of evaluation, a choice needs to be made regarding the type of data to be collected, with a mixture of qualitative and quantitative data often filling the need (12). The type of data to be collected should *always* be tied to the objectives and driven by their formatting and characteristics. Data collection should *never* drive the choice of objectives, which would result in squandered resources and data with little to no utility. For example, the presence of an existing survey or the desire to conduct interviews should never influence the objectives of the evaluation. In other words, you cannot answer questions that have not been asked, and you cannot evaluate change (collect data) unless you state intentions (objectives). Rather, the objectives that one develops should help guide decisions on the methods used to collect the data to assess those objectives. As a rule, objectives that seek to "determine the change" in something, "assess the number" engaging in a behavior, or "measure the difference between" groups tend to lend themselves to quantitative measures. Objectives that seek to "understand perspectives," "assess attitudes," or "establish histories" might be better suited to qualitative data collection. Regardless, a mixed-methods approach (both quantitative and qualitative methodologies) should be rigorously applied to increase the robustness of your evaluation.

Measurement Instruments

One of the biggest challenges to implementation monitoring is the lack of setting-specific measures to employ in the evaluation plan. For example, if an objective of your monitoring evaluation was to measure attendance at a senior exercise program, it would be relatively easy to design a check-in form to confirm attendance. However, if the level of engagement of the participants was of interest, it is likely that a new form would need to be developed to capture those data. When planning, it is important to identify all the instances where documentation will occur and whether new instruments exist or will need to be developed. It can take a considerable amount of time to develop, review, pilot test, revise, and finalize even a relatively simple tool and budgeting time to dedicate to this should be planned ahead.

BOX 21.2

Definitions

Validity: It refers to how well a measurement tool actually measures what it is intended to measure.

   Reliability: The degree to which a measurement tool is able to perform with consistency.

   Interrater reliability: It is used to assess how consistently data collectors are using a measurement tool by measuring the degree to which data are the same between different data collectors that are using the same measurement tool.

Sampling

As with other types of evaluation, it is important to develop a strategy that will capture a representative sample of the sites and intervention agents. Unless a project is very small (e.g., one site), it is unlikely that implementation monitoring will be conducted in the same manner at all locations at all times. For example, a worksite wellness program might be conducted across several sites where group exercise classes are offered during the lunch hour. While it would be allowable to collect information about attendance at all sites, it might not be possible to have observers in the classes to assess the quality of the instruction and adherence to the curriculum. In this example, it would be necessary to create a sampling strategy where each class was visited regularly in a systematic manner so that observations are conducted on different days and for each instructor. It is important that sampling is systematic (i.e., all worksites have an equal chance of being sampled), since (as in our example worksite wellness program) worksites and their workers can differ drastically in their willingness to participate in health promotion programming (13).

Data Collection Protocol

As with other types of evaluation, it is necessary to have a protocol and data collection tools to standardize the measurement of the constructs specified in your SMART objectives. As process data are often collected by those being intervened upon (e.g., staff at an after-school program), it is important to have clear instructions and training to ensure that data is collected correctly and uniformly. Preparing clear data collection protocols, instructions, and forms are very useful for staying organized and efficient in situations requiring you to depend on a number of different individuals to conduct the same tasks (e.g., when utilizing different volunteers or interns). As with any other materials, protocols should be piloted with a few different individuals who can comment on the clarity (readability and culturally appropriate), completeness, and accuracy of the materials. It should also be noted that evaluation is still research and should be treated with the same ethical precautions regarding confidential data and a plan to protect those data.

Barriers to Effective Implementation Monitoring

It probably comes as no surprise, but the most common barrier to effective evaluation is a lack of human and financial resources. While large, well-funded research projects can employ a large team of evaluation staff, most smaller projects orchestrated by community-based organizations lack full-time staff and a dedicated budget for evaluation. As such, evaluation may be conducted with the help of volunteers, "borrowed" staff, or student interns. When possible, budgets should be crafted to include sufficient funding for evaluation. When that is not possible, it is important to prioritize objectives so that the most important implementation constructs are assessed at the expense of those that would be nice to have, but a lack of resources prevent inclusion of low-priority constructs and objectives. Be mindful that insufficient planning for implementation monitoring can be a big contributor to the collection of less useful data, missing opportunities for data collection, or incomplete data collection. Needless to say, implementation monitoring should be prioritized in a manner such that sufficient resources, time, and personnel are dedicated to it. Do not allow common barriers to snowball into a poorly conducted evaluation. Identify your resources, recognize limitations, and optimize these components to plan and operationalize an evaluation that works for you.

◾ Conducting Implementation Monitoring

Once you have a solid implementation monitoring plan in place and the intervention begins, you can begin to implement your monitoring strategy. As with any other type of evaluation, implementation monitoring will require careful organization, scheduling, data entry/management processes, and analysis planning (see Chapter 20). The day-to-day conduct of intervention monitoring will depend on a number of factors including (but not limited to)

- ◾ Who will be conducting the monitoring
- ◾ The role of technology in the monitoring and storage of the data
- ◾ Availability of staffing
- ◾ The speed at which the monitoring results need to be returned to the intervention team

Data Collection

One of the key trade-offs when designing an implementation monitoring plan is whether data will be provided directly from participants, intervention agents, evaluation staff, or some combination of those sources. For example, something as simple as class attendance data could be self-reported from participants, or recorded by the teacher of the class, a staff member observing the class, or by a program that records attendance when participants swipe a membership card. Each of these will have benefits, challenges, and limitations. Participant data (self-report) is often the least valid, because it is very susceptible to bias. A method must also be developed to collect and enter it in a timely manner. Data from intervention agents can have similar challenges, and something as easy to develop as a sign-in sheet can present challenges for collection and data entry. Staff can provide more reliable and valid data if standard procedures are used, but they represent a huge expense that is outside the scope of most evaluation budgets. Technology is becoming more ubiquitous and might allow for automation of many tasks, which improves accuracy of data and reduces time for data entry. Unfortunately, many proprietary systems are not designed with data sharing in mind, and development of project-specific applications or mobile websites can be cost prohibitive. Regardless of how data are collected, they will need to be entered and stored to support fast retrieval.

Data Management

A key consideration that often gets overlooked until too late is the data management plan. A good data management plan will identify the roles and responsibilities of the staff (e.g., who will enter the data), detail how the data will be stored, how and when data will be backed up, how the data will be retrieved, and how documentation will occur and be stored. At a minimum, guidelines should be written to detail how files/versions will be named, how data should be entered and by whom, and how regularly they will be entered/reported. Additionally, all datasets should have a data dictionary that specifies the coding for each item to be stored and the units they represent (see Chapter 20).

Increasingly, data are being collected utilizing electronic methods (e.g., websites, text, cell phone applications, wearables), often saving time and increasing accuracy. These methods can be especially beneficial for implementation monitoring purposes if they decrease the time between collection and reporting, or if they allow for a more complete assessment of intervention activities. However, while they can reduce burden, they still require careful planning and some level of tech support to be utilized. For example, a survey from an online commercial provider may need to be downloaded and integrated with other data sources to be analyzed. If text messaging, mobile applications, or commercially available devices are to be used, an application programming interface (API) will often be necessary to aggregate or import data into a platform where they can be utilized for reporting or analyses. As such, time and money should be budgeted for data integration when electronic methods are proposed.

Using Implementation Monitoring Results

Before implementation monitoring data are available, it is important that thought be given to how and when they will be reported. Implementation monitoring data may be extremely useful during the intervention, especially for nonresearch projects where optimization of delivery is the priority. For example, if one were tasked with recruiting 20 schools from a large school district and wanted participation from as many schools serving low-income communities as possible, it would be important to report back to those responsible for recruitment on a regular basis. A simple report might list the interested schools along with the percentage of children eligible for free or reduced lunch. You would not want to simply collect those data, store them, and look at them at the end of the project. Similarly, persons implementing a program designed to train school staff to install colorful playground markings and active recess practices would want to regularly visit the schools to ensure that the markings were installed and observe the recess supervisors to confirm that they were delivering the active recess curriculum. It would be important that this information be reported back to the intervention team so that booster sessions could be provided (if feasible) to those schools where teachers were improperly delivering lessons, or a technical assistance call scheduled for the schools who are struggling with getting the playground markings in place.

Things to Consider

- Find a way to stay organized that works for you. It is of the utmost importance to maintain a clear view and command of the many moving parts during implementation monitoring.
- Be mindful to continuously document in detail all monitoring events and procedures. Data collected during implementation monitoring can reveal weaknesses in intervention delivery and lead to adjustments in implementation to improve the intervention. All changes need to be documented to inform all other monitoring activities extending from those changes as you move forward with the evaluation.
- Always have a backup plan. It never fails, when things are busiest, that your plans will come to a halt due to weather, electronics with dead batteries, a lack

of pens, or staff calling out sick. When planning out protocols and ordering supplies, always include extra of everything.

◼ Resources

- ◼ Saunders RP. *Implementation Monitoring and Process Evaluation.* Thousand Oaks, CA: Sage Publications; 2015.
  Program Evaluation for Public Health Programs: A Self-Study Guide: https://www.cdc.gov/eval/guide/index.htm

◼ References

1. Saunders RP, Evans MH, Joshi P. Developing a process-evaluation plan for assessing health promotion program implementation: a how-to guide. *Health Promot Pract.* 2005;6(2):134–147. doi:10.1177/1524839904273387
2. Wilson DK, Griffin S, Saunders RP, et al. Using process evaluation for program improvement in dose, fidelity and reach: the ACT trial experience. *Int J Behav Nutr Phys Act.* 2009;6(1):79. doi:10.1186/1479-5868-6-79
3. Weaver RG, Moore JB, Huberty J, et al. Process evaluation of making HEPA policy practice: a group randomized trial. *Health Promot Pract.* 2016;17(5):631–647. doi:10.1177/1524839916647331
4. Beets MW, Weaver RG, Turner-McGrievy G, et al. Are we there yet? Compliance with physical activity standards in YMCA afterschool programs. *Child Obes.* 2016;12(4):237–246. doi:10.1089/chi.2015.0223
5. McGoey T, Root Z, Bruner MW, et al. Evaluation of physical activity interventions in youth via the Reach, Efficacy/Effectiveness, Adoption, Implementation, and Maintenance (RE-AIM) framework: a systematic review of randomised and non-randomised trials. *Prev Med.* 2015;76:58–67. doi:10.1016/j.ypmed.2015.04.006
6. Saunders RP. *Implementation Monitoring and Process Evaluation.* Sage Publications; 2015.
7. Glasgow RE, Vogt TM, Boles SM. Evaluating the public health impact of health promotion interventions: the RE-AIM framework. *Am J Public Health.* 1999;89(9):1322–1327. doi:10.2105/AJPH.89.9.1322
8. Weaver RG, Beets MW, Webster C, et al. System for observing staff promotion of activity and nutrition (SOSPAN). *J Phys Act Health.* 2014;11(1):173–185. doi:10.1123/jpah.2012-0007
9. Yin Z, Hanes Jr, Moore JB, et al. An after-school physical activity program for obesity prevention in children: the Medical College of Georgia FitKid Project. *Eval Health Prof.* 2005;28(1):67–89. doi:10.1177/0163278704273079
10. Saunders RP, Wilcox S, Baruth M, et al. Process evaluation methods, implementation fidelity results and relationship to physical activity and healthy eating in the Faith, Activity, and Nutrition (FAN) study. *Eval Program Plann.* 2014;43:93–102. doi:10.1016/j.evalprogplan.2013.11.003
11. Pitts SB, Bringolf KR, Lloyd CL, et al. Formative evaluation for a healthy corner store initiative in Pitt County, North Carolina: engaging stakeholders for a healthy corner store initiative, part 2. *Prev Chronic Dis.* 2013;10:E120. doi:10.5888/pcd10.120319
12. Johnson RB, Onwuegbuzie AJ. Mixed methods research: a research paradigm whose time has come. *Education Research.* 2004;33(7):14–26. doi:10.3102/0013189X033007014
13. Jorgensen MB, Villadsen E, Burr H, et al. Does employee participation in workplace health promotion depend on the working environment? A cross-sectional study of Danish workers. *BMJ Open.* 2016;6(6):e010516. doi:10.1136/bmjopen-2015-010516

DISSEMINATION: MODELS AND METHODS

DANIELLE E. JAKE-SCHOFFMAN | ALICIA A. DAHL | JUSTIN B. MOORE

LEARNING OBJECTIVES

By the end of this chapter, the student should be able to

1. Define dissemination and its importance to physical activity (PA) promotion.
2. Describe the benefits of dissemination as it relates to public health practice and policy.
3. Describe the value of dissemination models and their utility in guiding dissemination efforts.
4. Describe the steps in developing a dissemination plan.
5. List and describe dissemination methods, and their relative strengths and limitations.

▓ Introduction

Dissemination, quite simply, is a purposeful process of sharing information across interested parties. At the dissemination stage in the process of physical activity (PA) interventions, researchers and practitioners have collected meaningful information to share in an effort to improve programs, processes, policies, or outcomes. Dissemination has been described as a planned process that includes considering project goals and the target audience in determining how best to distribute research findings to help ensure the research reaches public health and policy decision makers as needed (1). Dissemination (also called knowledge transfer) should be considered to be distinct from diffusion, which is a more passive process, and implementation, which involves the application of an evidence-based practice. Dissemination can be thought of as the beginning of the research to practice continuum once the research has been conducted, and a necessary,

© Springer Publishing Company DOI: 10.1891/9780826134592.0022

but not sufficient, aspect of adoption. In short, dissemination is a systematic, planned approach to transferring knowledge to individuals, and in many cases with the intention that they will take a prescribed action (Callout Box 22.1).

BOX 22.1

A Continuum: diffusion-dissemination-implementation

Dissemination can be thought of as part of a continuum of processes to spread research and practice, from most passive to most active (2):

- Diffusion: passive, untargeted, unplanned spread of research and practice
- Dissemination: active, targeted spread of research and practice to a target audience via planned strategies
- Implementation: active, targeted process of integrating new practices and policies into existing systems and structures

---

Benefits of Dissemination

The benefits of PA have been well established and accepted for decades, but PA levels remain low, along with the public health investments in research, infrastructure, programs, and policies (3). While much of the public is aware of the benefits of PA, this knowledge has not translated to concurrent changes in policies and environments necessary to change behavior on a population level (3) Similarly, while many who are trained in public health and medicine espouse the benefits of PA, the levers of change for policy, built environment, infrastructure, and design are held by those working in the political, urban planning, architecture, and civil engineering fields. Only through active dissemination of information and evidence concerning the opportunities, innovations, challenges, and successes can the field begin to have the broad impact that a robust public health endeavor requires. For example, it is insufficient that a physician understands and appreciates the benefits of counseling patients for PA if there is no policy in place for an insurer to reimburse the physician for the counseling costs for the patient, as is the case if the physician is counseling a patient about hypertension. This denial of coverage could create a financial burden for patients. Through dissemination of evidence of the effectiveness of clinical counseling for PA (4, 5), and the cost-effectiveness of this strategy (6), one can improve the probability of coverage of these services and generate a population-level impact.

Review of Dissemination Models

There are a number of models that can help guide dissemination planning and activities for PA programs and policies. Although not specific to PA research, two recent reviews provide a useful overview of the landscape of dissemination frameworks and guiding theories in health promotion. First, a review identified 33 frameworks to guide dissemination of research findings classifying the theoretical underpinnings of the frameworks and providing general information about the approaches taken to dissemination

(7). A second review categorized models of both dissemination and implementation, finding 11 models specific to dissemination (as opposed to a mix of dissemination and implementation), and providing information about the stated construct flexibility of the framework and socio-ecological levels targeted by the approach. While the frameworks reviewed vary in their specific approach to dissemination activities, they generally include guidelines to identify characteristics of the target audience, understand the type of message/information to be delivered (e.g., details of a new best practice for PA policy), and tailor the approach accordingly to maximize the potential impact of the dissemination approach (8). Further, the review articles provide a helpful overview to understanding the theoretical foundations and levels of approach that each framework takes, which is important information for PA researchers and practitioners looking to design a dissemination approach. Of the frameworks reviewed, two theories of dissemination most frequently served as part of the foundational approach (7): persuasive communication and Diffusion of Innovations theory.

Persuasive Communication

A persuasive communication approach describes both the inputs of communication that can impact message delivery and the outputs that can be used to measure the impact of the attempted communication. The five communication inputs to consider are source, message, recipient, channel, and context (setting for the communication), while the outputs are exposure, attention, interest, comprehension, acquisition, yielding, memory, retrieval, decision, action, reinforcement, and consolidation (9–11). These factors can be considered in a matrix, where each input could have an impact on each output. Techniques of persuasive communication have been applied in a variety of contexts, sometimes focusing on communication inputs for information dissemination. For example, the National Center for the Dissemination of Disability Research developed a framework (12) to guide the process of making research results more accessible, drawing on four characteristics of persuasive communication (source, message, recipient, channel) (13).

Diffusion of Innovations Theory

Diffusion of Innovations theory describes the spread of innovations through specific populations and social systems, resulting in the adoption of new ideas, behaviors, or products (14). Central to this theory are the five categories of adopters, used to describe people across a continuum from quick-to-adopt to slower and more conservative to try new things (innovators, early adopters, early majority, late majority, laggards). The theory proposes five phases that occur over time during the adoption of an innovation, from knowledge to persuasion, decision, implementation, and finally confirmation. Further, the theory outlines five factors that influence the adoption of innovations and need to be uniquely considered for each category of adopters: relative advantage (better than what is currently used), compatibility (aligned with the values and needs of adopters), complexity (difficult to use or understand), trialability (can be tested before adopted), and observability (produces tangible results). For example, one framework describes a six-step process for the international dissemination of research for PA promotion, specifically drawing upon the Diffusion of Innovations theory to describe necessary steps to successful dissemination (Callout Box 22.2) (15).

BOX 22.2

Best Practices for use of Dissemination Models

- Identify the target audience for the message.
- Consider characteristics of the message to be delivered.
- Determine the levels of socio-ecological influence to be targeted by the dissemination approach.
- Identify an appropriate framework to work from; when possible, work from an established dissemination framework (1, 7) and adapt as needed to fit the needs of the specific situation.
- Document adaptations to the framework to describe the approach for use in future dissemination campaigns.

Developing a Dissemination Plan

By definition, dissemination is an active process of spreading information to a target audience via planned strategies. Thus, a clear plan should be established to guide dissemination efforts across a project. There are several considerations that should factor into the dissemination plan, beginning with the choice of a guiding model if one will be used (see earlier for examples). Other considerations include characteristics of the target audience for the material, timeline for distribution, and budget, among other factors (Callout Box 22.3).

BOX 22.3

Developing a dissemination plan

- Select a dissemination model, if using one.
- Identify the target audience for the message.
- Determine the budget for the dissemination activities.
- Brainstorm about potential dissemination channels.
- Consult with stakeholders from the target audience to refine possible methods for dissemination.
- Draft a timeline for the dissemination activities.
- Develop dissemination materials.
- Consult with stakeholders from the target audience to refine dissemination materials.

A number of resources exist to help guide the development of a comprehensive plan for the dissemination of public health information. While these resources are not necessarily specific to PA, they can provide a useful framework from which to build a dissemination plan. The World Health Organization has an implementation research toolkit with a module dedicated to "Disseminating the Research Findings," with information on involving stakeholders in the dissemination and utilization of research results, developing a comprehensive dissemination plan, and tailoring dissemination tools for segments of the target audience. The Yale Center for Clinical Investigation Community Alliance for Research and Engagement also has a published guide on "Beyond Scientific Publication: Strategies for Disseminating Research Findings," with guidance on developing a dissemination plan, selecting strategies (e.g., media coverage, flyers, newsletters, local events), and sample documents to assist with developing dissemination materials. Other resources, such as tools from the Agency for Healthcare Research and Quality and a library of organizational links from the Centers for Disease Control and Prevention (CDC), are also available to guide public health professionals considering the development of a dissemination plan. A list of resources can be found at the end of this chapter.

Dissemination of information about evidence-based programs, practices, and PA guidelines can take place through a variety of methods, including press releases, journals, popular press, and social media (15, 16). Many dissemination plans include the use of a combination of outlets to achieve maximum spread of information. You will find more details on methods throughout the rest of the chapter (Callout Box 22.4).

BOX 22.4

Cultural considerations in dissemination

To have a broad impact on the target audience, it is critical to pay careful attention to the range of cultural and linguistic considerations that can impact the successful delivery and receipt of dissemination messages. Here are a few ways to incorporate these considerations into the development of a dissemination plan:

- When identifying the audience for the dissemination message, consider specific cultural and linguistic considerations that will be important for successful communication.
- Understand the needs of population and cultural expectations and perceptions around your goal (PA) to develop effective messaging.
- Involve stakeholders from the representative groups you hope to reach on the dissemination planning team.
- Ensure that dissemination materials include culturally appropriate language and images to resonate with the target audience.
- Use a range of communication methods in the dissemination plan and consider using nontraditional methods where needed to meet the cultural needs and norms of the target audience.
- Pilot test the dissemination package with individuals of the target audience prior to rollout.

Dissemination Methods

Peer-Reviewed Papers

Peer-reviewed papers in scientific journals are among the most widely used methods for academic researchers to disseminate their work and are an important part of academia.

Most motivation and reward for dissemination by an academic scientist is tied to peer-reviewed publication. However, the impact of publishing in a scientific journal from a dissemination perspective is limited because of the audience for the paper—many journals are not widely read outside of the academic setting and thus the results of successful research may not reach public health practitioners. Furthermore, the traditional publishing model requires the user to pay for the material in the form of subscription or pay-per-article fees. New publishing models such as open access, where the author pays to maintain copyright and distribution rights, has partially alleviated the latter concern. However, the technical nature of peer-reviewed publications remains a barrier to dissemination and adoption by a nonacademic audience or one with training in a field other than public health.

Policy Briefs

Policy briefs are concise summaries about a specific issue with a focus on the policy options to handle it as well as suggestions about the best option to pursue (17). The target audience of policy briefs is government policy makers and lobbyists, or others who are trying to influence policy formation or change. There are two main types of policy briefs—advocacy briefs that argue in favor of policy makers taking action toward a specific solution, and objective briefs that provide balanced information about a variety of potential solutions. The brief should be short in length but still include a sufficient overview of the evidence needed for the reader to understand the big picture implications of the information presented and come to a decision about his or her position on the issue. This format of dissemination has been used widely by nonprofit organizations, including scientific organizations like the Society of Behavioral Medicine and the American Council on Sports Medicine (18).

Press Releases

Press releases are brief, formal summaries of upcoming programming and other announcements that a media relations department and/or expert prepares (19). These are typically distributed to a variety of news and media outlets for their use in publishing an article or printing the information in their individual outlet. This format of dissemination has been used widely by universities, government offices, and nonprofit organizations. Governmental agencies such as the CDC often use press releases to spread the findings of their PA reports, such as results about levels of inactivity and public health guidelines for exercise. University media departments may also generate and distribute press releases to support the publication of new research articles about PA from their faculty and students; these can be circulated to the general media and to public health newsletters like the Association of Schools and Programs of Public Health's Friday Letter (see Box 22.1) (Callout Box 22.5).

BOX 22.5

Best practices for developing a press release

To develop an effective press release that will be well received by news organizations, there are a few things you can do to clearly and concisely deliver your message

---

(continued)

(continued)

- Use a catchy headline
- Be concise and to the point (~one page)
- Avoid jargon or specialized language
- Use a news style of third-person writing
- Use quotes from a trustworthy source
- Include contact information for one person for communications

---

BOX 22.6

More than one in four U.S. adults over 50 do not engage in regular PA.

Inactivity puts 31 million at risk of heart disease, diabetes, or cancer.

Press Release

Despite the many benefits of moderate physical activity, 31 million Americans (28 percent) age 50 years and older are inactive—that is, they are not physically active beyond the basic movements needed for daily life activities. This finding comes from a new study from the Centers of Disease Control and Prevention (CDC) published in today's *Morbidity and Mortality Weekly Report*.

"Adults benefit from any amount of physical activity," said Janet E. Fulton, Ph.D., chief of CDC's Physical Activity and Health Branch and one of the authors of the report. As Dr. Fulton puts it, "Helping inactive people become more physically active is an important step towards healthier and more vibrant communities."

Inactivity across the US

CDC researchers analyzed data from the 2014 Behavioral Risk Factor Surveillance System for all 50 states and the District of Columbia (D.C.) to examine patterns of inactivity among adults ages 50 and older by selected characteristics. The analysis showed:

- Inactivity was higher for women (29.4 percent) compared with men (25.5 percent).
- The percentage of inactivity by race and ethnicity varied: Hispanics (32.7 percent), non-Hispanic blacks (33.1 percent), non-Hispanic whites (26.2 percent), and other groups (27.1 percent).
- Inactivity significantly increased with age: 25.4 percent for adults 50–64 years, 26.9 percent for people 65–74 years, and 35.3 percent for people 75 years and older.
- More adults with at least one chronic disease were inactive (31.9 percent) compared with adults with no chronic disease (19.2 percent).
- By region, inactivity was highest in the South (30.1 percent) followed by the Midwest (28.4 percent) and in the Northeast (26.6 percent). Inactivity was lowest in the West (23.1 percent).
- By states and D.C., the percentage of inactivity ranged from 17.9 percent in Colorado to 38.8 percent in Arkansas.
- The percentage of inactivity decreased as education increased and also increased as weight status increased.

(continued)

(*continued*)

"This report helps us better understand and address differences in inactivity among adults 50 years and older," said Kathleen B. Watson, PhD, an epidemiologist in CDC's Division of Nutrition, Physical Activity, and Obesity and lead author of the report. "More work is needed to make it safer and easier for people of all ages and abilities to be physically active in their communities."

Helping older adults to be physically active

PA reduces the risk of premature death and can delay or prevent many chronic diseases, including heart disease, type 2 diabetes, dementia, and some cancers. As adults grow older, they are more likely to be living with a chronic disease and these diseases are major drivers of sickness and disability.

Noninstitutionalized adults ages 50 years and older account for $860 billion in healthcare costs each year; yet four in five of the costliest chronic conditions for this age group can be prevented or managed with PA. Noninstitutionalized adults are people not living in institutions such as correctional facilities, long-term care hospitals, or nursing homes and who are not on active duty in the Armed Forces.

Being physically active helps older adults maintain the ability to live independently and reduces the risk of falling and fracturing bones. Active older adults also have a reduced risk of moderate or severe limitations and are less likely to suffer from falls. Being physically active can also improve mental health and delay dementia and cognitive decline.

Everyone, including federal, state, and local governments, transportation engineers and community planning professionals, and community organizations can play a role in helping communities offer design enhancements and healthy lifestyle programs to create a culture that supports physical activity.

CDC is working with state health departments to increase physical activity by increasing the number of communities that have pedestrian and bike-friendly master transportation plans.

CDC is committed to helping adults of all physical ability levels become or remain physically active, including those with chronic conditions such as arthritis and diabetes. The CDC recommends several proven programs that can help people with chronic conditions be active and experience the benefits of physical activity despite physical limitations.

For more information on the CDC's efforts to promote physical activity: www.cdc.gov/physicalactivity/index.html and https://health.gov/paguidelines/second-edition/pdf/Physical_Activity_Guidelines_2nd_edition.pdf#page=66

U.S. Department of Health and Human Services, CDC

SOURCE: U.S. Department of Health and Human Services. More than 1 in 4 US adults over 50 do not engage in regular physical activity: Inactivity puts 31 million at risk of heart disease, diabetes, cancer. Press Release. September 15, 2016. Available at: https://www.cdc.gov/media/releases/2016/p0915-physical-activity.html

CDC, Centers for Disease Control and Prevention.

Infographics

Infographics (short for "informational graphics") are a more recent update to the press releases and graphical formats used in the past. They are visual representations of information that typically use pictures, tables, and graphs to succinctly present a rich array of data to the viewer, in a potentially more engaging format than traditional graphics (20). Infographics can be used as part of a press release, distributed through traditional media outlets, and can be printed as posters, posted on websites, or distributed through social media. A recent evaluation found that the infographics that received the most shares on social media contained just 396 words (20). A key component to creating effective infographics is replacing verbiage with visual representations of information so that readers can recall images later and retain the information (see Figure 22.1). To support the dissemination of the UK Chief Medical Officers' PA recommendations, the National Health Service released a series of infographics with information about the amount and type of physical activity needed for different age groups (e.g., pregnant women, young children, adults, and older people). The infographics were distributed widely to educate public health organizations and the public about PA recommendations and designing services to help support PA.

Workshops

Workshops are typically held as in-person trainings that might cover the release of new guidelines or could provide instructional support to supplement other information released through the media. For example, the release of new national guidelines for PA promotion are often accompanied by holding a series of workshops for public health practitioners.

Webinars

Webinars offer a similar presentation format to in-person workshops but can potentially reach a national or international audience. Webinars are commonly utilized by government departments and professional organizations as a platform to present on new PA guidelines, share information about successful programs, and to solicit input from PA practitioners and researchers on a variety of issues. Webinar engagement has been found to be meaningfully associated with uptake of PA guidelines. For example, the new Canadian Physical Activity and Sedentary Behavior Guidelines were released by the Canadian Society for Exercise Physiology, and the dissemination of the guidelines was supported by informational webinars (21). Researchers analyzed the content of public health organizations' websites to determine if they had updated their public websites to include the new guidelines, finding that organizations were more likely to post the new guidelines if they had a representative who had attended a webinar (21). The Active Living Research Network also regularly uses webinars as a way to share information about successful research and practice efforts, including topics on research to practice translation, walkability interventions, and policy issues.

Social Media

Over the past few years, the use of social media sites has become nearly ubiquitous for personal purposes, although research into the most effective way to use these networks for professional use is still nascent. Using social media offers the benefit of rapid dissemination and relative cost-effectiveness of each communication (e.g., post or tweet). Further, it is possible to reach a large potential audience with a single communication. For example, as of September 2017, the CDC has over 850,000 followers on Twitter. Social media has been used by a variety of stakeholders to disseminate PA information, including public health organizations sharing PA recommendations/guidelines, local governments sharing success stories of community projects, and individual researchers

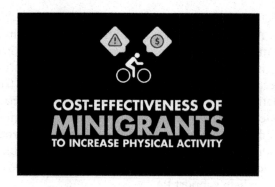

American youth are insufficiently active, and minigrant programs have been developed to facilitate implementation of evidence-based interventions in communities.

STUDY OBJECTIVE

DETERMINE COST-EFFECTIVENESS OF MINIGRANT PROGRAM.

While information about effectiveness of promotion strategies is important, cost-effectiveness and return on investment to support these strategies are equally important.

STUDY DESIGN

SETTING: 20 COUNTIES IN NORTH CAROLINA

20 community grantees were pair-matched and randomized to receive funding at the beginning of year 1 (2010-2011) or year 2 (2011-2012) to implement interventions to increase physical activity (PA) in youth.

METHODS

800 CHILDREN RANDOMLY SAMPLED FROM INTERVENTIONS.

Cost-effectiveness ratios (CERs) were calculated at the county and project levels to determine the cost per child-minute of moderate-to-vigorous PA (MVPA) increased by wave.

Analyses were conducted utilizing cost data from 20 community grantees and accelerometer-derived PA from the participating youth.

RESULTS

18 COUNTIES INCREASED YOUTH MVPA.

Of those 18 counties, the CER (US dollars/MVPA minutes per day) ranged from:

$0.02 to $1.86 in intervention year 1
$0.02 to $6.19 in intervention year 2
$0.02 to $0.58 across both years.

IMPLICATIONS

These results are important, as economic evaluations, such as cost-effectiveness analyses, are becoming increasingly important as policy makers make decisions regarding public health resource allocation and funding priorities.

FIGURE 22.1 Example of an infographic designed to communicate the results of a published study.

Source: Moore JB, Heboyan V, Oniffrey TM, et al. Cost-effectiveness of community-based minigrants to increase physical activity in youth. J Public Health Manag Pract. 2017;23(4):364-369. doi: 10.1097/PHH.0000000000000486, Reproduced with permission from Wolters Kluwer.

sharing their recent scientific publications. However, what is currently unknown is the representativeness of target audiences by social media platforms. While it is known that Facebook, Twitter, LinkedIn, and Instagram are demographically distinct (22), it is unclear how roles, professions, and priorities differ among users.

Other Considerations

There are benefits and drawbacks to the selection of any dissemination strategy and careful consideration of the target audience, timeline, and budget should factor into the design of a plan (23). A recent survey of PA practitioners and researchers reveals some insights into the ways that one sample of professionals prefer to receive and share information about PA (16). The results showed that, across professions, people used a range of sources to find and share PA information; the most common were websites, e-newsletters, webinars, and email listservs (16). Interestingly, while many respondents reported using social media (e.g., 53.5% use Facebook, 31.3% use ResearchGate), the other more traditional e-media sources were consistently ranked higher in terms of their professional appeal (16). Further, the survey revealed that most people preferred nonsocial media channels and would be reached using other methods as opposed to focusing on social media (16). These results demonstrate the complexity in selecting a dissemination plan and the need to evaluate the preferences of the intended audience and consider using a range of dissemination channels. Another example of this complexity is demonstrated with the example of the Canadian Physical Activity and Sedentary Behavior Guidelines (21). Due to budgetary constraints, the guidelines were supported by a webinar and not a comprehensive, multifaceted approach. While attendance at informational webinars was associated with organizational uptake of the new guidelines, adoption was not universal, suggesting that more active and tailored dissemination strategies are needed for future efforts to help overcome barriers to uptake (21).

Examples of Dissemination Plans

Past dissemination plans can also serve as a model for the development of an effective approach. There are a number of examples from the area of dissemination of national and regional PA guidelines that offer detailed and diverse approaches to reach stakeholders. For example, for the dissemination of the Pacific Physical Activity Guidelines for Adults, a guide for the promotion of PA in Pacific Island countries, leaders constructed a multistage plan to target various levels of the community with different activities (24). First, they targeted raising awareness of the guidelines at the country and regional levels through activities such as workshops, mailed copies of the guidelines, and newsletters. Next, they targeted more local professionals and agencies with materials that had regional examples and were distributed via mailed copies, another set of workshops, and website links on local health websites. Another example is the dissemination of evidence-based guidelines for PA promotion to U.S. health departments (25). To disseminate the best practices outlined in The Community Guide to Preventive Services, researchers held workshops, provided ongoing technical assistance, and distributed an instructional CD-ROM (25). Examining changes in knowledge of the Community Guide among local and state health department professionals before and after the dissemination plan, researchers concluded that more active strategies were needed to engage practitioners and sustain effects, and that a range of approaches should be included in a dissemination plan in order to engage practition-ers (25).

Case Studies

Case Study 1: National Physical Activity Plan

Despite the range of health benefits of regular PA (26), few Americans of any age group meet recommendations for weekly PA (27). In response to the need for innovative countrywide solutions, the National Physical Activity Plan (NPAP) Alliance was formed by a coalition of organizations to develop a healthy vision for promoting PA in the United States. The first NPAP was released in 2010 with an updated plan disseminated in 2016. The process of developing the NPAP was led by nine expert panels and relied on contributions from hundreds of professionals, researchers, and leaders working in public and private sectors. The overall goal of the NPAP is to provide strategies to improve health, prevent disease and disability, and enhance quality of life by providing and supporting opportunities for physically active lifestyles (28).

The NPAP Alliance was formed by representatives from over 20 organizations and is governed by a Board of Directors from nonprofit organizations, research institutions, and government entities (29). The 2016 NPAP involved a process for public comments and revision considerations as well. The target population of the NPAP includes all Americans and in recognizing the diversity of the population, the Alliance established a Diversity Committee to address the needs of persons of all racial, religious, cultural, ideological, sexual orientation, and gender identity groups to become more physically active.

The NPAP is grounded in a socio-ecological model of health behavior, understanding that PA is influenced by several factors operating at the personal, family, institutional, community, and policy levels. The NPAP Alliance works to advocate for and implement several overarching priorities that include a PA campaign to guide Americans toward places and programs for PA, developing and disseminating a national PA report card at regular intervals to evaluate the status of PA and promotion efforts, and increasing funding for PA promotion strategies of the NPAP (28).

Within the NPAP, there are recommendations for PA promotion organized into nine societal sectors:

1. Business and industry
2. Community, recreation, fitness, and parks
3. Education
4. Faith-based settings
5. Healthcare
6. Mass media
7. Public health
8. Sport
9. Transportation, land use, and community design

A study by Evenson et al. evaluated 2010 NPAP efforts through in-person interviews with 27 public health practitioners across 25 states (30). Reported reach and awareness of the NPAP was high with varying channels of communication (i.e., websites, newsletters, and webinars), indicating a continued need for wide breadth when communicating NPAP efforts (30). This study found inconsistencies with the dissemination of NPAP, as practitioners reported variation in frequency and extent of using NPAP (30). Furthermore, a study of 291 public health professionals found that half of the respondents reported awareness of NPAP in their respective organizations but only one quarter agreed that the leadership in their organization encouraged use and implementation of the plan (31). The 2016 plan provided specific guidance on the NPAP dissemination goals.

Each sector within the 2016 NPAP includes a set of specific strategies and tactics grounded in evidence-based research and practice models for the promotion of PA. Within the strategies, there are dissemination goals for increasing PA. For instance, the business and industry sector outlines a strategy that states "professional and scientific societies should create and widely disseminate a concise, powerful, and compelling business case for investment in physical activity promotion," specifically addressing the best tools for PA promotion and the reduction of prolonged sitting in the workplace (28). The public health sector proposes to "Disseminate physical activity-promoting practices and policies targeted at agencies and professional societies outside of public health (e.g., youth-serving social services, non-profits in underserved communities, transportation and planning, sports and recreation, education, environmental protection)" (28). With cultural and economic considerations in mind, the transportation, land use, and community design sector strategy proposes to "develop and disseminate policy tools to reduce the possible impacts of gentrification on low-income neighborhoods that adopt healthy design principles, as they become more desirable and experience rising home values" (28). Additional dissemination guidance is outlined in the NPAP, which is publicly available at www.physicalactivityplan.org.

Case Study 2: EnhanceFitness

The aging population is at increased risk for physical and mental disabilities compared to younger counterparts, and risk steadily increases with age (32). With the help of medical advances, humans are living longer life spans and managing chronic illnesses, which means the aging population is growing at a steady rate, putting more individuals at risk for impairments and disabilities (33). To address this growing public health concern, a multicomponent disability prevention program was developed through a collaboration of academic researchers, a health maintenance organization, and a nonprofit senior organization (34). The goal of EnhanceFitness was to provide routine exercise opportunities to help seniors maintain and improve cognitive, physical, and social well-being for living independent lives with lowered risk of disabilities. EnhanceFitness targeted older adults in senior communities and settings. The program was originally developed in 1994 by researchers at the University of Washington Health Promotion Research Center, Group Health Cooperative, and a nonprofit organization called Senior Services. After the initial pilot test of the program, Senior Services led the dissemination strategy. Stakeholders included leaders of senior centers, community dwellings, and service programs for older adults (34). Senior communities were optimal for disseminating the disability prevention program because of the established reputation and existing system for providing services to older adults. EnhanceFitness was first implemented at a senior living community in Washington State. Over the years, EnhanceFitness expanded its dissemination and implementation to hospitals, clinics, churches, senior centers, assisted living facilities, retirement communities, and fitness centers.

EnhanceFitness involves exercise classes led by certified fitness instructors three times per week in settings for older adults. The dissemination strategy of the EnhanceFitness program includes several phases. Senior Services holds the license for the program and provides new sites with training, manuals, implementation guidance, annual reports, marketing materials, workshops for instructors, and data collection and analysis (35). Dissemination of program materials is maintained through EnhanceFitness listservs, class DVDs, newsletters, website materials, site visits, grant-writing materials, and workshops (35, 36). Following the pilot study, the EnhanceFitness program was disseminated to 700 locations across 34 states between 1999 and 2014, serving over 45,000 participants (34). Participation in EnhanceFitness led to reduced hospital days, lower healthcare costs, and decreased mortality rate (37). Furthermore, healthcare cost savings increased with prolonged participation in EnhanceFitness (38).

In terms of health promotion programs, EnhanceFitness has been successful in demonstrating positive health outcomes at a low cost. Cost-effectiveness evaluations showed EnhanceFitness may have contributed to reduced healthcare costs for participants (37). Due to the maintained control over program implementation by an original partner, the program is replicable and consistent across program sites. EnhanceFitness has expanded its partnerships to include the American Council on Exercise and the Center for Medicaid and Medicare Services (34). However, there are weaknesses of the dissemination. Targeting senior centers and services for EnhanceFitness leaves out a large portion of older adults who may live independently or with family. The evaluations of EnhanceFitness rely on the number of classes attended by a participant, but may not capture other sources of cognitive and physical preventative services (38). Lastly, centers and services wishing to host EnhanceFitness may be limited in their capacity to pay licensing fees to Senior Services, limiting the reach of the program.

■ Summary

Dissemination should be a thoughtful, planned, and carefully executed part of PA promotion efforts. Much like the proverbial tree that falls in the woods, the good work of practitioners and researchers that lacks concurrent dissemination efforts will not make the "noise" or impact that it might with careful planning and execution. While organizations such as Active Living Research have wonderful dissemination resources (see activelivingresearch.org), efforts to produce research briefs, webinars, trainings, and tools are labor intensive and cannot be inclusive. Therefore, it is paramount for members of the practice and research community to disseminate success stories, evidence-based best practices, and emerging research (Callout Box 22.7).

BOX 22.7

Steps in dissemination of research and best practices

- Identify the target audience for the message.
- Craft the message to fit the priorities and interests of the target audience.
- Choose dissemination channels that are most appropriate for the target audience.
- Monitor reach (i.e., impressions, views) and uptake (i.e., downloads) of dissemination materials.

(continued)

(continued)

> ■ Diversify dissemination channels and messages based upon reach and uptake of target audience.

■ Things to Consider

- ■ Dissemination is a systematic and planned approach to transferring knowledge to individuals.
- ■ There are many potential outlets for information dissemination, including peer-reviewed papers, press releases, and social media.
- ■ Successful dissemination requires consideration of the target audience from the beginning of planning.
- ■ Involving stakeholders from the target group can help ensure effective methods for dissemination and appropriate use of language and messaging platforms for high impact.

■ Resources

- ■ Disseminating the Research Findings, World Health Organization Toolkit: http://www.who.int/tdr/publications/year/2014/participant-workbook5_030414.pdf
- ■ National Center for Chronic Disease Prevention and Health Promotion's Collection of Online Resources & Inventory Database: https://nccd.cdc.gov/coridor
- ■ Yale Center for Clinical Investigation, CARE: Community Alliance for Research and Engagement: https://depts.washington.edu/ccph/pdf_files/CARE_Dissemination_Strategies_FINAL_eversion.pdf
- ■ Rural Health Research Gateway, University of North Dakota Center for Rural Health: https://www.ruralhealthresearch.org/toolkit
- ■ Center for Dissemination and Implementation, Institute for Public Health at Washington University in St. Louis: https://publichealth.wustl.edu/dandi/di-resources

■ References

1. Wilson PM, Petticrew M, Calnan MW, et al. Disseminating research findings: what should researchers do? A systematic scoping review of conceptual frameworks. *Implement Sci.* 2010;5(1):91. doi:10.1186/1748-5908-5-91.
2. Rabin BA, Brownson RC. Developing the terminology for dissemination and implementation research. In: Brownson RC, Colditz GA, Proctor EK, eds. *Dissemination and Implementation Research in Health.* New York, NY: Oxford University Press; 2012:23–51.
3. King AC, Sallis JF. Why and how to improve physical activity promotion: lessons from behavioral science and related fields. *Prev Med.* 2009;49(4):286–288. doi:10.1016/j.ypmed.2009.07.007.

4. Albright CL, Steffen AD, Wilkens LR, et al. Effectiveness of a 12-month randomized clinical trial to increase physical activity in multiethnic postpartum women: results from Hawaii's Na Mikimiki Project. *Prev Med*. 2014;69:214–223. doi:10.1016/j.ypmed.2014.09.019.

5. Gallegos-Carrillo K, Garcia-Pena C, Salmeron J, et al. Brief counseling and exercise referral scheme: a pragmatic trial in Mexico. *Am J Prev Med*. 2017;52(2):249–259. doi:10.1016/j.amepre.2016.10.021.

6. Galaviz KI, Estabrooks PA, Ulloa EJ, et al. Evaluating the effectiveness of physician counseling to promote physical activity in Mexico: an effectiveness-implementation hybrid study. *Transl Behav Med*. 2017;7:1–10. doi:10.1007/s13142-017-0524-y.

7. Tabak RG, Khoong EC, Chambers DA, et al. Bridging research and practice: models for dissemination and implementation research. *Am J Prev Med*. 2012;43(3):337–350. doi:10.1016/j.amepre.2012.05.024.

8. Wilson PM, Petticrew M, Calnan MW, et al. Disseminating research findings: what should researchers do? A systematic scoping review of conceptual frameworks. *Implement Sci*. 2010;5(1):91. doi:10.1186/1748-5908-5-91.

9. McGuire WJ. The nature of attitudes and attitude change. In: Lindzey G, Aronson E, eds. *The Handbook of Social Psychology*. 2nd ed. Reading, MA: Addison-Wesley; 1969:136–314.

10. McGuire WJ. Input and output variables currently promising for constructing persuasive communications. In: McGuire WJ, Rice RE, Atkin CK, eds. *Public Communication Campaigns*. 3rd ed. Thousand Oaks, CA: Sage; 2001:22–48.

11. McGuire WJ. Theoretical foundations of campaigns. In: McGuire WJ, Rice R, Paisley W, eds. *Public Communication Campaigns*. Newbury Park, CA: Sage; 1989:43–65.

12. Huberman M. *A Review of the Literature on Dissemination and Knowledge Utilization*. U.S. National Center for the Dissemination of Disability Research (NCDDR); 1996.

13. Hughes M, McNeish D, Newman T, et al. *What Works? Making Connections: Linking Research and Practice*. Ilford, Essex, UK: Barnardo's; 2000.

14. Rogers EM. *Diffusion of Innovations*. 5th ed. New York, NY: Free Press; 2003.

15. Bauman AE, Nelson DE, Pratt M, et al. Dissemination of physical activity evidence, programs, policies, and surveillance in the international public health arena. *Am J Prev Med*. 2006;31(suppl 4):S57–S65. doi:10.1016/j.amepre.2006.06.026

16. Jake-Schoffman DE, Wilcox S, Kaczynski AT, et al. E-Media use and preferences for physical activity and public health information: results of a web-based survey. *J Public Health Manag Pract*. 2017;24:385–381. doi:10.1097/PHH.0000000000000638.

17. Agriculture and Economic Development Analysis Division. *Writing Effective Reports*. 2011.

18. Pratt SI, Jerome GJ, Schneider KL, et al. Increasing US health plan coverage for exercise programming in community mental health settings for people with serious mental illness: a position statement from the Society of Behavior Medicine and the American College of Sports Medicine. *Transl Behav Med*. 2016;6(3):478–481. doi:10.1007/s13142-016-0407-7.

19. Moore JB, Novick LF, Oniffrey TM. *Council of State and Territorial Epidemiologist (CSTE) Scientific Writing Toolkit*. Atlanta, GA: CSTE National Office; 2017.

20. Scott H, Fawkner S, Oliver C, et al. Why healthcare professionals should know a little about infographics. *Br J Sports Med*. 2017;50(18):1104–1105. doi:10.1136/bjsports-2016-096133.

21. Gainforth HL, Berry T, Faulkner G, et al. Evaluating the uptake of Canada's new physical activity and sedentary behavior guidelines on service organizations' websites. *Transl Behav Med*. 2013;3(2):172–179. doi:10.1007/s13142-012-0190-z.

22. Pew Research Center. Social media fact sheet; 2017. Available at: http://www.pewinternet.org/fact-sheet/social-media. Accessed October 17, 2017.

23. Brownson RC, Eyler AA, Harris JK, et al. Getting the word out: new approaches for disseminating public health science. *J Public Health Manag Pract*. 2017;24:102–111. doi:10.1097/PHH.0000000000000673.

24. *Pacific Physical Activity Guidelines for Adults: Framework for Accelerating the Communication of Physical Activity Guidelines*. Geneva, Switzerland: World Health Organization; 2008. Available at: http://www.who.int/dietphysicalactivity/publications/pacific_pa_guidelines.pdf.

25. Brownson RC, Ballew P, Brown KL, et al. The effect of disseminating evidence-based interventions that promote physical activity to health departments. *Am J Public Health.* 2007;97(10):1900–1907. doi:10.2105/AJPH.2006.090399.

26. Lee IM, Shiroma EJ, Lobelo F, et al. Effect of physical inactivity on major non-communicable diseases worldwide: an analysis of burden of disease and life expectancy. *Lancet.* 2012;380(9838):219–229. doi:10.1016/S0140-6736(12)61031-9.

27. President's Council on Sports Fitness & Nutrition. *Facts and Statistics: Physical Activity.* Rockville, MD: U.S. Departemnt of Health and Human Services. 2017. Available at: https://www.hhs.gov/fitness/blog/index.html.

28. National Physical Activity Plan Alliance. *National Physical Activity Plan.* Columbia, SC; 2018. Available at: http://physicalactivityplan.org/docs/2016NPAP_Finalforwebsite.pdf.

29. Bornstein DB, Pate RR, Buchner DM. Development of a National Physical Activity Plan for the United States. *J Phys Act Health.* 2014;11(3):463–469. doi:10.1123/jpah.2013-0358.

30. Evenson KR, Satinsky SB, Valko C, et al. In-depth interviews with state public health practitioners on the United States National Physical Activity Plan. *Int J Behav Nutr Phys Act.* 2013;10(1):72. doi:10.1186/1479-5868-10-72.

31. Evenson KR, Brownson RC, Satinsky SB, et al. The U.S. National Physical Activity Plan: dissemination and use by public health practitioners. *Am J Prev Med.* 2013;44(5):431–438. doi:10.1016/j.amepre.2013.02.002.

32. Grundstrom AC, Guse CE, Layde PM. Risk factors for falls and fall-related injuries in adults 85 years of age and older. *Arch Gerontol Geriatr.* 2012;54(3):421–428. doi:10.1016/j.archger.2011.06.008.

33. Centers for Disease Control and Prevention. Trends in aging—United States and worldwide. *MMWR Morb Mortal Wkly Rep.* 2003;52(6):101. Available at: https://www.cdc.gov/mmwr/preview/mmwrhtml/mm5206a2.htm

34. Snyder SJ, Thompson M, Denison P. EnhanceFitness: A 20-year dissemination history. *Front Public Health.* 2014;2(270):270. doi:10.3389/fpubh.2014.00270

35. Harris JR, Cheadle A, Hannon PA, et al. A framework for disseminating evidence-based health promotion practices. *Prev Chronic Dis.* 2012;9:E22. doi:10.5888/pcd9.110081

36. Belza B. *Moving Ahead: Strategies and Tools to Plan, Conduct, and Maintain Effective Community-Based Physical Activity Programs for Older Adults.* Atlanta, GA: Centers for Disease Control and Prevention; 2007.

37. Center for Medicare and Medicaid Services (CMS). *Report to Congress: The Centers for Medicare & Medicaid Services' Evaluation of Community-based Wellness and Prevention Programs under Section 4202 (b) of the Affordable Care Act.* 2013.

38. Ackermann RT, Williams B, Nguyen HQ, et al. Healthcare cost differences with participation in a community-based group physical activity benefit for Medicare managed care health plan members. *J Am Geriatr Soc.* 2008;56(8):1459–1465. doi:10.1111/j.1532-5415.2008.01804.x.

39. U.S. Department of Health and Human Services. More than 1 in 4 US adults over 50 do not engage in regular physical activity: Inactivity puts 31 million at risk of heart disease, diabetes, cancer. Press Release. September 15, 2016. Available at: https://www.cdc.gov/media/releases/2016/p0915-physical-activity.html

40. Moore JB, Heboyan V, Oniffrey TM, et al. Cost-effectiveness of community-based mini-grants to increase physical activity in youth. *J Public Health Manag Pract.* 2017;23(4):364–369. doi:10.1097/PHH.0000000000000486